Legionnaire's Disease

Editors

CHESTON B. CUNHA
BURKE A. CUNHA

INFECTIOUS DISEASE CLINICS OF NORTH AMERICA

www.id.theclinics.com

Consulting Editor
HELEN W. BOUCHER

March 2017 • Volume 31 • Number 1

ELSEVIER

1600 John F. Kennedy Boulevard • Suite 1800 • Philadelphia, Pennsylvania, 19103-2899.

http://www.theclinics.com

INFECTIOUS DISEASE CLINICS OF NORTH AMERICA Volume 31, Number 1
March 2017 ISSN 0891–5520, ISBN-13: 978-0-323-50979-4

Editor: Kerry Holland
Developmental Editor: Donald Mumford

Infectious Disease Clinics of North America (ISSN 0891–5520) is published in March, June, September, and December by Elsevier Inc., 360 Park Avenue South, New York, NY 10010-1710. Periodicals postage paid at New York, NY and additional mailing offices. Subscription prices are $301.00 per year for US individuals, $588.00 per year for US institutions, $100.00 per year for US students, $357.00 per year for Canadian individuals, $734.00 per year for Canadian institutions, $428.00 per year for international individuals, $734.00 per year for international institutions, and $200.00 per year for Canadian and international students. To receive student rate, orders must be accompained by name of affiliated institution, date of term, and the *signature* of program/residency coordinator on institution letterhead. Orders will be billed at individual rate until proof of status is received. Foreign air speed delivery is included in all *Clinics* subscription prices. All prices are subject to change without notice. **POSTMASTER**: Send address changes to *Infectious Disease Clinics of North America,* Elsevier Health Sciences Division, Subcription Customer Service, 3251 Riverport Lane, Maryland Heights, MO 63043. **Customer Service: 1-800-654-2452 (US). From outside of the US and Canada, call 1-314-447-8871. Fax: 1-314-447-8029. E-mail: JournalsCustomerService-usa@elsevier.com (print support) or JournalsOnlineSupport-usa@elsevier.com (online support).**

Infectious Disease Clinics of North America is also published in Spanish by Editorial Inter-Médica, Junin 917, 1er A 1113, Buenos Aires, Argentina.

Reprints. For copies of 100 or more, of articles in this publication, please contact the Commercial Reprints Department, Elsevier Inc., 360 Park Avenue South, New York, New York 10010-1710. Tel. 212-633-3874, Fax: 212-633-3820, E-mail: reprints@elsevier.com.

Infectious Disease Clinics of North America is covered in *MEDLINE/PubMed (Index Medicus), Current Contents/Clinical Medicine, Science Citation Alert, SCISEARCH,* and *Research Alert.*

Contributors

CONSULTING EDITOR

HELEN W. BOUCHER, MD, FIDSA, FACP
Director, Infectious Diseases Fellowship Program, Division of Geographic Medicine and Infectious Diseases, Tufts Medical Center, Associate Professor of Medicine, Tufts University School of Medicine, Boston, Massachusetts

EDITORS

CHESTON B. CUNHA, MD
Medical Director, Antimicrobial Stewardship Program, Division of Infectious Disease, Rhode Island Hospital, The Miriam Hospital, Assistant Professor of Medicine, Brown University Alpert School of Medicine, Providence, Rhode Island

BURKE A. CUNHA, MD, MACP
Chief, Infectious Disease Division, Winthrop-University Hospital, Mineola; Professor of Medicine, School of Medicine, State University of New York, Stony Brook, New York

AUTHORS

VIRGINIA ABELL, RN, BA
Director, Infection Prevention and Clinical Safety, Summa Akron City and St. Thomas Hospitals, Akron, Ohio

FLORENCE ADER, MD, PhD
CNR Legionelles, Inserm 1111 Centre International Recherche en Infectiologie (CIRI), Université Claude Bernard Lyon 1; Service des Maladies infectieuses et tropicales, Hospices Civils de Lyon, Lyon, France

SHANU AGARWAL, MD
Infectious Disease Division, Summa Health, Akron, Ohio; Associate Professor, Northeast Ohio Medical University, Rootstown, Ohio

EMILIO BOUZA, MD, PhD
Division of Clinical Microbiology; Chief, Division of Infectious Disease, Hospital General Universitario Gregorio Marañón, Instituto de Investigación Sanitaria Gregorio Marañón, Universidad Complutense de Madrid; CIBER de Enfermedades Respiratorias (CIBERES CB06/06/0058), Madrid, Spain

JOHN L. BRUSCH, BS, MD
Associate Chief, Medical Department; Consultant, Division of Infectious Disease; Regional Medical Director, Ambulatory Medicine, Cambridge Health Alliance, Cambridge, Massachusetts; Assistant Professor, Medicine, Harvard Medical School, Boston, Massachusetts

ALMUDENA BURILLO, MD, PhD
Divisions of Clinical Microbiology and Infectious Disease, Hospital General Universitario Gregorio Marañón, Instituto de Investigación Sanitaria Gregorio Marañón, Universidad Complutense de Madrid, Madrid, Spain

EMILIE CATHERINOT, MD, PhD
Service de pneumologie, Hopital Foch, Suresnes, France

ABDULLAH CHAHIN, MD
Critical Care Division, Miriam Hospital; Infectious Disease Division, Rhode Island Hospital, Brown University Alpert School of Medicine, Providence, Rhode Island

BURKE A. CUNHA, MD, MACP
Chief, Infectious Disease Division, Winthrop-University Hospital, Mineola; Professor of Medicine, School of Medicine, State University of New York, Stony Brook, New York

CHESTON B. CUNHA, MD
Medical Director, Antimicrobial Stewardship Program, Division of Infectious Disease, Rhode Island Hospital, The Miriam Hospital, Assistant Professor of Medicine, Brown University Alpert School of Medicine, Providence, Rhode Island

W. MICHAEL DUNNE Jr, PhD
Scientific Office, BioMérieux, Durham, North California

THOMAS M. FILE Jr, MD, MSc, MACP
Chair, Infectious Disease Division, Summa Health, Akron, Ohio; Professor, Internal Medicine; Master Teacher; Chair, Infectious Disease Section, Northeast Ohio Medical University, Rootstown, Ohio

MENACHEM GOLD, MD
Attending Neuroradiologist, Department of Radiology, Lincoln Hospital, Bronx, New York

JOHN J. HALPERIN, MD
Professor of Neurology and Medicine, Sidney Kimmel Medical College of Thomas Jefferson University, Philadelphia, Pennsylvania; Chair, Department of Neurosciences, Overlook Medical Center, Summit, New Jersey

LINDA B. HARAMATI, MD, MS, FACR
Professor of Clinical Radiology and Medicine, Departments of Radiology and Medicine, Montefiore Medical Center, Albert Einstein College of Medicine, Bronx, New York

TIN HAN HTWE, MD
Consultant Physician, Sentara Infectious Disease Specialists, Sentara Medical Group, Norfolk, Virginia

SOPHIE JARRAUD, MD, PhD
CNR Legionelles, Inserm 1111 Centre International Recherche en Infectiologie (CIRI), Université Claude Bernard Lyon 1, Lyon, France

DOUGLAS S. KATZ, MD, FACR
Vice Chair of Clinical Research and Education; Director of Body Imaging, Department of Radiology, Winthrop-University Hospital, Mineola; Professor of Radiology, Stony Brook University School of Medicine, Stony Brook, New York

NANCY M. KHARDORI, MD, PhD, FACP, FIDSA
Professor, Department of Internal Medicine; Director, Division of Infectious Diseases; Professor, Department of Microbiology and Molecular Cell Biology, Eastern Virginia Medical School, Norfolk, Virginia

FANNY LANTERNIER, MD, PhD
Service de Maladies Infectieuses et Tropicales, AP-HP, Hôpital Necker-Enfants malades, Centre d'Infectiologie Necker-Pasteur, IHU Imagine, Université Paris Descartes, Paris, France

ANN N. LEUNG, MD
Professor, Department of Radiology, Stanford University Medical Center, Stanford, California

OLIVIER LORTHOLARY, MD, PhD
Service de Maladies Infectieuses et Tropicales, AP-HP, Hôpital Necker-Enfants malades, Centre d'Infectiologie Necker-Pasteur, IHU Imagine, Université Paris Descartes, Paris, France

ELENI E. MAGIRA, MD, PhD
1st Department of Critical Care Medicine, Evaggelismos General Hospital, National and Kapodistrian University of Athens, Athens, Greece

SAMEER MITTAL, MD, MS
Radiology Resident, Department of Radiology, Winthrop-University Hospital, Mineola, New York

STEVEN M. OPAL, MD
Critical Care Division, Miriam Hospital; Infectious Disease Division, Rhode Island Hospital, Professor of Medicine, Brown University Alpert School of Medicine, Providence, Rhode Island

MARÍA LUISA PEDRO-BOTET, MD, PhD
Infectious Diseases Unit, Hospital Universitario German Trías i Pujol, Badalona, Spain; Universidad Autónoma de Barcelona, Madrid, Spain; CIBER de Enfermedades Respiratorias (CIBERES CB06/06/1089), Barcelona, Spain

NATHALIE PICOT, MSc
Innovation Group, Info Doc, BioMérieux, Marcy-l'Étoile, France

BENOIT PILMIS, MD
Service de Maladies Infectieuses et Tropicales, Sorbonne, Paris 6, AP-HP, Hôpital Necker-Enfants malades, Centre d'Infectiologie Necker-Pasteur, IHU Imagine, Université Paris Descartes, Paris, France

AYUSHI P. SINGH, DO
Medicine Resident, Department of Medicine, Maimonides Hospital, Brooklyn, New York

ALEX VAN BELKUM, PhD
Honorary Professor of Molecular Microbiology, Erasmus University, Rotterdam, The Netherlands; Chief Scientific Officer, BioMérieux, La Balme Les Grottes, France

SRYROS ZAKYNTHINOS, MD, PhD
1st Department of Critical Care and Pulmonary Services, Center of Sleep Disorders, Evangelismos General Hospital, National and Kapodistrian University of Athens, Athens, Greece

Contents

Preface: Legionnaire's Disease and Its Protean Clinical Manifestations: The Ongoing Challenges of the Most Interesting Atypical Pneumonia xiii

Cheston B. Cunha and Burke A. Cunha

Legionnaire's Disease Since Philadelphia: Lessons Learned and Continued Progress 1

Cheston B. Cunha and Burke A. Cunha

Legionnaire's disease has been recognized as a cause of severe community-acquired pneumonia (CAP). Legionnaire's disease has characteristic extrapulmonary findings that are the basis for a presumptive clinical diagnosis. The widespread use of *Legionella* culture, sputum DFA, serology, urinary antigen testing, and polymerase chain reaction have allowed earlier diagnosis of Legionnaire's disease. Excluding common source outbreaks, CAP caused by Legionnaire's disease is manifested as sporadic cases. In contrast, nosocomial Legionnaire's disease occurs in clusters or outbreaks from common *Legionella* species-contaminated water sources. Improved diagnostic tests have permitted accurate diagnosis. Bacterial coinfections with Legionnaire's disease are uncommon, but when present, are most often associated with bacteremic pneumococcal pneumonia.

Microbiology and Epidemiology of Legionnaire's Disease 7

Almudena Burillo, María Luisa Pedro-Botet, and Emilio Bouza

Legionnaire's disease (LD) is the pneumonic form of legionellosis caused by aerobic gram-negative bacilli of the genus *Legionella*. Individuals become infected when they inhale aerosolized water droplets contaminated with *Legionella* species. Forty years after the identification of *Legionella pneumophila* as the cause of the 1976 pneumonia outbreak in a hotel in Philadelphia, we have non–culture-based diagnostic tests, effective antibiotics, and preventive measures to handle LD. With a mortality rate still around 10%, underreporting, and sporadic outbreaks, there is still much work to be done. In this article, the authors review the microbiology, laboratory diagnosis, and epidemiology of LD.

Legionnaire's Disease and Immunosuppressive Drugs 29

Tin Han Htwe and Nancy M. Khardori

Immunosuppressive agents predispose patients to legionnaire's disease. Patients receiving tumor necrosis factor antagonists are generally not severely immunocompromised by the underlying disease. In patients with malignancy receiving immunosuppressive therapies, it is difficult to balance the underlying disease versus the therapy used. Transplant recipients are often on multiple drugs, including immunosuppressants. It seems that immunosuppressive drugs add to the risk for legionella infection. The index of suspicion should be high for legionella infection early

of Legionnaire's disease's. The pretest probability of Legionnaire's disease is increased if several characteristic extrapulmonary findings are present. Similarly, if certain key findings are absent, Legionnaire's disease may be eliminated from further diagnostic consideration. If characteristic clinical findings are present, then specific tests should be ordered to confirm or rule out Legionnaire's disease.

Legionnaire's Disease and its Mimics: A Clinical Perspective **95**

Burke A. Cunha and Cheston B. Cunha

Whenever the cardinal manifestations of a disorder occur in similar disorders, there is potential for a disease mimic. Legionnaire's disease has protean manifestations and has the potential to mimic or be mimicked by other community acquired pneumonias (CAPs). In CAPs caused by other than *Legionella* species, the more characteristic features in common with legionnaire's disease the more difficult the diagnostic conundrum. In hospitalized adults with CAP, legionnaire's disease may mimic influenza or other viral pneumonias. Of the bacterial causes of CAP, psittacosis and Q fever, but not tularemia, are frequent mimics of legionnaire's disease.

Severe Pneumonia Caused by *Legionella pneumophila*: Differential Diagnosis and Therapeutic Considerations **111**

Abdullah Chahin and Steven M. Opal

Severe legionella pneumonia poses a diagnostic challenge and requires early intervention. Legionnaire's disease can have several presenting signs, symptoms, and laboratory abnormalities that suggest that *Legionella pneumophila* is the pathogen, but none of these are sufficient to distinguish *L pneumophila* pneumonia from other respiratory pathogens. *L pneumophila* is primarily an intracellular pathogen and needs treatment with antibiotics that efficiently enter the intracellular space.

Legionnaire's Disease in Compromised Hosts **123**

Fanny Lanternier, Florence Ader, Benoit Pilmis, Emilie Catherinot, Sophie Jarraud, and Olivier Lortholary

Legionnaire's disease (LD) is mainly reported in apparently immunocompetent patients. Among them, risk factors include chronic lung disease and smoking. However, LD is also well reported among immunocompromised patients, particularly those treated with anti–tumor necrosis factor alpha therapy, patients with hematological malignancy, and transplant patients. This article discusses the available data on immunity against Legionella spp, epidemiology, clinical presentation, diagnosis, and treatment of LD in immunocompromised patients.

Legionnaire's Disease and Influenza **137**

Eleni E. Magira and Sryros Zakynthinos

Legionella pneumophila and influenza types A and B viruses can cause either community-acquired pneumonia with respiratory failure, or *Legionella* infection could attribute to influenza infection with potentially fatal prognosis. Copathogenesis between pandemic influenza and bacteria is characterized by complex interactions between coinfecting pathogens and the host. Understanding the underlying reason of the emersion of the secondary bacterial infection during an influenza infection is challenging. The dual infection has an impact on viral control and may delay viral clearance. Effective vaccines and antiviral therapy are crucial to increase resistance toward influenza, decrease the prevalence of influenza, and possibly interrupt the potential secondary bacterial infections.

Nosocomial (Health Care–Associated) Legionnaire's Disease 155

Shanu Agarwal, Virginia Abell, and Thomas M. File Jr

Nosocomial Legionnaire's disease is most frequently associated with presence of the organism in hospital water systems. Patients are often susceptible as a result of age, underlying comorbidities, or immunosuppression. Prevention focuses on reducing the reservoir within water systems and includes super heating, ultraviolent light, chlorination, silver-copper ionization, and distal filtration. This article reviews the epidemiology of health care–associated Legionnaire's disease, reviews characteristics of several health care–associated outbreaks, and discusses strategies to prevent health care–associated infection.

Laboratory Tests for Legionnaire's Disease 167

W. Michael Dunne Jr, Nathalie Picot, and Alex van Belkum

Legionella pneumophila is one of the more recently discovered bacterial pathogens of humans. The last 2 decades have seen tremendous progress in the evolution of diagnostic tests, for detection and characterization of this pathogen and for defining the host response to infection. This has generated several diagnostic tools that span the range from simple immunologic assays to modern genome sequencing. This review describes the state of affairs of this continuously evolving field regarding the diagnosis of Legionnaire's disease and covers detection, assessment of antibiotic susceptibility, and epidemiologic characterization of isolates of *L pneumophila* and other pathogenic species within the genus.

Antimicrobial Therapy for Legionnaire's Disease: Antibiotic Stewardship Implications 179

Cheston B. Cunha and Burke A. Cunha

Legionnaire's disease is a common cause of community-acquired pneumonia (CAP). Although no single clinical feature is diagnostic, if characteristic extrapulmonary findings are present a presumptive clinical syndromic diagnosis is possible. Depending on geographic location, season, and physician awareness, Legionnaire's disease may be included in the differential diagnosis of CAP. Some antibiotics effective against *Legionella* sp are also effective in treating the typical bacterial causes of CAP. From an antimicrobial stewardship program (ASP) perspective, monotherapy is preferred to double-drug therapy. From an ASP and pharmacoeconomic standpoint, monotherapy with doxycycline or a respiratory quinolone provides optimal cost effective therapy.

Index 193

INFECTIOUS DISEASE CLINICS OF NORTH AMERICA

FORTHCOMING ISSUES

June 2017
Bone and Joint Infections
Steven K. Schmitt, *Editor*

September 2017
Infections in the ICU
Naomi P. O'Grady and Sameer Kadri, *Editors*

December 2017
Infections in Older Adults
Robin L. Jump and David H. Canaday, *Editors*

RECENT ISSUES

December 2016
Infection Prevention and Control in Healthcare, Part II: Epidemiology and Prevention of Infections
Keith S. Kaye and Sorabh Dhar, *Editors*

September 2016
Infection Prevention and Control in Healthcare, Part I: Facility Planning and Management
Keith S. Kaye and Sorabh Dhar, *Editors*

June 2016
Antibacterial Resistance: Challenges and Opportunities
Richard R. Watkins and Robert A. Bonomo, *Editors*

RELATED INTEREST

Rheumatic Disease Clinics of North America, February 2017 (Vol. 43, Issue 1)
Infection and Malignancy in Rheumatic Diseases
Kevin L. Winthrop and Leonard H. Calabrese, *Editors*

Preface

Legionnaire's Disease and Its Protean Clinical Manifestations: The Ongoing Challenges of the Most Interesting Atypical Pneumonia

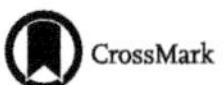

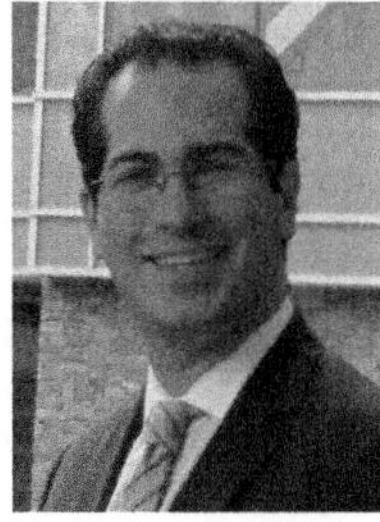

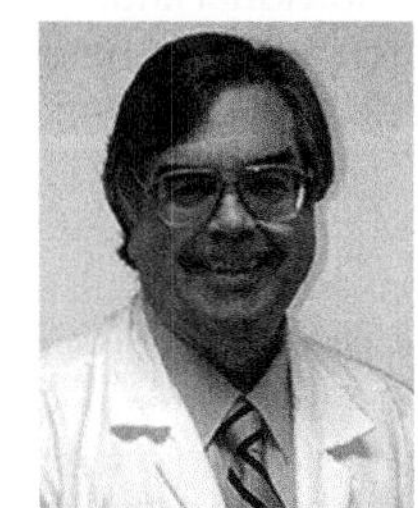

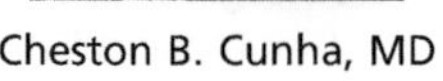

Cheston B. Cunha, MD Burke A. Cunha, MD, MACP
Editors

The *raison d'etre* of this issue on Legionnaire's disease is that not only is Legionnaire's disease the most interesting atypical pneumonia but also our knowledge of *Legionella* sp infections keeps expanding.[1–3]

Certainly, Legionnaire's disease existed before the 1976 Philadelphia outbreak, and when encountered by physicians, was likely considered an "unusual pneumonia" that was unlike other pneumonias. Often it takes an outbreak to galvanize investigative efforts to describe clinical features, devise diagnostic tests, and deduce effective therapy.[4,5] As the great imitator of other pneumonias, Legionnaire's disease does not disappoint.[6]

Classically, with the bacterial typical pneumonias, for example, *S pneumoniae*, *H influenzae*, *M catarrhalis*, clinical findings are limited to the lungs.[4] The term "atypical pneumonia" was introduced to describe pneumonias with extrapulmonary findings. Some argued the term "atypical pneumonia" was unhelpful since there already were other zoonotic pneumonias with extrapulmonary manifestations, for example, psittacosis, Q fever, tularemia, and each had a different pattern of extrapulmonary manifestations.[4,7,8] However, it was the recognition of *M pneumoniae* as the first nonzoonotic atypical pneumonia that resulted in widespread acceptance of the term "atypical pneumonia." *M pneumoniae* had its own set of extrapulmonary organ involvement with some distinctly unusual features, for example, meningoencephalitis (rarely), elevated cold agglutinins (commonly).[9] Early on, *M pneumoniae* was referred to as "cold agglutinin" pneumonia, and clinicians began to think about the patterns of extrapulmonary organ involvement with pneumonias.[10]

Infect Dis Clin N Am 31 (2017) xiii–xvi
http://dx.doi.org/10.1016/j.idc.2016.12.001
0891-5520/17/© 2016 Published by Elsevier Inc.

In 1976, a severe nonzoonotic atypical pneumonia, often fatal, with a distinctive pattern of extrapulmonary organ involvement was decided in the Philadelphia outbreak. The original reports of the characteristic clinical features of Legionnaire's disease were so well described and have not been improved on since.[11–13] Legionnaire's disease was clearly a "new" atypical pneumonia very different than *M pneumoniae* and from the other typical as well as the zoonotic atypical pneumonias.[14] The term "atypical pneumonia" remains clinically useful since it implies a pneumonia with extrapulmonary findings and a different clinical and diagnostic testing approach as well as a different therapeutic approach using antibiotics effective against atypical pneumonia pathogens.[15]

Given the many extrapulmonary manifestations of Legionnaire's disease, many investigators have tried to find a single pathognomonic finding that would be diagnostic of Legionnaire's disease.[16] However, no individual finding is indicative of Legionnaire's disease. Instead, clinicians should search for the characteristic findings of Legionnaire's disease, that is, "clinical predictors" that when considered together, make Legionnaire's disease highly likely.[17–19]

Since Legionnaire's disease often presents as a severe pneumonia, often requiring intensive care unit admission, clinicians need to recognize the characteristic pattern of extrapulmonary organ involvement of Legionnaire's disease so that diagnostic testing may be done, and anti-Legionella therapy added or included.[20,21] Clearly, all admitted adults with pneumonia should not be tested for Legionnaire's disease. Preferably, only those with severe pneumonia or those who have clinical predictors of Legionnaire's disease should be tested.[22] This selective approach has the effect of increasing the pretest probability of Legionnaire's disease and avoids "shotgun" overtesting.[23,24]

Decades after it was first described, Legionnaire's disease remains the most remarkable nonzoonotic atypical pneumonia with a multiple extrapulmonary manifestation, for example, fever with relative bradycardia, headache, mental confusion, watery diarrhea, abdominal pain, renal insufficiency.[4,22] As importantly, findings that are not associated with Legionnaire's disease (diagnostic eliminators) argue against the diagnosis, for example, no sore throat, eye, or ear involvement, no skin manifestations (*E multiforme*, Horder spots). Among the important nonspecific laboratory abnormalities of Legionnaire's disease are, otherwise unexplained, mildly elevated transaminases, hyponatremia, hypophosphatemia, highly elevated ferritin levels, elevated CPK, microscopic hematuria, and so forth.[22] Laboratory abnormalities that argue against a Legionnaire's disease diagnosis (diagnostic eliminators) include leukopenia, thrombocytopenia, thrombocytosis, or highly elevated cold agglutinin titers.[4]

The radiographic manifestations of Legionnaire's disease are nonspecific. The chest film is most helpful in ruling out other cause infiltrates, for example, CHF.[25] Similarly, chest CT scans provide greater resolution, but findings are not specific.[26] Given the unique ecological niche of *Legionella* sp in water, it is not surprising for Legionnaire's disease that there are more and more reports of various *Legionella* sp in aerosolized water sources that have caused Legionnaire's disease outbreaks in hospitals, chronic care facilities, and travelers.[1–3,27] Understanding the epidemiology of such outbreaks depends on suspicion as well as advanced diagnostic techniques, for example, PCR and molecular techniques to determine strain commonality.[5,28]

Recently, "new" zoonotic atypical pneumonias have emerged, for example, SARS, MERS.[4] The lessons learned from Legionnaire's disease in recognizing the pattern of extrapulmonary organ involvement have been useful in describing the clinical features of these "new" zoonotic atypical pneumonias.[4,29] Even the seasonal incidence of Legionnaire's disease depends somewhat on climate change, that is, related to precipitation patterns. With increased use of immunosuppressive drugs, we can expect more Legionnaire's disease in compromised hosts.[30-32] Legionnaire's disease still has much to teach us.

This issue of *Infectious Disease Clinics of North America* on Legionnaire's disease is a clinical compendium of the many interesting microbiologic, epidemiologic, and clinical aspects of Legionnaire's disease.[1–3] The contributors to this issue are internationally respected experts in their fields. Their articles provide clinicians worldwide with the benefit of their perspective, expertise, and clinical experience. The reader should enjoy this overview of the many fascinating aspects of Legionnaire's disease.

Cheston B. Cunha, MD
Antibiotic Stewardship Program
Division of Infectious Disease
Rhode Island Hospital
593 Eddy Street
Physicians Office Building
Suite #328
Providence, RI 02903, USA

Burke A. Cunha, MD, MACP
Infectious Disease Division
Winthrop-University Hospital
222 Station Plaza North, Suite #432
Mineola, NY 11501, USA

E-mail addresses:
ccunha@lifespan.org (C.B. Cunha)
bacunha@winthrop.org (B.A. Cunha)

REFERENCES

1. Honigsbaum M. Legionnaire's disease: revisiting the puzzle of the century. Lancet 2016;388:456–7.
2. Phin N, Parry-Ford F, Harrison T, et al. Epidemiology and clinical management of Legionnaire's disease. Lancet Infect Dis 2014;14:1011–21.
3. Cunha BA, Burillo A, Bouza E. Legionnaire's disease. Lancet 2016;387:376–85.
4. Cunha BA, editor. Pneumonia essentials. 3rd edition. Sudbury (MA): Jones & Bartlett; 2010.
5. Bouza E. Microbiology and epidemiology of Legionnaire's disease. Infect Dis Clin 2017;31(1):7–27.
6. Cunha BA, Cunha CB. Legionnaire's disease mimics: a clinical perspective. Infect Dis Clin 2017;31(1):95–109.
7. Cunha BA, Quintiliani R. The atypical pneumonias: a diagnostic and therapeutic approach. Postgrad Med 1979;66:95–102.
8. Cunha BA, Ortega AM. Atypical pneumonia. Extrapulmonary clues guide the way to diagnosis. Postgrad Med 1996;99:123–8.
9. Clyde WA Jr. Clinical overview of Mycoplasma pneumoniae infections. Clin Infect Dis 1993;1:s32–6.
10. Cunha CB. The first atypical pneumonia: the history of the discovery of Mycoplasma pneumoniae. Infect Dis Clin N Am 2010;24:1–5.
11. Lattimer GL, Rhodes LV 3rd. Legionnaires disease. Clinical findings and one-year follow-up. JAMA 1978;240:169–71.

12. Woodhead MA, Macfarlane JT. The protean manifestations of Legionnaires disease. J R Coll Physicians Lond 1985;19:224–30.
13. Woodhead MA, Macfarlane JT. Legionnaires disease: a review of 79 community acquired cases in Nottingham. Thorax 1986;41:635–40.
14. Cunha BA. Legionnaire's disease: clinical differentiation from typical and other atypical pneumonias. Infect Dis Clin N Am 2010;24:73–105.
15. Cunha BA. Atypical pneumonias: current clinical concepts focusing on Legionnaires disease. Curr Opin Pulm Med 2008;14:183–94.
16. Woodhead MA, Macfarlane JT. Comparative clinical and laboratory features of legionella with pneumococcal and mycoplasma pneumonias. Br J Dis Chest 1987; 81:133–9.
17. Strampfer MA, Cunha BA. Clinical and laboratory aspects of Legionnaire's disease. Semin Respir Infect 1987;2:228–34.
18. Cunha BA. Clinical features of legionnaires disease. Semin Respir Infect 1998;13: 116–27.
19. Cunha BA. The clinical diagnosis of Legionnaires disease: the diagnostic value of combining non-specific laboratory tests. J Infect 2008;56:395–7.
20. Opal S. Severe pneumonia: Legionnaire's disease: differential diagnosis considerations. Infect Dis Clin 2017;31(1):111–21.
21. Carratala J, Carcia-Vidal C. An update on Legionella. Curr Opin Infect Dis 2010; 23:152–7.
22. Cunha BA, Wu G, Raza M. Clinical diagnosis of Legionnaire's disease: six characteristic criteria. Am J Med 2015;128:e21–2.
23. Cunha BA. Characteristic predictors that increase the pretest probability of Legionnaires disease: "don't' order a test just because you can" revisited. South Med J 2015;108:761.
24. Den Boer JW, Yzerman PF. Diagnosis of Legionella infection of Legionnaire's disease. Eur J Clin Microbiol Infect Dis 2004;23:871–8.
25. Coletta FS, Fein AM. Radiological manifestations of Legionella/Legionella-like organisms. Semin Respir Infect 1998;13:109–15.
26. Katz D. Radiologic features of Legionnaire's disease. Infect Dis Clin 2017;31(1): 43–54.
27. File T. Nosocomial Legionnaire's disease. Infect Dis Clin 2017;31(1):155–65.
28. Dunne WM Jr, Picot N, Van Belkum A. Laboratory tests for Legionnaire's disease. Infect Dis Clin 2017;31(1):167–78.
29. Cunha CB, Opal SM. Middle East respiratory syndrome (MERS): a new zoonotic viral pneumonia. Virulence 2014;5:650–4.
30. Khardori N. Legionnaire's disease and immunosuppressive drugs. Infect Dis Clin 2017;31(1):29–42.
31. Lortholary O. Legionnaire's disease in compromised hosts. Infect Dis Clin 2017; 31(1):123–35.
32. Iannuzzi M, De Robertis E, Piazza O, et al. Respiratory failure presenting in H1N1 influenza with Legionnaires disease: two case reports. J Med Case Rep 2011;5: 520–5.

Legionnaire's Disease Since Philadelphia

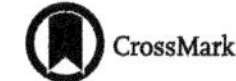

Lessons Learned and Continued Progress

Cheston B. Cunha, MD[a,*], Burke A. Cunha, MD, MACP[b,c]

KEYWORDS

- Atypical pneumonias • Legionnaire's disease • Legionella
- Community-acquired pneumonia

KEY POINTS

- After the Philadelphia outbreak, Legionnaire's disease was recognized as a newly described cause of severe community-acquired pneumonia (CAP).
- Legionnaire's disease has characteristic extrapulmonary findings, which, when considered together, are the basis for a presumptive clinical diagnosis.
- The widespread use of *Legionella* culture, sputum DFA, serology, urinary antigen testing, and polymerase chain reaction (PCR) have allowed earlier diagnosis of Legionnaire's disease.
- Excluding common source outbreaks (eg, from water towers), CAP caused by Legionnaire's disease is manifested as sporadic cases. In contrast, nosocomial Legionnaire's disease, which clinically has the same features as community-acquired Legionnaire's disease, occurs in clusters or outbreaks from common *Legionella* species-contaminated water sources.
- Improved diagnostic tests have permitted accurate diagnosis, which allows Legionnaire's disease mimics to be differentiated from *Legionella* species CAP. Bacterial coinfections with Legionnaire's disease are uncommon, but when present, are most often associated with bacteremia pneumococcal pneumonia.

THE PHILADELPHIA OUTBREAK AND EARLY CASES

There are many clinical lessons that came from the Philadelphia outbreak and early cases.[1] When it was finally determined that the new atypical pneumonia in Philadelphia was due to Legionnaire's disease, 2 clinical varieties were described. The usual clinical manifestation of Legionnaire's disease was that of an atypical pneumonia (ie, a

[a] Division of Infectious Disease, Rhode Island Hospital, Miriam Hospital, Brown University Alpert School of Medicine, Providence, RI 02903, USA; [b] Division of Infectious Disease, Winthrop-University Hospital, Mineola, NY 11501, USA; [c] School of Medicine, State University of New York, Stony Brook, NY 11794, USA
* Corresponding author.
E-mail address: ccunha@lifespan.org

Infect Dis Clin N Am 31 (2017) 1–5
http://dx.doi.org/10.1016/j.idc.2016.10.001 id.theclinics.com
0891-5520/17/

pneumonia with extrapulmonary manifestations). In some cases, there was an acute febrile illness without pneumonia, which was termed Pontiac fever. There has been little progress in the understanding of why *Legionella* uncommonly presents as Pontiac fever, while most cases of *Legionella* manifest as Legionnaire's disease.[2] When it was finally established that Legionnaire's disease was caused by to a gram-negative intracellular pathogen in alveolar microphages, tests were developed to diagnose Legionnaire's disease by a variety of methods. First sputum culture on selective media was developed, followed by DFA and serologic methods.[2]

The initial clinical descriptions of Legionnaire's disease remain among the best classic descriptions in the history of newly described infectious diseases.[3–5] Virtually all of the characteristic clinical findings of Legionnaire's disease were so well described in the early cases, (eg, high fever with relative bradycardia, mental confusion, watery diarrhea, abdominal pain, relative lymphopenia, hypophosphatemia, hyponatremia, and renal insuffiency).[6–10] Although Legionnaire's disease was recognized as a new atypical pneumonia, it had distinctive extrapulmonary clinical features. Many investigators tried to find individual clinical findings that would be diagnostic of Legionnaire's disease to no avail. Rather, it is the pattern of extrapulmonary organ involvement that is characteristic in Legionnaire's disease, not isolated findings (eg, degree of fever, pulmonary symptoms, and hyponatremia). Key Legionnaire's disease clinical findings, considered together as a diagnostic pattern, are the basis of presumptive clinical syndromic diagnosis.[11–13] Also, still underappreciated is that all Legionnaire's disease characteristic findings do not have the same diagnostic weight or diagnostic significance.[14,15] It is important to realize the diagnostic importance relative diagnostic weights of Legionnaire's disease clinical findings (eg, in CAP patients, hyponatremia is common and consistent with the diagnosis of *Legionella* disease, but otherwise unexplained hypophosphatermia, when present, has much more diagnostic weight as a prediction of Legionnaire's disease).[15] Similarly, in a hospitalized adult with zoonotic atypical pneumonias that can be reasonably excluded by negative history, CAP, a fever greater than 102°F, and an otherwise unexplained pulse deficit (ie, relative bradycardia), limit diagnostic possibilities to Legionnaire's disease. This key finding also eliminates the other causes of typical bacterial pneumonias and other non-zoonotic atypical pneumonias, *Mycoplasma pneumoniae, Chlamydophila pneumonia*.[15,16]

HOST FACTORS

Initially, it was thought that Legionnaire's disease was primarily to be a disease of the elderly and compromised hosts. It is now appreciated that Legionnaire's disease is a common cause of severe pneumonias in normal hosts.[12] With the widespread use of immunosuppresive medications, there is increased awareness that Legionnaire's disease is not uncommon in these patients.[17] It is now known that impaired cell meditated immunity (CMI) is the host defense defect that predisposes to Legionnaire's disease.[18] Given the increasing use of immunosuppressive therapies, more Legionnaire's disease is to be expected in the future.

MICROBIOLOGY AND EPIDEMIOLOGY

Legionella species are fresh water microorganisms with the ability to survive in biofilms, which has important implications for outbreak investigations and disinfection of water systems containing *Legionella* species like other microbes, are profoundly affected by temperature. Optimal growth of *Legionella* species is between 20°C and 40°C, and *Legionella* species growth is inhibited by temperatures of 40° to 70°C.

Because *Legionella* species are water organisms, if the *Legionella* species in water are present in sufficient concentrations pathogenic for people, it is not surprising that inhaled aerosolized contaminated water has been linked to an amazing variety of water sources in Legionnaire's disease outbreaks.[16,19–21] Community-acquired Legionnaire disease, excluding common source exposures, presents as sporadic cases. In contrast, nosocomial or nursing home Legionnaire's disease always occurs in clusters or outbreaks due to a common contaminated water source. In the community, it may be difficult to determine the common source of an outbreak (eg, water towers) when cases vary in geographic location or patients are admitted to different hospitals. Expectedly, there have been increasing reports of travel-related Legionnaire's disease outbreaks.[20] The common denominator in travel-related Legionnaire's disease is a common exposure to *Legionella* species-containing water.[16]

Epidemiologically, Legionnaire's disease outbreaks have been traced to a wide variety of water sources (eg, windshield wiper fluid, sprays from water puddles, planting soil/compost, vegetable misters in food markets, air conditioning, humidifiers, and hot tubs). There will be more reports of travel-related Legionnaire's disease as potential sources are recognized. Molecular methods have been a major advance in identifying and tracing outbreaks in travel and related nosocomial outbreaks.[16,19,20]

The importance of climate change on the frequency and seasonality of Legionnaire's disease has only recently been appreciated. Traditionally, Legionnaire's disease has peaked in the late summer/early fall. With climate change affecting precipitation patterns, Legionnaire's disease is now not uncommon in the spring with increased rainfall.

DIAGNOSTIC METHODS

Sputum cultures, DFA of sputum, and *Legionella* titers traditionally were the mainstay of Legionnaire's disease diagnosis. The next important advance in diagnostic testing was the *Legionella* urinary antigen test. Urinary antigen testing has been useful in the diagnosis of Legionnaire's disease in those with a nonproductive cough or without titer elevations. Because Legionella antigenesis persists for weeks, cases of suspected Legionnaire's disease may be diagnosed weeks after the illness. Fortunately, the most common species causing Legionnaire's disease is *L pneumophila* (serotype I). The main limitation of *Legionella* urinary antigen testing is that it may not be present early and detects only *L pneumophila* (serotype I). Speciation may be done by serology polymerase chain reaction.[20,22]

LEGIONNAIRE'S DISEASE MIMICS

As the clinical features of Legionella disease are appreciated, some other causes of severe CAP may have features is common with Legionnaire's disease (ie, may be considered Legionnaire's disease mimics). Most common mimics of Legionnaire's disease are *Streptococcus pneumoniae*, Q fever, influenza, some influenza like illness (ILI) viruses (eg, RSV, hMPV, HPIV-3, or adenovirus). Viral PCR of respiratory secretions have helped to accurately diagnose ILI viral mimics of Legionnaire's disease.[23,24] Legionnaire's disease mimics are likely to continue to be recognized and reported.

ANTIMICROBIAL THERAPY

The initial Philadelphia cases were a common source of outbreak at a center city hotel, during a Legionnaire's convention.[1] The outbreak prompted clinicians to carefully describe the clinical aspects of Legionnaire's disease to determine what effective therapy was. In the early years of Legionnaire's disease treatment, erythromycin and tetracycline were found to be effective, and β-lactam antibiotics were found to be ineffective.[12] Later, other antibiotics were also found to be effective against Legionnaire's disease (eg, quinolones, azithromycin, rifampin, TMP-SMX, and tigecycline). The mainstay of antibiotic therapy of Legionnaire's disease is with doxycycline, quinolones, or azithromycin.[25] Combination therapy with previously mentioned antibiotics plus rifampin or TMP-SMX can be used for severe Legionnaire's disease. Because these agents have a high degree of anti-Legionella activity and achieve high concentrations in alveolar macrophages. it is unlikely that additional antibodies to treat Legionnaire's disease will be needed.

SUMMARY

Since the Philadelphia outbreak, Legionnaire's disease has recognized as a newly described cause of non-zootonic atypical pneumonia. Since early clinical descriptions of this new infectious disease entity, little has been added to the knowledge of additional extrapulmonary features of Legionnaire's disease. The most progress in Legionnaire's disease has been made in the areas of microbiology and epidemiology. Given its unique aquatic ecological niche, Legionnaire's disease has been increasingly recognized as a cause of nosocomial and travel-related outbreaks, and the mainstay of antibiotic therapy in Legionnaire's disease remains doxycycline, quinolones, and azithromycin. There have been few new effective anti-*Legionella* antibiotics. With the widespread presence of antibiotic stewardship programs (ASPs), empiric single-versus double-drug therapy, and widespread utilization of intravenous to oral route switch therapy, there has been an attempt to decrease drug costs and hospital length of stay in therapy of Legionnaire's disease and to streamline therapy.

REFERENCES

1. Fraser DW, Tsai TR, Orenstein W, et al. Legionnaire's disease: description of an epidemic of pneumonia. N Engl J Med 1977;297:1189–97.
2. McDade JE, Shepard CC, Fraser DW, et al. Legionnaire's disease: isolation of a bacterium and demonstration of its role in other respiratory disease. N Engl J Med 1977;297:1197–203.
3. Lattimer GL, Rhodes LV 3rd. Legionnaire's disease. Clinical findings and one-year follow up. JAMA 1978;240:169–71.
4. Tsai TF, Finn DR, Plikaytis BD, et al. Legionnaire's disease: clinical features of the epidemic in Philadephia. Ann Intern Med 1979;90:509–17.
5. Woodhead MA, Macfarlane JT. Legionnaire's disease: a review of 79 community acquired cases in Nottingham. Thorax 1986;41:635–40.
6. Strampfer MA, Cunha BA. Clinical and laboratory aspects of Legionnaire's disease. Semin Respir Infect 1987;2:228–34.
7. Cunha BA, Quintiliani R. The atypical pneumonias: a diagnostic and therapeutic approach. Postgrad Med 1979;66:95–102.
8. Cunha BA, Ortega AM. Atypical pneumonia. Extrapulmonary clues guide the way to diagnosis. Postgrad Med 1996;99:123–8.
9. Cunha BA. Legionnaire's disease: clinical differentiation from typical and other atypical pneumonias. Infect Dis Clin North Am 2010;24:73–105.
10. Cunha BA. Characteristic predictors that increase the pretest probability of Legionnaires disease: "don't order a test just because you can" revisited. South Med J 2015;108:761.

11. Cunha BA. The clinical diagnosis of Legionnaires disease: the diagnostic value of combining non-specific laboratory tests. J Infect 2008;56:395–7.
12. Edelstein PH. Legionnaire's disease. Clin Infect Dis 1993;16:741–7.
13. Cunha BA. Atypical pneumonias: current clinical concepts focusing on Legionnaire's disease. Curr Opin Pulm Med 2008;14:183–94.
14. Cunha BA. Severe Legionella Pneumonia: rapid presumptive clinical Diagnosis with Winthrop-University Hospital's Weighted Point Score System (Modified). Heart Lung 2008;37:312–21.
15. Cunha BA, Wu G, Raza M. Clinical diagnosis of Legionnaire's disease: six characteristic criteria. Am J Med 2015;128:e21–2.
16. Phin N, Parry-Ford F, Harrison T, et al. Epidemiology and clinical management of Legionnaire's disease. Lancet Infect Dis 2014;14:1011–21.
17. Lortholary O. Legionnaire's disease in compromised hosts. Infectious Disease Clinics 2017;31(1):123–35.
18. Khardori N. Legionnaire's disease & Immunosuppresive drugs. Infectious Disease Clinics 2017;31(1):29–42.
19. Cunha BA, Burillo A, Bouza E. Legionnaire's disease. Lancet 2016;387:376–85.
20. Bouza E. Microbiology & Epidemiology of Legionnaire's disease. Infectious Disease 2017;31(1):7–27.
21. File T. Nosocomial Legionnaire's disease. Infectious Disease Clinics 2017;31(1): 155–65.
22. Van Belkum A. Laboratory tests for Legionnaire's disease. Infectious Disease Clinics 2017;31(1):167–78.
23. Cunha BA, Cunha CB. Legionnaire's disease Mimics: a clinical perspective. Infectious Disease Clinics 2017;31(1):95–109.
24. Opal S. Severe pneumonia: Legionnaire's disease: differential diagnosis considerations. Infectious Disease Clinics 2017;31(1):111–21.
25. Edelstein PH. Antimicrobial chemotherapy for Legionnaires disease: a review. Clin Infect Dis 1995;21(Supply 3):S265–7.

Microbiology and Epidemiology of Legionnaire's Disease

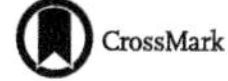

Almudena Burillo, MD, PhD[a,b,c],
María Luisa Pedro-Botet, MD, PhD[d,e,f], Emilio Bouza, MD, PhD[a,b,c,g,*]

KEYWORDS

- *Legionella* • Legionnaire's disease • Legionnaire's disease epidemiology
- Legionnaire's diseases microbiology • Legionnaire's diseases diagnosis

KEY POINTS

- Microorganisms of the genus *Legionella*, discovered in 1976-77, are particular gram negative rods with special growth requirements. Currently, 58 species and over 70 distinct serogroups of *Legionella* have been identified. It mainly causes pneumonia.
- *Legionella* spp are ubiquitous in aquatic environments and water distribution systems. LD is transmitted from the environment to humans mainly through inhalation of contaminated aerosols. There has been one case of probable human-to-human transmission of *Legionella* spp.
- The incidence of the disease has important geographic variations and ranges from 2 cases/million inhabitants in Ontario (Canada) or some European countries to 18 cases/million inhabitants in Australia. True incidence is probably underestimated.
- Host risk factors for LD include male sex, age over 50 years, smoking, alcohol abuse, certain chronic diseases, hematological malignancies, and immunosuppression.
- The gold standard for diagnosis is culture isolation from clinical samples, but this only is achieved in a low percentage of cases. Alternative diagnostic techniques include the detection of urinary antigen (for *Legionella pneumophila* serogroup 1), seroconversion or nucleic acid amplification tests.

Continued

Transparency Declarations: Nothing to disclose.

[a] Division of Clinical Microbiology and Infectious Diseases, Hospital General Universitario Gregorio Marañón, Doctor Esquerdo 46, 28007 Madrid, Spain; [b] Instituto de Investigación Sanitaria Gregorio Marañón, Doctor Esquerdo 46, 28007 Madrid, Spain; [c] Departamento de Medicina, Facultad de Medicina, Universidad Complutense de Madrid, Plaza Ramón y Cajal s/n, 28040 Madrid, Spain; [d] Infectious Diseases Unit, Hospital Universitario German Trías i Pujol, Carretera de Canyet s/n, 08916 Badalona, Spain; [e] Departamento de Medicina, Area de Medicina, Universidad Autónoma de Barcelona, Plaza Cívica, Campus de la UAB, 08193 Bellaterra, Sardañola del Vallés (Barcelona), Spain; [f] CIBER de Enfermedades Respiratorias (CIBERES CB06/06/1089), Instituto de Salud Carlos III, Monforte de Lemos 3-5, Pabellón 11, 28029 Madrid, Spain; [g] CIBER de Enfermedades Respiratorias (CIBERES CB06/06/0058), Instituto de Salud Carlos III, Monforte de Lemos 3-5, Pabellón 11, 28029 Madrid, Spain
* Corresponding author. Division of Infectious Disease, Hospital General Universitario Gregorio Marañón, Doctor Esquerdo 46, Madrid 28007, Spain.
E-mail address: ebouza@pdi.ucm.es

Infect Dis Clin N Am 31 (2017) 7–27
http://dx.doi.org/10.1016/j.idc.2016.10.002
id.theclinics.com
0891-5520/17/

Continued

- The incidence of the disease has important geographic variations and ranges from 2 cases per million inhabitants in Ontario (Canada) or some European countries to 18 cases per million inhabitants in Australia. True incidence is probably underestimated.
- Host risk factors for Legionnaire's disease (LD) include male sex, older than 50 years, smoking, alcohol abuse, certain chronic diseases, hematological malignancies, and immunosuppression.
- Source factors linked to the risk of infection are bacterial load, virulence of the colonizing bacteria, dissemination efficiency, and aerosol type. Cumulative exposure to a source of LD is a risk factor for disease acquisition.
- Because *Legionella* is an intracellular pathogen, direct in vitro susceptibilities to antibiotics are difficult to interpret. Intracellular or animal models seem to correlate better with clinical response to treatment.
- Genotyping of strains is helpful to establish the environmental source of the disease.

INTRODUCTION

Legionellosis is caused by aerobic gram-negative bacilli of the genus *Legionella*. Currently, 58 species and more than 70 distinct serogroups of *Legionella* have been identified. Although all species are potentially pathogenic, legionellosis is most often caused by *Legionella pneumophila* serogroup 1 (Lp1). Other species of *Legionella* commonly identified as agents of disease in humans are *Legionella micdadei*, *Legionella bozemanae*, *Legionella dumoffii*, and *Legionella longbeachae*.

Legionellosis may present as Pontiac fever or Legionnaire's disease (LD). Pontiac fever is a mild, self-limiting flulike illness, which resolves in 2 to 5 days and does not benefit from antibiotic treatment. LD is the pneumonic form of legionellosis, with a case fatality rate of around 10%. Mortality is higher in nosocomial and immunosuppressed patients (more than 25%).

Legionella spp are present worldwide and are found in natural water bodies and water distribution systems. Susceptible individuals become infected when they inhale aerosolized water droplets contaminated with *Legionella* spp. The increased use of engineering products that create aerosols has increased the risk of human exposure to this microorganism.

LD is an important public health problem with notification rates that are still low. Outbreaks are the result of deficiencies in the keeping of water systems. Both LD and Pontiac fever are notifiable diseases in the United States, Canada, and Singapore. LD is also notifiable in the European Union, Israel, Japan, Australia, and New Zealand.

Laboratory testing for the detection of *Legionella* spp may include respiratory culture, urine antigen testing, serum antibody testing, and other molecular methods (eg, polymerase chain reaction [PCR]). Respiratory culture is the gold standard for a diagnosis of legionellosis and permits species identification. Although urine antigen detection is increasingly used among clinicians, this method is only able to diagnose Lp1. PCR is increasingly being used in several countries, and it is currently the only approach valid for a rapid diagnosis of LD caused by non-Lp1 and non–*Legionella pneumophila* spp.

Most cases of LD are sporadic and community acquired (more than 70%), followed by those travel associated (more than 20%) or health care related (around 10%). Over the past decade, incidence rates for legionellosis have been increasing in the United States, Canada, Europe, Israel, and Japan, though it is underestimated globally. Risk factors for *Legionella* spp infection include male sex, more than 40 years of age, smoking, alcohol abuse, certain chronic diseases (eg, diabetes, chronic heart/lung diseases, chronic renal failure), immunocompromised (eg, corticosteroids, chemotherapy, transplant recipients), hematological malignancy, iron overload, and/or a history of recent travel.

In this article, the authors discuss the microbiology, laboratory diagnosis, and epidemiology of LD.

Disease description

- Legionellosis is caused by aerobic gram-negative bacilli of the genus *Legionella*. Currently, 58 species and more than 70 distinct serogroups of *Legionella* have been identified.
- The most frequent cause is Lp1. Other species of *Legionella* associated with disease in humans include *L micdadei*, *L bozemanae*, *L dumoffii*, and *Legionella longbeachae*.
- Susceptible individuals become infected when they inhale aerosolized water droplets contaminated with the bacteria. There has been one case of probable human-to-human transmission of *Legionella* spp. It is an intracellular pathogen.
- There are 2 main clinical presentations: Pontiac fever or LD.
- Pontiac fever is a mild, self-limiting flulike illness that resolves in 2 to 5 days and does not benefit from antibiotic treatment.
- LD is the pneumonic form of legionellosis, with a case fatality rate of around 10%. Mortality is higher in nosocomial and immunosuppressed patients (more than 25%).
- LD occurs worldwide. Over the past decade, incidence rates for legionellosis have been increasing. It follows seasonal and geographic variability. Most cases are sporadic and community acquired (more than 70%), followed by those travel associated (more than 20%) or health care related (around 10%).
- It is a significant public health problem with still low notification rates.

MICROBIOLOGY

Legionella is the only genus of the family *Legionellaceae* and consists of 59 species and 3 subspecies (http://www.bacterio.net/legionella.html). All species have been discovered in aquatic environments.[1] Some 30 species are known to cause human infection, mostly lower respiratory tract (LRT) infections.

Legionella spp are small to filamentous gram-negative rods with strict growth requirements.[2] On solid media, both selective and nonselective,[2,3] colonies are usually appreciable after 3 to 5 days of incubation. Young colonies are 0.5 to 1.0 mm in diameter, flat, smooth, and self-contained and have a typical ground-glass appearance and iridescent hue. Older colonies appear opaque, with a white center and poorly defined opalescent margins. When *Legionella* is suspected, colonies should be gram stained to check for negative rods and plated onto 2 different media with and without L-cysteine to confirm the bacterium's requirement of this amino acid.

To identify the species of *Legionella*, more sophisticated tests are needed, including phenotypic characteristics; growth requirements; agglutination or fluorescent antibody techniques for serologic identification; fatty acid, carbohydrate, or ubiquinone analysis; protein profiling; and molecular techniques.[4]

Today, *Legionella* spp are identified by comparing their 16S ribosomal RNA or macrophage infectivity potentiator (*mip*) genes with known sequences available respectively at GenBank (www.ncbi.nlm.nih.gov) or the UK Health Protection Agency (http://www.hpa-bioinfotools.org.uk/mip_help.html).[5–8] The reader is referred to a recently updated flowchart describing the identification of *Legionella* spp isolates.[3]

Several methods are available to subtype *Legionella* spp.[9] So far, these methods have been mostly used on *L pneumophila* and to compare clinical and environmental isolates when investigating an outbreak.

Monoclonal antibodies (MAbs) directed against lipopolysaccharide epitopes (LPS) on the bacterial cell surface have been useful to identify Lp1 and to detect strains that express the virulence-associated epitope recognized by MAb 3/1 of the Dresden panel (MAb 2 of the international panel).[10] In addition, the MAb method has been long used to select *Legionella* strains for genotyping[11,12] and recently used to subtype urinary antigen-positive urine samples.[13]

Some *Legionella* spp designated *Legionella*-like amoebal pathogens (LLAP) do not grow on routinely used culture media. One such LLAP was isolated by ameba enrichment from the sputum of a patient with pneumonia.[14] Other LLAP strains may also be human pathogens, but this remains to be clearly demonstrated.[15] The optimal growth temperature for most LLAP is 35°C.

LABORATORY DIAGNOSIS

The laboratory diagnosis of LD can be based on either culture or nonculture techniques.

Nonculture Techniques

Legionella spp are difficult to detect by microscopy examination of gram-stained patient samples.[2] Staining with 0.1% basic fuchsin solution rather than safranin is more effective; but even so, it is hard to visualize them. *L pneumophila* can be identified in clinical samples by fluorescent microscopy. However, the sensitivity of this method is low because of its high dependence on staining quality, operator skill, and the necessity of a high bacterial load.[16] In addition, the existence of cross-staining non-*Legionella* organisms has determined that this diagnostic method is rarely used.

The first-line non–culture-based diagnostic test for LD is urinary soluble antigen detection, which picks up a component of the *L pneumophila* cell wall LPS. This method is the fastest method, though it is limited to Lp1.[3,17] In Europe, cases diagnosed using the urinary antigen method have significantly increased since 1998 (15% in 1995 vs more than 90% in 2006), accompanying the increase in the use of this test. Patients return a positive test result within 48 to 72 hours of symptom onset and may continue to test positive for several weeks to months. Test sensitivity is 56% to 99%,[3,18] meaning it may miss as many as 40% of cases of LD.[19] The method is most sensitive for Lp1 MAb 3/1 subtypes. A lower sensitivity of around 40% has been observed for other subtypes. Test sensitivity has been correlated with LD severity.[20] Sensitivity is also lower in patients with nosocomial infection or under immunosuppression because of a greater likelihood of infections caused by Lp1 MAb 3/1 negative strains or by *Legionella* spp other than *L pneumophila*.[17]

A minority of patients with Pontiac fever may also test positive for the urinary antigen. If epidemiologic and clinical findings in these patients indicate Lp1-associated Pontiac fever, the test could serve to confirm cases and the occurrence of an outbreak.[21,22]

IDSA-ATS guidelines on the management of community-acquired pneumonia (CAP) in adults recommend urinary antigen testing in patients not responding to outpatient antibiotic treatment; those with severe pneumonia, especially if they require intensive care; immunocompromised hosts; patients actively abusing alcohol; those who have traveled within the past 2 weeks; those with pleural effusions; those with pneumonia in the setting of an LD outbreak; and those with suspected health care–associated pneumonia.[23]

When to perform urinary antigen testing for *Legionella* in patients with CAP

- Patients not responding to outpatient antibiotic treatment
- Patients with severe pneumonia, especially if they require intensive care
- Immunocompromised hosts
- Patients actively abusing alcohol
- Patients who have traveled within the past 2 weeks
- Patients with pleural effusions
- Patients with pneumonia in the setting of an LD outbreak
- Patients with suspected health care–associated pneumonia

Molecular techniques can improve a diagnosis of LD because they detect different serogroups and species. These techniques also feature a higher sensitivity (around 30%) than culture methods.[7,24,25] Nucleic acid amplification-based methods have successfully identified *Legionella* spp, especially *Legionella pneumophila*, in urine, sputum, and blood. Six commercial assays exist, but only one has received approval from the US Food and Drug Administration (BD ProbeTec ET *L pneumophila* amplified DNA assay, Becton, Dickinson and Company, Franklin Lakes, NJ), though it is not marketed in the United States at the time of writing this article.[2,26] For LRT secretions, serum, and urine, molecular test sensitivities of 80% to 100%, 30% to 80%, and 0% to 90%, respectively, have been reported.[2,24] At most laboratories, the *mip* gene is targeted for *L pneumophila* identification.[24,27]

Serologic methods are not too effective. High antibody titers detected in acute-phase serum samples are not diagnostic because antibodies from prior subclinical *Legionella* spp infection or cross-reacting antibodies from heterologous bacterial infections may be present. Moreover, in most patients with culture-confirmed LD, seroconversion is not detectable until 3 weeks after infection at the very earliest. In up to a quarter of patients with culture-confirmed disease, there is no detectable seroconversion. Further, many immunosuppressed patients never produce antibodies.[16] Moreover, acute-phase serum samples with a high antibody titer are not diagnostic given that 1% to 16% of healthy adults have titers greater than 1:256.[28,29]

To diagnose Pontiac fever, an immune response to the bacterium is usually looked for, though the sensitivity of this method varies and it is often nonspecific. To effectively detect this mild legionellosis, serologic positivity rates need to be compared in a large group of people with symptoms of Pontiac fever exposed to a common source and in a control population.[30]

Culture-Based Techniques

LRT sample culture is still the gold standard for detecting LD.[3]

Samples for culture obtained in the acute infection phase should be quickly transported to the laboratory, preferably before starting antimicrobial therapy.

For optimal yields of *Legionella* spp, samples are diluted to limit growth inhibition by tissue and serum factors or antibiotics. To minimize commensal respiratory microbiota, samples are pretreated with a heat shock or an acid-wash solution.[3] Initial isolation requires special culture media containing L-cysteine, iron, and alpha-ketoglutarate (eg, buffered charcoal-yeast extract [BYCE] agar); pH should be kept at 6.7 to 6.9.[2,3,31] BYCE medium supplemented with 0.1% alpha-ketoglutarate is commonly used to isolate and grow *Legionella* spp. This medium can be made selective by adding antibiotics.

The routine use of this technique is highly recommended as it enables the diagnosis of all *Legionella* spp and the investigation of an outbreak and further epidemiologic study.[32] In addition, LRT secretion cultures can be used for antimicrobial susceptibility testing.

The culture of nonrespiratory samples is recommended only if the disease is suspected to affect other anatomic sites.[2] In a small proportion of episodes, nonrespiratory legionellosis manifestations may occur accompanied or not by pneumonia. Extrarespiratory infections are protean and may include splenomegaly and spleen rupture,[33] pericarditis,[34] myocarditis,[35] wound infections,[36] endocarditis,[37,38] arthritis,[39,40] and central nervous system infections.[41,42]

Culture plates are incubated at 35°C in conditions of high humidity. An atmosphere of 2% to 5% carbon dioxide can improve the growth of some species on solid media.[43] The sensitivity of culturing respiratory samples is 20% to 80% and varies with the sample type.[3,44,45] Infection severity has a strong impact on culture yield. Patients with severe pneumonia show much higher sputum bacterial concentrations than those who are not as ill.[25,46] A low sensitivity is sometimes attributed to patients frequently producing insufficient sputum, prior antibiotic therapy, fastidious growth requirements of the causative strain, and the technical expertise required for its isolation.[47,48] Moreover, respiratory samples are infrequently obtained from patients with suspected LD.[24,49]

Both in the United States and Europe, there has been a decline in the culture-based diagnosis of LD. Currently, 5% to 12% of cases of LD are culture confirmed in these countries, with the exception of Denmark where as many a third of cases are culture proven.[50,51]

Investigating Outbreaks

When investigating an outbreak, several steps need to be taken.[4,52,53] These steps include case definition, gathering epidemiologic information, and testing environmental samples for *Legionella* spp. Very importantly, a confirmatory epidemiologic investigation is also required. For a list of environmental sites commonly sampled for *Legionella* spp along with details of the sampling and sample processing techniques to be used, the reader is referred to the report by Kozak and colleagues.[54]

Culture remains the gold standard for the detection of *Legionella* spp in the environment.[54] The culture method is complex, and considerable losses of *Legionella* spp may occur during its multiple steps. Viable but nonculturable (VBNC) cells incapable of multiplying on artificial media also exist.

Nonculture methods, such as quantitative PCR, are more sensitive for the identification of *Legionella* spp in the environment.[53] Molecular methods, on the other hand, have the drawback of not being able to differentiate between live and dead bacteria. A quantitative PCR method has been developed for the rapid simultaneous detection and identification of Lp1 in both clinical and environmental samples with a high negative predictive value.[55] This technique has proved useful to quickly detect or eliminate potential sources.

Once *Legionella* spp strains are recovered, different isolates of the same species are discriminated using typing methods to establish the source of an outbreak.

Monoclonal antibody subtyping is useful to exclude environmental strains not related to patient isolates from further investigation.

Genotyping of strains isolated from patients serves to identify the strain that originated the outbreak, and this strain can then be looked for in environmental samples using culture techniques. The genotyping methods most frequently used are pulsed-field gel electrophoresis and amplified fragment length polymorphisms (AFLPs) for all *Legionella* spp and sequence-based typing (SBT) for *L pneumophila*.[9,56,57] In the SBT method, the strain to be identified is assigned to a sequence type or allele profile, which can be compared with known sequence types defined in the European Working Group for *Legionella* Infections SBT database for *L pneumophila* (http://www.hpa-bioinformatics.org.uk/legionella/legionella_sbt/php/sbt_homepage.php). SBT is usually performed directly on culture isolates, though it has proved successful on nucleic acids extracted from human samples.[58]

Genotyping methods have several limitations. Studies have shown that AFLPs alone can lead to erroneous conclusions regarding the outbreak source. Further, some sequence types are common to many strains, limiting the discrimination capacity of the SBT method. Other sequence types are rare or restricted to local areas. Likewise, several unrelated strains might be indistinguishable using any one method. Accordingly, a combination of strategies is recommended to determine the identity or nonidentity of isolates, including spoligotyping, microarrays, high-resolution melt curve analysis, or whole-genome sequencing (WGS).[9,59] Indeed, WGS can narrow down the possible point source of exposure, identify *Legionella* to the species level, and establish relatedness between isolates.[60]

Environmental testing also serves to monitor the effectiveness of decontamination procedures and is of particular importance in centers caring for high-risk patients, such as bone marrow or organ transplant patients.[54,61]

Prompt reporting of suspected or confirmed cases of LD to public health authorities is essential to identify outbreaks and is legally required in many regions.[46]

Recommendations for LD risk assessment and outbreak management are available from the World Health Organization, Centers for Disease Control and Prevention (CDC) (*Legionella* Web sites) and the European Center for Disease Prevention and Control (ECDC) (ECDC legionellosis health topic Web site).[4] From 2000 to 2014, the CDC participated in 38 field investigations of LD[62]; 9 in 10 investigations showed almost all outbreaks were caused by problems preventable with more effective water management. The CDC has just released a tool kit for building owners and managers: "Developing a Water Management Program to Reduce *Legionella* Growth & Spread in Buildings: A Practical Guide to Implementing Industry Standards" (http://www.cdc.gov/*legionella*/maintenance/wmp-toolkit.html). Based on the American Society of Heating, Refrigerating, and Air Conditioning Engineers Standard 188, a document for building engineers, the tool kit provides a checklist to help identify if a water management program is needed, examples to help identify where *Legionella* spp could grow and spread in a building, and ways to reduce the risk of *Legionella* spp contamination.

Finally, antibody tests on paired serum samples may be useful to track outbreaks.

Antimicrobial Susceptibility Testing

Interpreting *Legionella* spp susceptibilities to antibiotics is difficult; there is no standardized test, and in vitro results often conflict with clinical outcomes.[63,64] The 3 methods currently used are extracellular susceptibility tests (standard dilutions in agar or broth or Epsilon-test), in vitro intracellular models, and animal infection models.[63,65] Conventional broth or agar-based methods are insufficiently reliable to predict the clinical activity of drugs. BYCE agar used for *Legionella* spp binds antibiotics limiting their activity.[66] Further, the susceptibility of *L pneumophila* grown in broth or on agar may lack clinical significance; because of its intracellular location, not all antibiotics can access the bacterium.[2,63]

In vitro intracellular models take into account the intracellular concentrations and activities of antibiotics. Several cell models, such as alveolar macrophages,[67] human monocytes,[68] or neutrophils,[69] exist, along with tissue culture models, including HeLa[70] or Human promyelocytic leukemia cell line-60[71] cells, among others. Once the given cell line is infected with *Legionella* spp, antibiotics are then added. To determine the capacity of an agent to block the intracellular growth of the bacterium, bacterial concentrations are measured over time. The time until bacterial regrowth after drug removal is taken to indicate the drug's intracellular activity. Based on this procedure, Edelstein classified antibiotics as noninhibitory, reversibly inhibitory, or capable of killing or causing prolonged intracellular growth inhibition after drug removal.[72]

Generally, intracellular or animal models correlate well with human disease.[73] However, these methods have the drawback that they are technically demanding and costly. Moreover, pharmacokinetics vary between animals and humans, and several strains or drugs cannot be tested at the same time. Consequently, today they are only used for research purposes.

LD treatment failure does not seem to be associated with resistance to the drugs used. In effect, only one clinical *L pneumophila* isolate resistant to ciprofloxacin has been reported.[74]

EPIDEMIOLOGY

Incidence

LD global incidence is unknown nowadays, mainly because it is grossly underdiagnosed and underreported[75] and because countries differ in their level of awareness, diagnostic methods, and investigation efforts.[4]

In spite of this, the available information concerning this disease has greatly improved in the past 20 years, because the disease is diagnosed more frequently and notifications have increased.

There are some data concerning the frequency of *Legionella* spp as a cause of CAP. It is estimated that this is the causative agent of 2% to 9% of these cases.[76]

There are incidence data available from the United States and Canada, Europe, some countries from Southeast Asia (Japan, Singapore), and from Australia and New Zealand (**Table 1**). LD is a notifiable disease in all these countries.

About 5000 cases of LD are now reported each year in the United States. The CDC has just communicated that LD increased by 286% from 2000 to 2014 (http://www.cdc.gov/*legionella*/surv-reporting.html).[77]

In the United States, in the 2000s, there was a general increasing trend in LD. Factors contributing to this increase included a true increase in the number of cases, greater use of diagnostic testing, and increased reporting. During this period, the incidence of legionellosis increased by 200%. The number of reported cases increased from 1110 to 3346 (0.39–1.09 cases per 100,000 persons).[50,78] Cases were more frequent in persons aged 50 years or older (74%), 64% of patients were male, and an increasing population of older affected individuals and persons at high risk of infection was identified. The period from June to October accounted for 62% of cases reported each year. Twenty-four percent of cases were travel associated. Only 4% of cases were linked to a known outbreak or cluster. In 97% of cases, the diagnostic method was urinary antigen detection. Only 5% of cases were culture confirmed.

The most recent data available from the United States are from the year 2013, with an incidence rate of 1.4 cases per 100,000 persons.[79,80]

Table 1
Incidence of Legionnaire's disease worldwide

Reference	Year	Area	Rate/Million Inhabitants	Type (%)	Peak Incidence Months	Mortality (%)
Ozeki et al,[116] 2012	2009	Japan	6.0	—	June–November February–May	—
Lam et al,[83] 2011	2009	Singapore	3.8	—	—	2.2
CDC,[50] 2011	2009	United States	11.5	TALD 24	June–October	8.0
Rota et al,[117] 2013	2010	Italy	17.5	CA 7.0; TALD 13.5; HCR 11.0	—	11.8
Farnham et al,[118] 2014	2011	New York	27.4	—	Summer–early fall	12.8
Moran-Gilad et al,[119] 2014	2006–2011	Israel	6.7	CA 21%; TALD 8%; HCR 24%	July–November	12.6
Graham et al,[84] 2012	2012	New Zealand	14.0[a] 25.0[b]	46% *L longbeachae*	September–November and March–May	5.1
Public Health Ontario,[120] 2014	2013	Ontario, Canada	2.0	—	July	10.2
Campese et al,[88] 2015	2013	France	19.4	—	—	12.2
Stypulkowska-Misiurewicz & Czerwinski,[121] 2015	2013	Poland	0.29	—	—	45
Dooling et al,[80] 2015	2013	United States	14.0	—	—	9.4
NNDSS Annual Report Working Group,[122] 2016	2014	Australia	18.0	*L pneumophila* 54% *L longbeachae* 45%	*L pneumophila* April–May *L longbeachae* October	4
ECDC,[51] 2016	2014	Europe (European Union & Norway)	13.5	*CA* 74, *TALD* 18, *HCR* 7	August–November	8
		Austria	15.9	74, 3, 20	—	9
		Belgium	17.4	28, 13, 60	—	NA
		Bulgaria	0.1	0, 100, 0	—	100
		Croatia	5.9	72, 12, 16	—	0

(*continued on next page*)

Table 1
(continued)

Reference	Year	Area	Rate/Million Inhabitants	Type (%)			Peak Incidence Months	Mortality (%)
ECDC,[51] 2016	2014	Cyprus	7.0	0	0	100	—	0
		Czech Republic	10.5	75	5	20	—	17
		Denmark	28.1	61	11	28	—	8
		Estonia	6.1	75	13	13	—	25
		Finland	1.8	70	0	30	—	NA
		France	20.5	64	10	19	—	9
		Germany	10.3	65	7	28	—	4
		Greece	2.5	74	15	11	—	12
		Hungary	3.2	0	55	45	—	6
		Ireland	1.7	50	0	50	—	NA
		Italy	24.3	83	6	10	—	NA
		Latvia	19.0	100	0	0	—	16
		Lithuania	2.7	50	25	25	—	14
		Luxembourg	9.1	—	—	—	—	0
		Malta	18.8	—	—	—	—	11
		Netherlands	20.7	54	3	43	—	4
		Norway	10.0	41	0	59	—	NA
		Poland	0.3	0	50	25	—	25
		Portugal	56.4	95	2	3	—	5
		Romania	0.1	100	0	0	—	0
		Slovakia	2.6	71	21	7	—	7
		Slovenia	28.6	95	0	5	—	0
		Spain	19.9	86	8	6	—	NA
		Sweden	14.1	—	—	—	—	13
		United Kingdom	5.8	47	2	51	—	7

Data were incorporated when contain episodes per 1,000,000 inhabitants in a country. If several years were reported, the authors took the most recent year for which information was available.

Abbreviations: CA, community acquired; HCR, health care related; NA, not applicable (≥25% of outcomes were unknown); NNDSS, National Notifiable Diseases Surveillance System; TALD, travel-associated Legionnaire's diseases.

[a] Notified cases.

[b] Laboratory-confirmed cases only.

To illustrate the point of underreporting, in a multicenter study conducted by the German Competence Network for CAP in 2008, a standardized extensive testing microbiology protocol was used to diagnose *Legionella* spp pneumonia.[49] The reported incidence was 180 to 360 cases per million inhabitants, and a similar incidence was observed for outpatients and inpatients (3.8%). Extrapolating these data to the United States, cases of LD reported to the CDC are likely less than 5% of actual cases.

Data from Canada (1978–2006) have shown a decline in LD in this country since 1998. Reported data indicate a lower incidence compared with the United States (0.5 cases per 100,000 inhabitants in 2006). Only 66% of culture-confirmed isolates were Lp1,[81] whereas Lp1 was remarkably frequent in environmental samples (52%).[82]

Reported figures for Singapore indicate a declining incidence of LD to 2.8 cases per million inhabitants in 2009, much lower than in Europe.[83] Notwithstanding, rates of imported cases of LD increased from 6% in 2000 to 2004 to 27% in 2005 to 2009. The most likely explanation for this is more travel and better reporting.

In New Zealand, approximately 30% to 50% of LD cases were attributed to *Legionella longbeachae* and *L pneumophila* each in every year of the period 1979 to 2009.[84] An environmental risk was identified in 52% of cases. However, 60% of cases linked to environmental exposure were associated with compost, whereas travel-associated LD was much less frequent. This finding suggests that LD has a characteristic epidemiologic pattern in this country.

In Europe, the number of notifications per million inhabitants has grown steadily in Europe since 1995, when the reported incidence was 4 cases per million inhabitants. In 2014, 6941 cases of LD were reported to the European Legionnaire's Disease Surveillance Network. This figure translates to an incidence of 13.5 cases per million inhabitants.[51]

In the recent European report, LD showed marked geographic and seasonal variation in cases (**Fig. 1**). Seventy-four percent of these cases occurred in 5 countries: France, Germany, Italy, Portugal, and Spain. In Eastern European countries, reported numbers of cases were very low and likely do not reflect the true LD burden. There was one peak of disease in August and another in November. The distribution of cases by setting of infection remained unchanged since 2008 and was, as in the United States, community acquired 74%, travel associated 18%, and health care related 7%. Globally, the incidence of reported travel-associated LD in Europe was 21% higher than in 2013. The same risk factors found in US cases were present in European cases: affected individuals were older than 50 years in 80% of all cases and the male to female ratio was 2.6. Only 14% of cases were reported as part of a cluster. The case mortality rate was similar to that found in America and did not vary from previous years (overall 9%, community acquired 8%, nosocomial 29%, travel associated 5.5%). As in the United States, most cases (87%) were confirmed by urinary antigen detection and few reported cases were culture detected, though rates varied widely across countries (0%–45%). In the European report, *L pneumophila* and its serogroup 1 were responsible for 95% of all cases and 85% of culture-confirmed cases. MAb 3/1 positive (85%) and negative (15%) subtype distributions were maintained through the reporting period and were similar to those already found in Europe in 2002. Over a 7-year period, the number of PCR-diagnosed cases reported grew from less than 2% in 2008% to 8% in 2014. Other reported species were *L longbeachae* (2%), *L micdadei* (1%), *L bozemanae* (<1%), *L maceachernii* (<1%), and *L sainthelensi* (<1%). Only in 32% of cases of patients known not to have traveled outside their country within the incubation period was an environmental investigation conducted. In only 9% of the 666 cases linked to positive environmental sample tests could isolates be matched with clinical isolates.

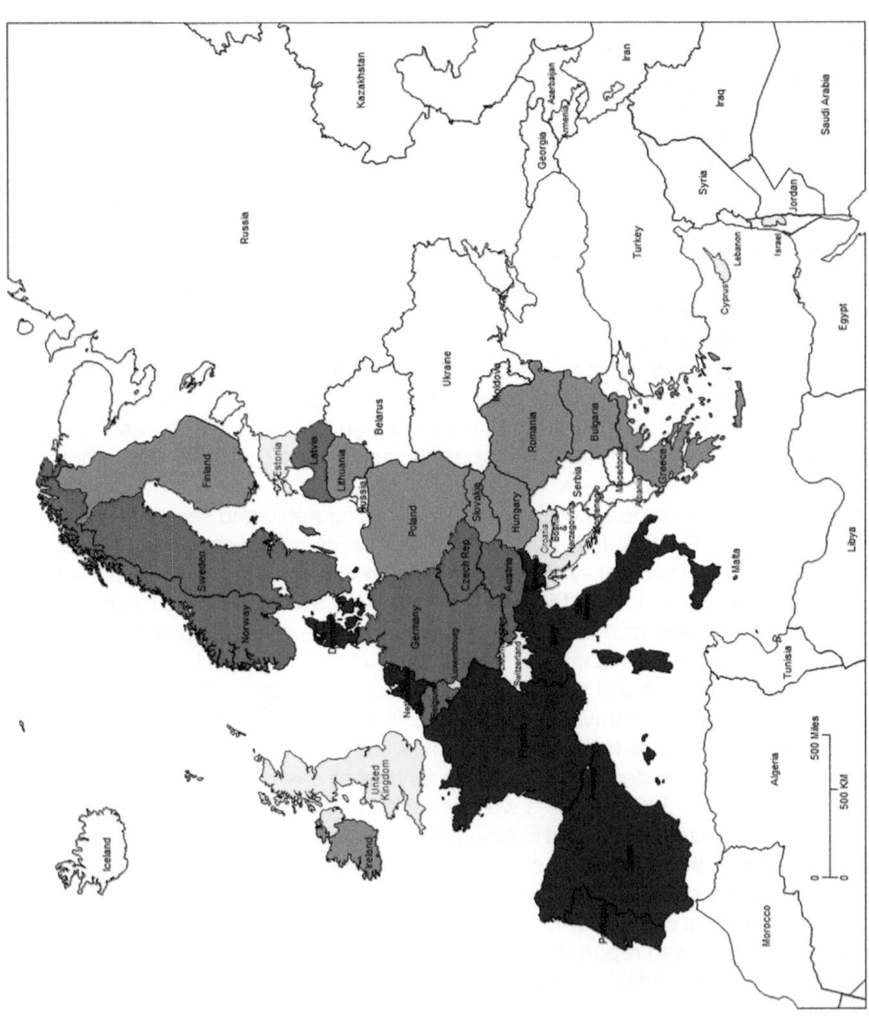

Fig. 1. Reported cases and notifications of LD per million inhabitants, European economic area. Notification rate. ≥20.0; 10.0–19.9; 5.0–9.9; <5.0. (*From* European Centre for Disease Prevention and Control. Legionnaire's disease in Europe, 2014. Stockholm: ECDC; 2016.)

In Europe, in 2014, a large community outbreak involving more than 400 cases occurred in Vila Franca de Xira near Lisbon, Portugal.

Distribution of Species, Serogroups, Monoclonal Antibody Subgroups, and DNA Sequence Types

Among all *Legionella* species, Lp1 is the most virulent and has most commonly been implicated in human disease.[76] It seems that most cases of LD are caused by only a few sequence types of Lp1.

A European-wide study of *L pneumophila* has serotyped 1335 cases of LD. Approximately 67% were serogroup 1 MAb 3/1 positive, and 12% were MAb 3/1 negative. Of MAb 3/1-negative strains, 53.5% were isolated from nosocomial infections, 27% from community-acquired infections, and 14% from travel-associated infections.[85]

In a recent US study of the prevalence of Lp1 and of its sequence types in clinical and environmental isolates from 1982 to 2012, the types found in both outbreak-associated and sporadic cases were ST1, ST35, ST36, ST37, and ST222.[86]

In Great Britain, among isolates collected in England and Wales from 2000 to 2008, 98% of clinical isolates were Lp1, 92% were MAb 3/1 positive, and 46% were ST47, ST37, and ST62.[87] Of the environmental isolates, only 56% were Lp1, 8% were MAb 3/1 positive, and 34% were ST1 or ST79. Little overlap was detected between the two types of isolates. Sequence types commonly found in patients were infrequently found in the environment and vice versa.

The main clinical sequence types detected in England and Wales were also identified as causing infection in France and The Netherlands.

In France, ST23, ST1, and ST47 cause 39% of LD cases with an identified strain; ST1 is widely distributed in the environment.[88]

However, unlike the other countries, the most frequent clinical sequence type in Germany was ST1.

In Japan, Lp1 was the most frequently recovered in clinical samples (80%), 80% of isolates being MAb 3/1 positive, as in Europe. With the exception of ST1, the most common sequence types detected (ST1, ST306, ST120, and ST138) differed from those found in Western Europe.[89]

A higher genetic diversity among environmental isolates compared with clinical isolates, and the presence of specific clones of *L pneumophila* overrepresented in human disease, have been identified worldwide thanks to newer typing methods.[90] Collectively, reported data suggest distinctive trends and patterns of legionellosis in the different world regions.

Non–*L pneumophila* species are isolated more frequently in immunocompromised individuals. After *L pneumophila*, most *Legionella* spp infections in immunosuppressed patients are caused by *L micdadei*, *L bozemanae*, and *L dumoffii*.

Combined infections with different *Legionella* spp strains are rare. In effect, only 17 such cases were reported in Europe for the period 2002 to 2012.[91] These infections are more likely with less virulent strains and in immunocompromised hosts.

Host Risk Factors

Established risk factors for LD are chronic lung disease, smoking,[92] aged more than 50 years,[93] glucocorticoid treatment,[94] hematologic malignancy under cytotoxic chemotherapy,[95] hairy cell leukemia,[96] solid tumor,[97] and anti-(TNF)-alpha treatment.[98] Among the biological TNF-alpha blockers, lower LD incidences have been related to etanercept (3×) than adalimumab (38×) or infliximab (15×).

LD can occur any time after organ transplant,[99,100] though it frequently coincides with rejection episodes and increases morbidity/mortality.[101] Neutropenia does not predispose a patient to *Legionella* spp infection.[102] Human immunodeficiency virus infection has not been established so far as a risk factor for LD.[103]

Risk factors for LD

- Male sex
- Aged more than 50 years
- Smoking (current or historical)
- Alcohol abuse
- Certain chronic diseases (eg, diabetes, chronic heart/lung diseases, chronic renal failure)
- Immunosuppression (eg, corticosteroids, chemotherapy, transplant recipient)
- Hematological malignancies
- Iron overload
- Anti–TNF-alpha treatment
- History of recent travel

Reservoir

Legionella spp are ubiquitous in aquatic environments and water distribution systems.[4] *L pneumophila* withstands temperatures of 50°C, yet cannot proliferate at less than 20°C.[4,104] In these aquatic environments, *Legionella* bacteria exist as intracellular parasites of amebae, ciliated protozoa, or slime molds.[19] Parasitized amebae have been detected in naturally occurring microbial communities forming biofilms.[4]

Once a biofilm becomes established it is difficult to eliminate such that prevention is an important control measure against the proliferation of *Legionella* spp. The risk factors identified so far for biofilm formation are the presence of nutrients (both in the water and materials composing the system), scale and corrosion, a warm water temperature, and low-flow or stagnant water.

In low-nutrient environments, *Legionella* spp are found in a VBNC metabolic state. This state makes their isolation difficult and probably renders them more resistant to biocides.[46,105]

Hospital-acquired LD has often been related to the presence of the organism in the hospital water supply.[106,107] *Legionella* spp have been reported to colonize the hot water supply in 12% to 70% of hospitals.[108]

Transmission Mechanisms

LD is transmitted from the environment to humans mainly through inhalation of contaminated aerosols.[109] Less common routes of infection are microaspiration of colonized water or the inoculation of surgical wounds.[110,111] The nature of the infectious form is still unknown.[46] A probable case of transmission between humans has recently been reported.[112]

Practically all water systems that produce aerosols have been linked to LD cases and outbreaks. These systems include cooling towers, hot tubs, industrial equipment, domestic plumbing, hot spas, drains, or respiratory devices/nebulizers or nasogastric tubes in hospitals.[4,46] Cumulative exposure to a source of LD is a risk factor for disease acquisition.[46] Source factors linked to the risk of infection are bacterial load, virulence of the colonizing bacteria, dissemination efficiency, and aerosol type. The *Legionella* spp count alone does not indicate whether a source will or will not cause infection.[4]

Recent evidence exists that *L pneumophila* can be air spread from at least 6 km from its source. French scientists reviewed the details of an LD epidemic in Pas-de-Calais, northern France, produced in 2003 to 2004. There were 86 confirmed cases and 18 deaths related to the pathogen. The source of infection was a cooling tower in a petrochemical plant, and some affected individuals lived 6 km from the plant.[113]

Several cases of LD caused by *L longbeachae* have been linked to potting soil and soil amendments containing the bacterium, not hand-washing after gardening, and to dripping hanging flower pots.[114] However, the transmission mode of *L longbeachae* remains unclear.[4,115]

Pontiac fever is originated by inhalation of a water aerosol containing *Legionella* spp and their toxins. However, the cause and pathogenesis of Pontiac fever remain unknown.[21,46]

REFERENCES

1. *Legionella.* LPSN bacterio net. List of prokaryotic names with standing in nomenclature. 2015. Available at: http://www.bacterio.net/legionella.html. Accessed November 3, 2016.
2. Edelstein PH. Legionella. In: Versalovic J, Carroll KC, Funke G, et al, editors. Manual of clinical microbiology, vol. 1, 10th edition. Washington, DC: American Society of Microbiology Press; 2011. p. 770–85.
3. Jarraud S, Descours G, Ginevra C, et al. Identification of *legionella* in clinical samples. Methods Mol Biol 2013;954:27–56.
4. Hornei B, Ewig S, Exner M, et al. Laboratory aspects of *Legionella.* Chapter 11. In: Bartram J, Chartier Y, Lee JV, et al, editors. *Legionella* and the prevention of legionellosis. 1st edition. Geneva: World Health Organization; 2007. p. 175–92. Available at. http://www.who.int/water_sanitation_health/emerging/legionella.pdf. Accessed November 3, 2016.
5. Fry NK, Warwick S, Saunders NA, et al. The use of 16S ribosomal RNA analyses to investigate the phylogeny of the family *Legionella*ceae. J Gen Microbiol 1991; 137(5):1215–22.
6. Ratcliff RM, Lanser JA, Manning PA, et al. Sequence-based classification scheme for the genus *Legionella* targeting the mip gene. J Clin Microbiol 1998;36(6):1560–7.
7. Ratcliff RM. Sequence-based identification of *legionella.* Methods Mol Biol 2013; 954:57–72.
8. Mentasti M, Kese D, Echahidi F, et al. Design and validation of a qPCR assay for accurate detection and initial serogrouping of *Legionella pneumophila* in clinical specimens by the ESCMID Study Group for *Legionella* Infections (ESGLI). Eur J Clin Microbiol Infect Dis 2015;34(7):1387–93.
9. Luck C, Fry NK, Helbig JH, et al. Typing methods for *legionella.* Methods Mol Biol 2013;954:119–48.
10. Dournon E, Bibb WF, Rajagopalan P, et al. Monoclonal antibody reactivity as a virulence marker for *Legionella pneumophila* serogroup 1 strains. J Infect Dis 1988;157(3):496–501.
11. Joly JR, McKinney RM, Tobin JO, et al. Development of a standardized subgrouping scheme for *Legionella pneumophila* serogroup 1 using monoclonal antibodies. J Clin Microbiol 1986;23(4):768–71.
12. Helbig JH, Kurtz JB, Pastoris MC, et al. Antigenic lipopolysaccharide components of *Legionella pneumophila* recognized by monoclonal antibodies:

possibilities and limitations for division of the species into serogroups. J Clin Microbiol 1997;35(11):2841–5.
13. Helbig JH, Jacobs E, Luck C. *Legionella pneumophila* urinary antigen subtyping using monoclonal antibodies as a tool for epidemiological investigations. Eur J Clin Microbiol Infect Dis 2012;31(7):1673–7.
14. Fry NK, Rowbotham TJ, Saunders NA, et al. Direct amplification and sequencing of the 16S ribosomal DNA of an intracellular *Legionella* species recovered by amoebal enrichment from the sputum of a patient with pneumonia. FEMS Microbiol Lett 1991;67(2):165–8.
15. Marrie TJ, Raoult D, La Scola B, et al. *Legionella*-like and other amoebal pathogens as agents of community-acquired pneumonia. Emerg Infect Dis 2001; 7(6):1026–9.
16. Edelstein PH, Meyer RD, Finegold SM. Laboratory diagnosis of Legionnaire's disease. Am Rev Respir Dis 1980;121(2):317–27.
17. Helbig JH, Uldum SA, Bernander S, et al. Clinical utility of urinary antigen detection for diagnosis of community-acquired, travel-associated, and nosocomial Legionnaire's disease. J Clin Microbiol 2003;41(2):838–40.
18. Shimada T, Noguchi Y, Jackson JL, et al. Systematic review and metaanalysis: urinary antigen tests for legionellosis. Chest 2009;136(6):1576–85.
19. Fields BS, Benson RF, Besser RE. *Legionella* and Legionnaire's disease: 25 years of investigation. Clin Microbiol Rev 2002;15(3):506–26.
20. Yzerman EP, den Boer JW, Lettinga KD, et al. Sensitivity of three urinary antigen tests associated with clinical severity in a large outbreak of Legionnaire's disease in The Netherlands. J Clin Microbiol 2002;40(9):3232–6.
21. Edelstein PH. Urine antigen tests positive for Pontiac fever: implications for diagnosis and pathogenesis. Clin Infect Dis 2007;44(2):229–31.
22. Burnsed LJ, Hicks LA, Smithee LM, et al. A large, travel-associated outbreak of legionellosis among hotel guests: utility of the urine antigen assay in confirming Pontiac fever. Clin Infect Dis 2007;44(2):222–8.
23. Mandell LA, Wunderink RG, Anzueto A, et al. Infectious Diseases Society of America/American Thoracic Society consensus guidelines on the management of community-acquired pneumonia in adults. Clin Infect Dis 2007;44(Suppl 2):S27–72.
24. Mentasti M, Fry NK, Afshar B, et al. Application of *Legionella pneumophila*-specific quantitative real-time PCR combined with direct amplification and sequence-based typing in the diagnosis and epidemiological investigation of Legionnaire's disease. Eur J Clin Microbiol Infect Dis 2012;31(8):2017–28.
25. Murdoch DR, Podmore RG, Anderson TP, et al. Impact of routine systematic polymerase chain reaction testing on case finding for Legionnaire's disease: a pre-post comparison study. Clin Infect Dis 2013;57(9):1275–81.
26. Cho MC, Kim H, An D, et al. Comparison of sputum and nasopharyngeal swab specimens for molecular diagnosis of *Mycoplasma pneumoniae, Chlamydophila pneumon*iae, and *Legionella* pneumophila. Ann Lab Med 2012;32(2): 133–8.
27. Nazarian EJ, Bopp DJ, Saylors A, et al. Design and implementation of a protocol for the detection of *Legionella* in clinical and environmental samples. Diagn Microbiol Infect Dis 2008;62(2):125–32.
28. Guidelines for prevention of nosocomial pneumonia. Centers for Disease Control and Prevention. MMWR Recomm Rep 1997;46(RR-1):1–79.
29. Rudbeck M, Molbak K, Uldum S. High prevalence of antibodies to *Legionella* spp. in Danish blood donors. A study in areas with high and average incidence of Legionnaire's disease. Epidemiol Infect 2008;136(2):257–62.

30. Edelstein PH. Legionnaire's disease: history and clinical findings. In: Heuner K, Swanson M, editors. Legionella. Molecular microbiology. 1st edition. Norfolk (United Kingdom): Caister Academic Press; 2008. p. 1–18.
31. Chatfield CH, Cianciotto NP. Culturing, media, and handling of *legionella*. Methods Mol Biol 2013;954:151–62.
32. Pasculle AW, McDevitt D. *Legionella* cultures. In: Garcia LS, editor. Clinical microbiology procedures handbook, vol. 1, 3rd edition. Washington, DC: American Society for Microbiology Press; 2010. p. 3.11.14.11–13.11.14.15.
33. Saura P, Valles J, Jubert P, et al. Spontaneous rupture of the spleen in a patient with legionellosis. Clin Infect Dis 1993;17(2):298.
34. Mayock R, Skale B, Kohler RB. *Legionella pneumophila* pericarditis proved by culture of pericardial fluid. Am J Med 1983;75(3):534–6.
35. Armengol S, Domingo C, Mesalles E. Myocarditis: a rare complication during *Legionella* infection. Int J Cardiol 1992;37(3):418–20.
36. Brabender W, Hinthorn DR, Asher M, et al. *Legionella pneumophila* wound infection. JAMA 1983;250(22):3091–2.
37. McCabe RE, Baldwin JC, McGregor CA, et al. Prosthetic valve endocarditis caused by *Legionella pneumophila*. Ann Intern Med 1984;100(4):525–7.
38. Menasalvas A, Bouza E. Infective endocarditis caused by unusual microorganisms. Rev Esp Cardiol 1998;51(Suppl 2):79–85 [in Spanish].
39. Loveridge P. Legionnaire's disease and arthritis. CMAJ 1981;124(4):366–7.
40. Fernandez-Cruz A, Marin M, Castelo L, et al. *Legionella micdadei*, a new cause of prosthetic joint infection. J Clin Microbiol 2011;49(9):3409–10.
41. Heath PD, Booth L, Leigh PN, et al. *Legionella* brain stem encephalopathy and peripheral neuropathy without preceding pneumonia. J Neurol Neurosurg Psychiatry 1986;49(2):216–8.
42. Andersen BB, Sogaard I. Legionnaire's disease and brain abscess. Neurology 1987;37(2):333–4.
43. Winn WC Jr. *Legionella* and the clinical microbiologist. Infect Dis Clin North Am 1993;7(2):377–92.
44. Breiman RF, Butler JC. Legionnaire's disease: clinical, epidemiological, and public health perspectives. Semin Respir Infect 1998;13(2):84–9.
45. Cloud JL, Carroll KC, Pixton P, et al. Detection of *Legionella* species in respiratory specimens using PCR with sequencing confirmation. J Clin Microbiol 2000; 38(5):1709–12.
46. Edelstein PH, Cianciotto NP. Legionella. In: Mandell GL, Bennett JE, Dolin R, editors. Mandell, Douglas and Bennett's principles and practice of infectious diseases, vol. 2, 7th edition. Philadelphia: Churchill Livingstone Elsevier; 2010. p. 2969–84.
47. Viasus D, Di Yacovo S, Garcia-Vidal C, et al. Community-acquired *Legionella pneumophila* pneumonia: a single-center experience with 214 hospitalized sporadic cases over 15 years. Medicine 2013;92(1):51–60.
48. Yu VL, Stout JE. Community-acquired legionnaires disease: implications for underdiagnosis and laboratory testing. Clin Infect Dis 2008;46(9):1365–7.
49. von Baum H, Ewig S, Marre R, et al. Community-acquired *Legionella* pneumonia: new insights from the German competence network for community acquired pneumonia. Clin Infect Dis 2008;46(9):1356–64.
50. Centers for Disease Control and Prevention (CDC). Legionellosis -- United States, 2000-2009. MMWR Morb Mortal Wkly Rep 2011;60(32):1083–6.
51. European Centre for Disease Prevention and Control. Legionnaire's disease in Europe, 2014. 2016. Available at: http://ecdc.europa.eu/en/publications/Publications/legionnares-disease-europe-2014.pdf. Accessed July 31, 2016.

52. Joseph C. Investigation of outbreaks: epidemiology. Methods Mol Biol 2013; 954:73–86.
53. Lee S, Lee J. Outbreak investigations and identification of *legionella* in contaminated water. Methods Mol Biol 2013;954:87–118.
54. Kozak NA, Lucas CE, Winchell JM. Identification of *legionella* in the environment. Methods Mol Biol 2013;954:3–25.
55. Merault N, Rusniok C, Jarraud S, et al. Specific real-time PCR for simultaneous detection and identification of *Legionella pneumophila* serogroup 1 in water and clinical samples. Appl Environ Microbiol 2011;77(5):1708–17.
56. Gaia V, Fry NK, Afshar B, et al. Consensus sequence-based scheme for epidemiological typing of clinical and environmental isolates of *Legionella pneumophila*. J Clin Microbiol 2005;43(5):2047–52.
57. Ratzow S, Gaia V, Helbig JH, et al. Addition of neuA, the gene encoding N-acylneuraminate cytidylyl transferase, increases the discriminatory ability of the consensus sequence-based scheme for typing *Legionella pneumophila* serogroup 1 strains. J Clin Microbiol 2007;45(6):1965–8.
58. Luck PC, Ecker C, Reischl U, et al. Culture-independent identification of the source of an infection by direct amplification and sequencing of *Legionella pneumophila* DNA from a clinical specimen. J Clin Microbiol 2007;45(9):3143–4.
59. Mercante JW, Winchell JM. Current and emerging *Legionella* diagnostics for laboratory and outbreak investigations. Clin Microbiol Rev 2015;28(1):95–133.
60. Graham RM, Doyle CJ, Jennison AV. Real-time investigation of a *Legionella pneumophila* outbreak using whole genome sequencing. Epidemiol Infect 2014;142(11):2347–51.
61. Lin YE, Stout JE, Yu VL. Prevention of hospital-acquired legionellosis. Curr Opin Infect Dis 2011;24(4):350–6.
62. Garrison LE, Kunz JM, Cooley LA, et al. Vital signs: deficiencies in environmental control identified in outbreaks of Legionnaire's disease - North America, 2000-2014. MMWR Morb Mortal Wkly Rep 2016;65(22):576–84.
63. Edelstein PH. Antimicrobial chemotherapy for Legionnaire's disease: a review. Clin Infect Dis 1995;21(Suppl 3):S265–76.
64. Sabria M, Pedro-Botet ML, Yu V, et al. *Legionella* species (Legionnaire's disease) In: Yu V, Burdette SD, editors. Manual of infectious diseases; 2013. Available at: http://www.antimicrobe.org/b118rev.asp#9. Accessed July 31, 2016.
65. Rhomberg PR, Bale MJ, Jones RN. Application of the Etest to antimicrobial susceptibility testing of *Legionella* spp. Diagn Microbiol Infect Dis 1994;19(3): 175–8.
66. Pohlod DJ, Saravolatz LD, Quinn EL, et al. The effect of inoculum, culture medium and antimicrobial combinations on the in-vitro susceptibilities of *Legionella pneumophila*. J Antimicrob Chemother 1981;7(4):335–41.
67. Edelstein PH, Edelstein MA. In vitro activity of azithromycin against clinical isolates of *Legionella* species. Antimicrob Agents Chemother 1991;35(1):180–1.
68. Vilde JL, Dournon E, Rajagopalan P. Inhibition of *Legionella pneumophila* multiplication within human macrophages by antimicrobial agents. Antimicrob Agents Chemother 1986;30(5):743–8.
69. Anderson R, Joone G, van Rensburg CE. An in-vitro evaluation of the cellular uptake and intraphagocytic bioactivity of clarithromycin (A-56268, TE-031), a new macrolide antimicrobial agent. J Antimicrob Chemother 1988;22(6):923–33.
70. Goldoni P, Castellani Pastoris M, Cattani L, et al. Effect of monensin on the invasiveness and multiplication of *Legionella pneumophila*. J Med Microbiol 1995; 42(4):269–75.

71. Stout JE, Arnold B, Yu VL. Comparative activity of ciprofloxacin, ofloxacin, levofloxacin, and erythromycin against *Legionella* species by broth microdilution and intracellular susceptibility testing in HL-60 cells. Diagn Microbiol Infect Dis 1998;30(1):37–43.
72. Edelstein PH, Edelstein MA. In vitro extracellular and intracellular activities of clavulanic acid and those of piperacillin and ceftriaxone alone and in combination with tazobactam against clinical isolates of *Legionella* species. Antimicrob Agents Chemother 1994;38(2):200–4.
73. Chiaraviglio L, Kirby JE. High-throughput intracellular antimicrobial susceptibility testing of *Legionella pneumophila*. Antimicrob Agents Chemother 2015; 59(12):7517–29.
74. Bruin JP, Koshkolda T, IJzerman EP, et al. Isolation of ciprofloxacin-resistant *Legionella pneumophila* in a patient with severe pneumonia. J Antimicrob Chemother 2014;69(10):2869–71.
75. Garrison LE, Shaw KM, McCollum JT, et al. On-site availability of *Legionella* testing in acute care hospitals, United States. Infect Control Hosp Epidemiol 2014;35(7):898–900.
76. Stout JE, Yu VL. Legionellosis. N Engl J Med 1997;337(10):682–7.
77. Legionella (Legionnaire's Disease and Pontiac Fever). In: Centers for Disease Control and Prevention. 2016. Available at. http://www.cdc.gov/legionella/surv-reporting.html. Accessed November 3, 2016.
78. Centers for Disease Control and Prevention (CDC). Summary of notifiable diseases–United States, 2010. MMWR Morb Mortal Wkly Rep 2012;59(53):1–111.
79. Adams DA, Jajosky RA, Ajani U, et al. Summary of notifiable diseases–United States, 2012. MMWR Morb Mortal Wkly Rep 2014;61(53):1–121.
80. Dooling KL, Toews KA, Hicks LA, et al. Active bacterial core surveillance for legionellosis - United States, 2011-2013. MMWR Morb Mortal Wkly Rep 2015; 64(42):1190–3.
81. Ng V, Tang P, Jamieson F, et al. Laboratory-based evaluation of legionellosis epidemiology in Ontario, Canada, 1978 to 2006. BMC Infect Dis 2009;9:68.
82. Reimer AR, Au S, Schindle S, et al. *Legionella pneumophila* monoclonal antibody subgroups and DNA sequence types isolated in Canada between 1981 and 2009: laboratory component of national surveillance. Eur J Clin Microbiol Infect Dis 2010;29(2):191–205.
83. Lam MC, Ang LW, Tan AL, et al. Epidemiology and control of legionellosis, Singapore. Emerg Infect Dis 2011;17(7):1209–15.
84. Graham FF, White PS, Harte DJ, et al. Changing epidemiological trends of legionellosis in New Zealand, 1979-2009. Epidemiol Infect 2012;140(8):1481–96.
85. Helbig JH, Bernander S, Castellani Pastoris M, et al. Pan-European study on culture-proven Legionnaire's disease: distribution of *Legionella pneumophila* serogroups and monoclonal subgroups. Eur J Clin Microbiol Infect Dis 2002; 21(10):710–6.
86. Kozak-Muiznieks NA, Lucas CE, Brown E, et al. Prevalence of sequence types among clinical and environmental isolates of *Legionella pneumophila* serogroup 1 in the United States from 1982 to 2012. J Clin Microbiol 2014;52(1):201–11.
87. Harrison TG, Afshar B, Doshi N, et al. Distribution of *Legionella pneumophila* serogroups, monoclonal antibody subgroups and DNA sequence types in recent clinical and environmental isolates from England and Wales (2000-2008). Eur J Clin Microbiol Infect Dis 2009;28(7):781–91.
88. Campese C, Descours G, Lepoutre A, et al. Legionnaire's disease in France. Med Mal Infect 2015;45(3):65–71.

89. Amemura-Maekawa J, Kura F, Helbig JH, et al. Characterization of *Legionella pneumophila* isolates from patients in Japan according to serogroups, monoclonal antibody subgroups and sequence types. J Med Microbiol 2010; 59(Pt 6):653–9.
90. Gomez-Valero L, Rusniok C, Buchrieser C. *Legionella pneumophila*: population genetics, phylogeny and genomics. Infect Genet Evol 2009;9(5):727–39.
91. Wewalka G, Schmid D, Harrison TG, et al. Dual infections with different *Legionella* strains. Clin Microbiol Infect 2014;20(1):O13–9.
92. Doebbeling BN, Wenzel RP. The epidemiology of *Legionella pneumophila* infections. Semin Respir Infect 1987;2(4):206–21.
93. England AC 3rd, Fraser DW, Plikaytis BD, et al. Sporadic legionellosis in the United States: the first thousand cases. Ann Intern Med 1981;94(2):164–70.
94. Hofflin JM, Potasman I, Baldwin JC, et al. Infectious complications in heart transplant recipients receiving cyclosporine and corticosteroids. Ann Intern Med 1987;106(2):209–16.
95. Kugler JW, Armitage JO, Helms CM, et al. Nosocomial Legionnaire's disease. Occurrence in recipients of bone marrow transplants. Am J Med 1983;74(2): 281–8.
96. Radaelli F, Langer M, Chiorboli O, et al. Severe *Legionella pneumophila* infection in a patient with hairy cell leukemia in partial remission after alpha interferon treatment. Hematol Oncol 1991;9(3):125–8.
97. Marston BJ, Lipman HB, Breiman RF. Surveillance for Legionnaire's disease. Risk factors for morbidity and mortality. Arch Intern Med 1994;154(21):2417–22.
98. Tubach F, Ravaud P, Salmon-Ceron D, et al. Emergence of *Legionella pneumophila* pneumonia in patients receiving tumor necrosis factor-alpha antagonists. Clin Infect Dis 2006;43(10):e95–100.
99. Myerowitz RL, Pasculle AW, Dowling JN, et al. Opportunistic lung infection due to "Pittsburgh Pneumonia Agent". N Engl J Med 1979;301(18):953–8.
100. Singh N, Stout JE, Yu VL. Prevention of Legionnaire's disease in transplant recipients: recommendations for a standardized approach. Transpl Infect Dis 2004; 6(2):58–62.
101. Ampel NM, Wing EJ. *Legionella* infection in transplant patients. Semin Respir Infect 1990;5(1):30–7.
102. Yu VL. *Legionella pneumophila* (Legionnaire's disease). In: Mandell GL, Bennett JE, Dolin R, editors. Mandell, Douglas and Bennett's principles and practice of infectious diseases, vol. 2, 7th edition. Philadelphia: Churchill Livingstone Elsevier; 2000. p. 2424–35.
103. Sandkovsky U, Sandkovsky G, Suh J, et al. *Legionella* pneumonia and HIV: case reports and review of the literature. AIDS Patient Care STDs 2008;22(6):473–81.
104. Fliermans CB, Soracco RJ, Pope DH. Measure of *Legionella pneumophila* activity in situ. Curr Microbiol 1981;6:89–94.
105. Steinert M, Emody L, Amann R, et al. Resuscitation of viable but nonculturable *Legionella pneumophila* Philadelphia JR32 by *Acanthamoeba castellanii*. Appl Environ Microbiol 1997;63(5):2047–53.
106. Stout J, Yu VL, Vickers RM, et al. Ubiquitousness of *Legionella pneumophila* in the water supply of a hospital with endemic Legionnaire's disease. N Engl J Med 1982;306(8):466–8.
107. Allen JG, Myatt TA, Macintosh DL, et al. Assessing risk of health care-acquired Legionnaire's disease from environmental sampling: the limits of using a strict percent positivity approach. Am J Infect Control 2012;40(10):917–21.

108. Lin YS, Stout JE, Yu VL, et al. Disinfection of water distribution systems for *Legionella*. Semin Respir Infect 1998;13(2):147–59.
109. Fraser DW. Legionellosis: evidence of airborne transmission. Ann N Y Acad Sci 1980;353:61–6.
110. Johnson JT, Yu VL, Best MG, et al. Nosocomial legionellosis in surgical patients with head-and-neck cancer: implications for epidemiological reservoir and mode of transmission. Lancet 1985;2(8450):298–300.
111. Marrie TJ, Haldane D, MacDonald S, et al. Control of endemic nosocomial Legionnaire's disease by using sterile potable water for high risk patients. Epidemiol Infect 1991;107(3):591–605.
112. Correia AM, Ferreira JS, Borges V, et al. Probable person-to-person transmission of Legionnaire's disease. N Engl J Med 2016;374(5):497–8.
113. Nguyen TM, Ilef D, Jarraud S, et al. A community-wide outbreak of Legionnaire's disease linked to industrial cooling towers–how far can contaminated aerosols spread? J Infect Dis 2006;193(1):102–11.
114. Steele TW, Lanser J, Sangster N. Isolation of *Legionella longbeachae* serogroup 1 from potting mixes. Appl Environ Microbiol 1990;56(1):49–53.
115. O'Connor BA, Carman J, Eckert K, et al. Does using potting mix make you sick? Results from a *Legionella longbeachae* case-control study in South Australia. Epidemiol Infect 2007;135(1):34–9.
116. Ozeki Y, Yamada F, Saito A, et al. Seasonal patterns of legionellosis in Saitama, 2005-2009. Jpn J Infect Dis 2012;65(4):330–3.
117. Rota MC, Caporali MG, Bella A, et al. Legionnaire's disease in Italy: results of the epidemiological surveillance from 2000 to 2011. Euro Surveill 2013;18(23):1–9.
118. Farnham A, Alleyne L, Cimini D, et al. Legionnaire's disease incidence and risk factors, New York, New York, USA, 2002-2011. Emerg Infect Dis 2014;20(11): 1795–802.
119. Moran-Gilad J, Mentasti M, Lazarovitch T, et al. Molecular epidemiology of Legionnaire's disease in Israel. Clin Microbiol Infect 2014;20(7):690–6.
120. Public Health Ontario. Monthly infectious diseases surveillance report. 2014;3(5):1–14. Available at: http://www.publichealthontario.ca/en/DataAndAnalytics/Documents/PHO_Monthly_Infectious_Diseases_Surveillance_Report_-_May_2014.pdf. Accessed July 31, 2016.
121. Stypulkowska-Misiurewicz H, Czerwinski M. Legionellosis in Poland in 2013. Przegl Epidemiol 2015;69(2):235–7, 357–238.
122. NNDSS Annual Report Working Group. Australia's notifiable disease status, 2014: annual report of the National Notifiable Diseases Surveillance System. Commun Dis Intell Q Rep 2016;40(1):E48–145.

Legionnaire's Disease and Immunosuppressive Drugs

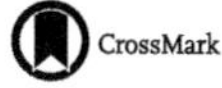

Tin Han Htwe, MD[a,*], Nancy M. Khardori, MD, PhD[b]

KEYWORDS

- Legionnaire's disease • *Legionella pneumophila* • Immunosuppressive agents
- Tumor necrosis factor antagonists • Chemotherapeutic agents • Antirejection agents

KEY POINTS

- Immunosuppressive drugs predispose patients to legionnaire's disease.
- Tumor necrosis factor antagonists are the most recent and common agents that currently put patients at risk for opportunistic infections, including legionnaire's disease.
- The role of immunosuppressive agents, such as chemotherapy agents, corticosteroids, and antirejection agents, is more difficult to determine because of more severe immunocompromising underlying conditions and more complex pharmacotherapy in these patient populations, but they seem to add to the risk for legionnaire's disease.

INTRODUCTION

Immunosuppression is a major risk factor for legionnaire's disease and includes use of immunosuppressive agents like tumor necrosis factor (TNF) antagonists, corticosteroids, and chemotherapy for malignancy, especially hairy cell leukemia, and antirejection agents for organ transplant. Elderly patients with myelodysplastic syndrome and postsplenectomy patients have impairment of both cellular and humeral immune functions and are predisposed to legionellosis.[1] Its association with human immunodeficiency virus (HIV) infection is still unclear. Immunosuppression is commonly associated with nosocomial infection with legionella (90%) compared with community-acquired cases. Legionnaire's disease involves multiple organs but pneumonia is the commonest presentation, especially in immunocompromised patients. Among *Legionella* species, *Legionella pneumophila* serotype 1 is the most virulent and most common species responsible for human infections.[2]

Disclosure: None.

[a] Sentara Infectious Diseases Specialists, Sentara Medical Group, 850 Kempsville Road, Norfolk, VA 23502, USA; [b] Department of Microbiology and Molecular Cell Biology, Eastern Virginia Medical School, Hofheimer Hall, 825 Fairfax Avenue, Norfolk, VA 23507, USA
* Corresponding author. 941 Brittlebank Drive, Virginia Beach, VA 23462.
E-mail address: TinHanHtwe@gmail.com

Infect Dis Clin N Am 31 (2017) 29–42
http://dx.doi.org/10.1016/j.idc.2016.10.003

Complications like pleural effusion and cavitation can occur in this patient population despite appropriate antibiotic therapy. In immunosuppressed populations, legionella pneumonia tends to progress to abscess formation, which is not common otherwise. Yu and colleagues[3] were able to analyze 62 out of 79 case reports of lung abscess caused by *Legionella* species. Of these, 45% were nosocomial and 27% died. The most common type was *L pneumophila* serotype 1. A large number of patients (69%) were receiving corticosteroids, 35% of patients had received solid organ transplants, and 11% had hematologic malignancy. In patients with neutropenia, abscesses were diagnosed during the recovery phase. The investigators hypothesized that progression to abscess formation was related to impairment of host defenses rather than virulence of the organism.[3] In a review of 8 patients with legionella pneumonia from Henry Ford hospital in Detroit, Michigan, over a 7-month period (between December 1977 and June 1978), all of the patients were immunosuppressed. Corticosteroid therapy was the most common risk factor (7 out of 8 patients), and 4 patients were on additional immunosuppressive therapy. Hematologic malignancy was present in 4 of the patients and renal transplant in 2. Most of the patients responded well to intravenous antibiotic therapy and only 1 died. Five patients required open lung biopsy to establish diagnosis.[4] In a review of 87 patients from Iowa over a 10-year period (July 1970 to June 1980), 31% were receiving corticosteroid chemotherapy or other immunosuppressive agents. Most patients (70%) had underlying medical comorbidities, including malignancy, renal failure, and chronic lung disease. The case fatality rate (70%) in nosocomial cases was higher than for disease acquired in the community (22%).[5]

Legionellosis can present with several extrapulmonary manifestations. The first case of *L pneumophila* serotype 1 pericarditis was reported in an allogeneic bone marrow recipient by Scerpella and colleagues[6] in 1994. A total of 12 cases of legionella pericarditis were included in that review with 1 each of liver transplant, bronchial carcinoma, and Hodgkin disease. *L pneumophila* serotype 1 septic arthritis and suspected endocarditis with mobile vegetations on anterior mitral valve leaflet leading to severe mitral valve insufficiency has been reported in a patient with lymphocyte-rich thymoma with presumed secondary thymoma-associated immunoglobulin deficiency.[7] A rare case of *L pneumophila* serotype 3 pericarditis has been reported in a patient with newly diagnosed bronchial carcinoma.[8] *Legionella* species rarely cause skin and soft tissue infections. So far only 19 case of subcutaneous legionella infection have been reported in the literature. Of these, 9 were caused by *L pneumophila* and most of the patients were immunocompromised. A pneumonitis presentation followed by cutaneous abscesses involving the right lower extremity 3 weeks later was reported in a patient with rectal adenocarcinoma and lung metastasis. The growth from the skin abscess was noted on chocolate agar and confirmed by polymerase chain reaction (PCR) assay.[9] On rare occasions, *Legionella* species can be seen as acid-fast positive bacilli and this can lead to misdiagnosis in immunosuppressed patients, mimicking mycobacterial infections.[10]

Legionella micdadei is the second most common species associated with legionella pneumonia. This species has been found to be associated with more immunosuppressed patients than *L pneumophila*. It is seen more often in solid organ transplant recipients in the early postoperative period compared with bone marrow transplant recipients. In a review of a nosocomial outbreak of *L micdadei* infection, 12 cases of pneumonia were diagnosed over a 3-month period among 38 kidney and heart transplant recipients, and these were related to hot water sources, including patients' shower and sinks and a water heating system in the recirculation loop. A year later, after a 3-week period of malfunctioning chlorinating system, a second outbreak of 5 culture-confirmed cases of *L micdadei* infection occurred. *L micdadei* is not identified by first-line screening test (legionella urinary antigen), therefore it is important to peruse specific legionella cultures to identify *Legionella* species other than *L pneumophila*, especially in immunocompromised patients.[11,12] In an analysis of 104 consecutive renal allografts in 103 patients over 28 months following a nosocomial outbreak of *L micdadei*, infection occurred during the early posttransplant period when patients were severely compromised. Seroconversion for *L pneumophila* or *L micdadei* was noted in 21 of 89 recipients during the 6 months after transplant and initiation of immunosuppressive therapy. These patients included those with definitive pneumonia, patients with febrile pneumonitis suspected to be related to legionella pneumonia, and 6 asymptomatic patients.[13] *L micdadei* has also been reported to cause prostatic valve endocarditis. So far, 12 cases have been reported in the literature and most patients were immunosuppressed. A renal transplant recipient on immunosuppressive therapy with cyclosporine A and prednisone was diagnosed with prosthetic valve endocarditis after a year of valve replacement. He was successfully treated with valve replacement and placed on lifelong antibiotic therapy.[14]

Legionella longbeachae was reported to cause severe legionnaire's disease with multiorgan failure in a long-term renal transplant recipient who was 26 years posttransplant and maintained on long-term immunosuppression therapy with cyclosporine A, mycophenolic acid, and prednisone. She presented with fever, headache, and gastrointestinal complaints; progressed to multiorgan failure; and, after a third bronchoscopy, the culture grew *Legionella* species. She was successfully treated with a prolonged course of azithromycin. She gave a history of extensive exposure to potting soil (an usual source of *L longbeachae*) before the onset of illness. It is recommended that long-term transplant recipients wear protective clothing, including mask and goggles, while handling soil-related products, and wash hands frequently.[15]

Legionella feeleii has been reported to cause severe pneumonia in an elderly allogeneic bone marrow transplant recipient. The diagnosis was established from lung tissue histopathology and confirmed by PCR. Literature review revealed 10 cases of *L feeleii* infection, and most of these patients were immunosuppressed, including transplant recipients and patients with HIV infection, systemic lupus erythematosus, non-Hodgkin lymphoma, and breast carcinoma.[16] The first reported case of *Legionella bozemanii* pulmonary abscess was reported in a pediatric stem cell transplant recipient 6 months after transplant. A splenic nodule was suspected to be an abscess but culture was not sent.[17]

LEGIONNAIRE'S DISEASE AND TUMOR NECROSIS FACTOR ANTAGONISTS

Infection with *Legionella* induces both cellular and humoral immune responses but the former play a major role in protection. Activated mononuclear phagocytes prevent the multiplication of *L pneumophila* intracellularly. Mononuclear cells from patients recovered from legionnaire's disease respond to *L pneumophila* antigens with the production of cytokines that activate monocytes and macrophages.[18] In vitro data from mice showed that TNF-alpha is crucial in inducing resistance of macrophages to infection with *L pneumophila*. Treatment with anti–TNF-alpha antagonists renders macrophages susceptible to *L pneumophila* infection and diminishes its clearance by macrophages.[19]

One-year review of consecutive case series of 10 patients from France who developed legionella pneumonia while on anti-TNF agents showed that the disease was severe but mostly curable. The investigators recommended that first-line antibiotics for pneumonia for this patient population should include agents with activity against *L pneumophila*. Of the 10 described in this study, 8 were receiving anti-TNF therapy for rheumatoid arthritis, 1 for psoriasis, and 1 for pyoderma gangrenosum. The agents used were adalimumab in 6 patients, etanercept in 2 patients, and infliximab in the other 2 patients. Corticosteroids were being used in 80% of patients and 60% received methotrexate concomitantly. Relative risk for legionellosis in this population compared with general population in France was estimated to be between 16.5 and 21.0. One patient developed a second episode of legionella infection following reintroduction of treatment with a TNF antagonist.[20]

Over the last 2 decades, TNF antagonist agents are being used increasingly in inflammatory conditions, including rheumatoid arthritis, Crohn disease, ankylosing spondylitis, and psoriasis with and without arthritis. Their increased use has led to an increase in infections caused by intracellular organisms. *Mycobacterium tuberculosis*, *Listeria monocytogenes*, *L pneumophila*, *Coccidioides immitis*, *Histoplasma capsulatum*, *Aspergillus* spp, *Nocardia* spp, and *Pneumocystis jiroveci* are among the species encountered most frequently in this patient population.

There are 3 prototypes of TNF antagonists: infliximab (chimeric), adalimumab (human anti–TNF-alpha monoclonal antibodies), and etanercept (soluble TNF-alpha receptor P75 fusion protein that binds to soluble TNF only). In a prospective French study over 3 years (February 2004 to January 2007), 27 cases of *L pneumophila* infection were identified. Overall annual incidence of *L pneumophila* infection in patients receiving anti–TNF-alpha treatment, adjusted for age and sex, was 46.7 per 100,000 patient years. Overall incidence ratio was higher in patient receiving infliximab and adalimumab compared with etanercept. Note that the corticosteroids did not add to the risk for legionellosis in this study even though most patients received concomitant therapy with corticosteroids.[21]

The first case of legionellosis in a patient on an anti–TNF-alpha agent was reported from the Netherlands in 2004. The case was of a patient with rheumatoid arthritis receiving infliximab therapy. The patient developed fever with respiratory symptoms and diarrhea after her visit to various parts of United States during summer months. None of her travel companions developed infection. The patient was treated with intravenous erythromycin and recovered without complication. The infliximab therapy was resumed after 6 weeks.[22] The first case of *L pneumophila* serotype 1 infection associated with the use of TNF antagonists in the United States was reported from Hawaii in a patient receiving long-term treatment with adalimumab for rheumatoid arthritis who presented with severe right-sided pneumonia and parapneumonic effusion. Diagnosis was confirmed by positive urine *Legionella* antigen test and positive direct immunofluorescence antibody (DFA) stain and growth of *Legionella* from bronchoalveolar lavage.[23]

Treatment with TNF antagonists puts the patients at risk for other intracellular infections; for example, *M tuberculosis*, *L monocytogenes*, *C immitis*, *H capsulatum*, *Aspergillus* species, *Nocardia* species, and *P jiroveci*. *L pneumophila* infection was reported in a patient receiving infliximab treatment of Behçet disease. This patient developed pulmonary tuberculosis before legionella infection. This case provides further evidence that TNF-alpha is critical in the control and containment of intracellular organisms, attracts inflammatory cells to sites of infection, is involved in the process of granuloma formation/maintenance, and promotes bactericidal activity of macrophages.[24]

Case series have been reported with associated use of the anti-TNF agent infliximab in Crohn disease presenting with severe pneumonia and resulting in acute respiratory distress syndrome. Several other cases of legionellosis have been reported in patients on infliximab therapy for Crohn disease, including in a pregnant woman. Based on the review of literature, legionellosis is rare in patients with autoimmune and inflammatory bowel disease receiving other immunosuppressive therapies. However, when TNF antagonists are added to the existing immunosuppressive agents, risk for legionellosis increases.[25–27]

A fatal legionella infection case was reported in a patient who received a second course of infliximab infusion for severe psoriasis that had not responded to prolonged corticosteroid therapy.[28] Another case of fatal legionella pneumonia was documented in a Japanese patient treated with adalimumab and methotrexate for rheumatoid arthritis for 2 years. The patient presented with severe pneumonia and despite treatment he progressed to respiratory failure with septic shock and died 8 hours after admission. The blood culture was later reported to have grown *L pneumophila* serotype 1.[29]

There are individual case reports for severe legionella pneumonia leading to pulmonary necrosis and cavity lesions in patients with rheumatoid arthritis receiving adalimumab. French researchers reported that increased risk of infection from intracellular organisms is higher in recipients of adalimumab or infliximab compared with recipients of etanercept. The investigators reported 11 cases of *Legionella* species infection in association with the use of adalimumab.[30] A review published in 2012 reported 30 cases of legionellosis in patients receiving TNF antagonists and included both hospital-acquired and community-acquired infections. This series described 2 cases of nosocomial legionellosis that occurred during a hospital construction project.[31]

It is clear that patients presenting with respiratory symptoms who are receiving TNF antagonists should be screened for legionella pneumonia and initially given an antibiotic regimen that provides coverage against legionellosis.

LEGIONNAIRE'S DISEASE, MALIGNANCY, AND CHEMOTHERAPEUTIC AGENTS

Patients with malignancy are more susceptible to infection by *Legionella* because of impaired cellular immune defenses, concomitant immunosuppressive therapy, and comorbidities. A retrospective review of legionella pneumonia in 49 patients with cancer over 13 years (1991–2003) showed that 82% of patients had hematologic malignancy and 37% were bone marrow transplant recipients. Associated features included lymphopenia (47%), corticosteroid use (41%), and chemotherapy use (63%). Malignant disease was active in 80% of infected patients, 37% had a complicated course, and the case fatality rate was 31%.[32] An earlier retrospective study in 1986 reviewed a total of 151 patients with legionellosis over a 4-year period and 24% (36 patients) of patients had malignancy. Of these, 42% had hematologic malignancy and 22% had lung cancer. The overall mortality in patients with cancer with legionella infection was 53%. The use of corticosteroids before onset of pneumonitis and neutropenia was the significant factor associated with legionella infection.[33]

Of the hematological malignancies, hairy cell leukemia has been reported to have the highest association with legionellosis. In a review of 33 cases of acute pneumonitis in a hematology department, 4 patients were diagnosed with legionellosis and 3 of them had underlying hairy cell leukemia. Severe monocytopenia is a unique feature of hairy cell leukemia resulting in reduced monocyte activation and decrease in macrophage numbers, both leading to susceptibility to intracellular pathogens such as *M tuberculosis* and *L pneumophila*.[34]

Recently a case of persistent pulmonary legionellosis in an elderly patient with hairy cell leukemia was diagnosed with high immunoglobulin M titer against *L pneumophila* (serogroups 1–8) with repeatedly negative urinary legionella antigen test who was treated with a prolonged course of antibiotic therapy.[35] Legionellosis can present with severe pulmonary disease in patients with hairy cell leukemia following partial remission with interferon alfa therapy, indicating persistence of monocyte and macrophage dysfunction.[36]

Fatal legionella pneumonia has been reported in a child with acute lymphoblastic leukemia undergoing chemotherapy.[37] Another fatal incident has been documented in a patient with lymphoma who was receiving corticosteroid and cytotoxic chemotherapy. The patient presented with acute pneumonia caused by *L pneumophila* serotype 3 and extrapulmonary evidence of infection was found by positive direct immunofluorescence stain in liver and splenic tissue.[38]

In patients with chronic lymphocytic leukemia, treatment with nucleoside analogues can lead to impaired T-cell immunity and increased susceptibility to intracellular infections such as legionellosis. Fatal pneumonia has been reported in a patient receiving fludarabine for the treatment of chronic lymphocytic leukemia.[39] Another case of fatal pneumonia was encountered in a patient with disseminated adenocarcinoma of lungs with persistent positive DFA stain for *L pneumophila* despite prolonged treatment with antimicrobial therapy. The patient had been initiated on immunosuppressant therapy with cyclophosphamide, vincristine sulfate, and doxorubicin hydrochloride.[40]

A recent retrospective review of legionella cases in patients with cancer receiving cytotoxic chemotherapy and stem cell transplant over a 15-year study period (January 1999 to December 2013) was published from Memorial Sloane Kettering Cancer Center. A total of 40 cases of legionella pneumonia were identified, of which 77.5% (31 out of 40) were caused by *L pneumophila* and the remaining 9 cases were caused by non-*pneumophila* species. Non-*pneumophila* infections tend to present with nodular infiltrates (50%), which makes differentiation from invasive fungal infections, tuberculosis, atypical mycobacterial infections, and nocardia infections difficult, but the clinical presentation is much milder and patients can be asymptomatic. In addition, 90% (8 out of 9) of non-*pneumophila* infections occurred in patients with hematologic malignancy and stem cell transplant recipients who were severely immunosuppressed. Of the patients who presented with atypical features, only 1 had underlying lung carcinoma. Only 1 case of coinfection was found with aspergillosis diagnosed from biopsy of a pulmonary nodule from a stem cell transplant recipient.[41]

A recent analysis of microbiological and clinical features of 33 consecutive cases of legionella infection that occurred at MD Anderson Cancer Center, Houston, Texas (2001–2014), again revealed *L pneumophila* subspecies *pneumophila* as the most common *Legionella* species to cause pneumonia. Other species of legionella recovered included *Legionella donaldsonii*, *L micdadei*, *L bozemanii*, *L feeleii*, *Legionella gormanii*, *L longbeachae*, *Legionella maceachernii*, *Legionella parisiensis*, *Legionella sainthelensi*, and *Legionella* sp strain D5382. Out of 33 patients, 27 patients had underlying hematologic malignancies, 6 patients were allogeneic hematopoietic stem cell transplant recipients, and 23 patients had leukopenia. *L donaldsonii* and *Legionella* sp D5382 were reported to be human pathogens for the first time.[42]

P jiroveci is a well-known pathogen in patients with HIV infection and malignancy, transplant recipients, and patients receiving immunosuppressive therapy for various reasons. Coinfection with *L pneumophila* and *P jiroveci* has been reported in patients with chronic lymphocytic leukemia and adult T-cell leukemia.[43,44] Three case reports with concomitant infection caused by *L pneumophila* and *Cryptococcus neoformans* were found on review of the literature. The patients involved were a heart transplant recipient on cyclosporine for immunosuppression, a second patient with chronic lymphocytic leukemia, and a third patient with Hodgkin disease and autoimmune hemolytic anemia receiving corticosteroid, azathioprine, and danazol. The patients responded to initial antibacterial and antifungal therapy. However, the heart transplant recipient died before the completion of therapy.[45]

LEGIONNAIRE'S DISEASE, TRANSPLANT RECIPIENTS, AND ANTIREJECTION AGENTS

Legionellosis has been recognized as an important infection in solid organ (heart, kidney, lungs) and bone marrow transplant recipients with increased severity of disease and higher mortality. More cases have been reported in renal, heart, and bone marrow transplant recipients than in those receiving liver and lung transplants. The incidence of legionellosis was reported to be 7.7% in heart, 23.6% in kidney, and 1.2% in liver transplant recipients. These data were based on positive serology results. Mortality caused by legionellosis also varies among various transplant populations. A large prospective study of legionellosis over 8 years (January 1986 to December 1994) at Presbyterian University Hospital, Pittsburg, Pennsylvania, reported a total of 40 cases of legionella infection. Of these, 30% were organ transplant recipients. The most common species was *L pneumophila* serotype 1 (29 out of 40). Most of the transplant recipients (57%) acquired legionella infection from nosocomial sources, mortality was 43%, and 5 out of 6 patients died of legionella infection. Solid organ recipients were noted to have less severe clinical course and fewer complications. Tacrolimus use is associated with a lower rate of bacterial and fungal infections compared with cyclosporine A and in this study 12 out of 14 patients were receiving cyclosporine A for immunosuppression. Nosocomial origin, respiratory failure requiring ventilator support, pulmonary complications (lung abscess, empyema, and pleural effusion) were independent risk factors for increased mortality.[46] Legionella infection has been classified as fatal pneumonia because of an unknown causal agent since before its discovery in 1976. In the fall of 1975, 3 renal transplant patients were diagnosed with gram-negative pneumonia during autopsy and *Legionella* was later identified with direct fluorescent antibody test.[47] In a prospective study in the summer of 1978 in Burlington, Vermont, out of 86 episodes of pneumonia, 9 cases of legionella were identified. Out of 9 patients, 3 were recent cadaver renal transplant recipients on immunosuppressive therapy. Two of these patients survived with antibiotic management and titration of dose of immunosuppressive therapy. Two out of 7 patients developed lung abscess.[48]

Cavitary legionella pneumonia is a common presentation in renal transplant recipients. Over an 18-month review period, a total of 17 renal transplant patients developed legionella pneumonia and 5 of them had cavitary disease. In contrast with the high reported mortality in this patient population, all of the patients in this report were successfully treated with prolonged antibiotic therapy. The young age of patients, lack of underlying cardiopulmonary disease, and early empiric therapy including erythromycin were thought to contribute to better outcomes.[49]

From January 1976 to March 1982 (>74 months), 28 episodes of pneumonia were reviewed in 26 renal transplant recipients and overall mortality was as high as 46%. *L pneumophila* accounted for 2 of the cases, and both of these patients survived. The immunosuppressive agents involved were azathioprine, prednisone, and cyclosporine A.[50]

Over the course of several years, several nosocomial outbreaks of legionellosis in transplant patient populations have been reported from the United States and Europe. The outbreaks have been linked to water distribution, drinking systems, shower equipment, and even decorative water fountains. A cluster of 5 nosocomial legionella pneumonia cases was reported in a transplantation unit in Stockholm, Sweden, between September 1981 and December 1982. Of the 5 patients, 4 were renal transplant recipients and 1 had combination of renal and pancreas transplant. *L pneumophila* serogroup 6 was isolated from sputum and pleural effusion in 2 of the patients. Diagnosis was confirmed in all the patients by serology. The immunosuppression regimens included cyclosporine, azathioprine, and prednisone. All of the patients had received several doses of intravenous corticosteroid for rejection before the onset of legionella infection. All patients survived but 2 of the patients rejected their transplants before the onset of legionella infection and another 2 rejected them after the infection after reduction of immune suppressive therapy as a part of treatment. The intervals from the start of rejection to radiological diagnosis of pneumonia ranged from 6 to 15 days. *Legionella* species found in the water distribution system in the transplant ward was the same as the infecting species.[51]

The outbreaks have also occurred in pediatric transplant units. A combination of a retrospective and prospective review reported 5 cases of legionella infection in the pediatric nephrology ward (August 1994 to December 1998) in Barcelona, Spain. Renal transplant recipients on immunosuppression constituted 4 of the group and 1 patient had systemic lupus erythematosus with renal involvement. *L pneumophila* serogroup 6 was identified in bronchial specimens of 4 of the patients. The source of infection was thought to be the shower facility and equipment.[52]

Although most of the legionella infections in transplant recipients have been reported to be nosocomial, a case of community-acquired culture-proven legionnaire's disease caused by *L pneumophila* serogroup 10 was reported in a renal transplant recipient. The clinical course in this patient was further complicated by cytomegalovirus pneumonia, invasive aspergillosis, failed transplanted kidney, and death from multiorgan failure 4 months after initial diagnosis with legionella pneumonia.[53]

Dual infection with different strains of *Legionella* has been reported in series of cases from Denmark, the United Kingdom, and Germany. Cases were reported through the European national *Legionella* reference laboratories system between 2002 and 2012. A total of 15 cases were identified; 3 were solid organs transplant recipients and 3 were hematologic and bronchial cancer. Diagnosis was obtained mostly by cultures from respiratory sites (12 from respiratory samples, 1 from lung tissue, 1 from pericardial fluid, and 1 from blood culture). From a total of 29 isolates, 14 (48.3%) were dual infections, including 5 cases of *L pneumophila* serogroup 1 with different monoclonal antibody types. The non-*pneumophila* isolates included *L bozemanii*, *Legionella dumoffii*, and *L longbeachae*. Nine cases (60% of cases) were assumed to be of nosocomial origin and 5 of them were linked to the water system in the hospital. The same strains of *Legionella* were found in the water system of the hospital. More than half the patients (53.3%) were women. Case fatality rate was as high as 40% in this case series, compared with a reported annual rate of 6.6% to 10.8% in European countries. The higher mortality in patients with dual-strain infection may be related to more severe immunocompromise compared with single-strain infections.[54]

A cluster of nosocomial legionella infections reported from the National Institutes of Health (Bethesda, Maryland) was linked to a decorative water fountain despite decontamination equipment in place. Two patients with hematologic malignancy undergoing myeloablative conditioning for allogenic stem cell transplant were diagnosed with *L pneumophila* serotype 1 infection in November 2007.[55]

HEART TRANSPLANT

The first 2 cases of legionnaire's disease in cardiac transplant patients were reported in the early 1980s from Tucson, Arizona. Both cases developed cavitary lesions and one of them progressed to bronchopleural fistula. Both cases were successfully treated with antimicrobial therapy in combination with surgical intervention for bronchopleural fistula.[56] In heart transplant recipients, the incidence has been reported to vary from 3% (in patients receiving azathioprine and corticosteroids) to 5% (in patients receiving cyclosporine A and corticosteroids). In a review of 20 legionnaire's disease cases among heart transplant recipients in Germany over a 2-year period, the incidence was 17%, compared with 4.7% in the control group (postoperative cardiac patients without immunosuppressive therapy). *Legionella* urine antigen test was positive in all patients. Only 9 patients developed pneumonia, nodular infiltrates were seen in 5 patients, and the remaining patients had only fever. The time to urinary antigenuria varied from 10 to 179 days and the period of antigen shedding was prolonged despite appropriate therapy. It is suggested that frequent screening for *Legionella* urinary antigen might help in early diagnosis.[57]

A nosocomial outbreak of 3 cases of legionella pneumonia was reported from Denmark in 3 transplant (2 heart and 1 lung) recipients receiving immunosuppressive therapy. *L pneumophila* (2 serotype 1 and 1 serotype 6) grew from the bronchial lavage specimens. The source was identified as a contaminated ice machine located in the intensive care unit.[58]

A case of *L pneumophila* serotype 6 infection has been reported to cause ascending aortitis presenting with pseudoaneurysm of the aorta 16 months after transplant. The surveillance culture of the hospital water supply system proved that a nosocomial source was a possibility and it was hypothesized that the infection occurred through the contamination of the wound during the posttransplant period. A Teflon ring that was implanted during transplant procedure was assumed to be responsible for unusually deep-seated infection. The patient was successfully treated with surgical intervention and prolonged antibiotic treatment followed by lifelong antibiotic suppression.[59] A fatal legionella pneumonia case has been reported in the early posttransplant period in a patient receiving highly immunosuppressive therapy with corticosteroid, cyclosporine A, and mycophenolic mofetil. *L pneumophila* was detected by direct immunofluorescence assay and cultured from tracheal aspirates. Despite aggressive measures and appropriate antimicrobial therapy, the patient expired on day 25 after transplant. The potable hospital water supply was suspected to be the source of legionella infection.[60]

LUNG TRANSPLANT

A patient with double lung transplant was reported to have a complicated postoperative course with pulmonary emboli, acute renal failure, and *Clostridium difficile* colitis. Two months after transplant, he presented with fever and gastrointestinal symptoms and was diagnosed with disseminated cytomegalovirus infection and recurrent *C difficile* colitis. He progressed to respiratory failure and eventually died. Autopsy revealed multilobar pneumonia and *L pneumophila* serogroup 4 infection.[61]

LIVER TRANSPLANT

The first reported case of *L pneumophila* serogroup 1 infection was a 2-month-old orthotropic liver transplant patient in 1992 who died of infection despite antimicrobial therapy. Because of drug interaction with immunosuppressants used in liver transplant recipients, fluoroquinolones are the preferred antibiotic choice in this patient population.[62] Cavitary pneumonia caused by *L pneumophila* in a liver transplant recipient after 7 years was reported by Fraser and colleagues[63] and treated with surgical resection and antimicrobial therapy. Literature review showed that non-*pneumophila* species (*L micdadei* and *L bozemanii*) have also been reported to cause cavitary pneumonia in these patients. Singh and colleagues[64] postulated that tacrolimus use is more likely to be associated with legionella and fungal infections than cyclosporine A. Cytomegalovirus infection suppresses humeral and cellular immunity in vitro and in vivo. Halkic and colleagues[65] reported an unusual case of recurrent cytomegalovirus disease that required intravenous ganciclovir therapy followed by intravenous forscarnet and precipitated visceral leishmaniasis and legionella pneumonia in a liver transplant recipient. The immunosuppressive therapy for this patient was tacrolimus and prednisone. He presented with cytomegalovirus infection initially 1 month after liver transplant from a cytomegalovirus-positive donor followed by visceral leishmaniasis and legionella pneumonia. He was successfully treated with antimicrobial therapy.[65] In a large prospective review of pulmonary infection in 101 consecutive liver transplant recipients on tacrolimus, 15% of patients had 19 episodes of bacterial pneumonia; legionella accounted for 27%; and 12 were nosocomial infections, which included 1 case of legionella pneumonia. Because legionella cases can be easily overlooked, *Legionella*-specific cultures on diagnostic specimens and routine surveillance of hospital water supplies for the legionella contamination should be done routinely in centers caring for immunocompromised patients.[66] In a review of 700 liver transplants, simultaneous splenectomy during liver transplant procedures significantly increased the risk of opportunistic pneumonia during the posttransplant period.[67]

BONE MARROW TRANSPLANT

A retrospective review of 10 cases of legionella pneumonia in bone marrow transplant recipients over a 6-year period ending in 1993 in Washington state reported that 7 cases were caused by non-*pneumophila* species, 5 patients survived, and all 3 patients with *L pneumophila* died. One patient had relapse or persistent infection after 3 weeks of antimicrobial therapy, suggesting that prolonged antibiotic treatment is likely to be of benefit in this patient population.[68] Schindel and colleagues[69] reported a patient with persistent legionella pneumonia that progressed to pulmonary abscess with cavity formation over a 12-week period in a bone marrow transplant recipient receiving cyclosporine A and prednisone. The species was *L pneumophila* serotype 1 and lung abscess was superinfected by *Prevotella* species. Cure was achieved by surgical resection.

SUMMARY

It is clear from this extensive review of the literature that immunosuppressive agents predispose patients to legionnaire's disease. The role is clear for TNF antagonists because the patients receiving this class of agents are generally not severely immunocompromised by the underlying disease. In patients with malignancy receiving immunosuppressive therapies, it is difficult to balance the role of the underlying disease versus the therapy used. Transplant recipients are often on multiple drugs, including immunosuppressants. It seems that immunosuppressive drugs add to the risk for legionella infection with quantitative difference among the agents. Other than known immunologic defects that lead to increased susceptibility to other intracellular organisms, the literature review does not provide evidence of a specific relationship of these agents to the pathogens involved in legionnaire's disease.

Because atypical presentations are common in patients on immunosuppressive agents, the index of suspicion should be high and diagnostic testing and presumptive therapy should be added for legionella infection early during a compatible clinical syndrome. The significance of nosocomial acquisition and environmental acquisition, in particular water sources in the hospital, is shown by evidence from multiple reports. The control of *Legionella* species in the environment and prevention of transmission should clearly be the first and foremost goal in protecting susceptible patient populations from morbidity and mortality associated with legionnaire's disease.

REFERENCES

1. Cunha BA, Hage JE. *Legionella pneumophila* community-acquired pneumonia (CAP) in a post-splenectomy patient with myelodysplastic syndrome (MDS). Heart Lung 2012;41(5):525–7.
2. Cunha BA, Burillo A, Bouza E. Legionnaire's disease. Lancet 2016;387(10016): 376–85.
3. Yu H, Higa F, Koide M, et al. Lung abscess caused by *Legionella* species: implication of the immune status of hosts. Intern Med 2009;48(23):1997–2002.
4. Saravolatz LD, Burch KH, Fisher E, et al. The compromised host and Legionnaire's disease. Ann Intern Med 1979;90(4):533–7.
5. Helms CM, Viner JP, Weisenburger DD, et al. Sporadic Legionnaire's disease: clinical observations on 87 nosocomial and community-acquired cases. Am J Med Sci 1984;288(1):2–12.
6. Scerpella EG, Whimbey EE, Champlin RE, et al. Pericarditis associated with Legionnaire's disease in a bone marrow transplant recipient. Clin Infect Dis 1994; 19(6):1168–70.
7. Thurneysen C, Boggian K. *Legionella pneumophila* serogroup 1 septic arthritis with probable endocarditis in an immunodeficient patient. J Clin Rheumatol 2014;20(5):297–8.
8. Lück PC, Helbig JH, Wunderlich E, et al. Isolation of *Legionella pneumophila* serogroup 3 from pericardial fluid in a case of pericarditis. J Infect 1989;17(6): 388–90.
9. Barigou M, Cavalie L, Daviller B, et al. Isolation on chocolate agar culture of *Legionella pneumophila* isolates from subcutaneous abscesses in an immunocompromised patient. J Clin Microbiol 2015;53(11):3683–5.
10. Bentz JS, Carroll K, Ward JH, et al. Acid-fast-positive *Legionella pneumophila*: a possible pitfall in the cytologic diagnosis of mycobacterial infection in pulmonary specimens. Diagn Cytopathol 2000;22(1):45–8.
11. Knirsch CA, Jakob K, Schoonmaker D, et al. An outbreak of *Legionella micdadei* pneumonia in transplant patients: evaluation, molecular epidemiology, and control. Am J Med 2000;108(4):290–5.
12. Muder RR, Stout JE, Yu VL. Nosocomial *Legionella micdadei* infection in transplant patients: fortune favors the prepared mind. Am J Med 2000;108(4):346–8.
13. Dowling JN, Pasculle AW, Frola FN, et al. Infections caused by Legio*nella micdadei* and *Legionella pneumophila* among renal transplant recipients. J Infect Dis 1984;149(5):703–13.
14. Patel MC, Levi MH, Mahadevi P, et al. *L. micdadei* PVE successfully treated with levofloxacin/valve replacement: case report and review of the literature. J Infect 2005;51(5):e265–8.

15. Wright AJ, Humar A, Gourishankar S, et al. Severe Legionnaire's disease caused by *Legionella longbeachae* in a long-term renal transplant patient: the importance of safe living strategies after transplantation. Transpl Infect Dis 2012; 14(4):E30–3.
16. Lee J, Caplivski D, Wu M, et al. Pneumonia due to *Legionella feeleii*: case report and review of the literature. Transpl Infect Dis 2009;11(4):337–40.
17. Miller ML, Hayden R, Gaur A. *Legionella bozemanii* pulmonary abscess in a pediatric allogeneic stem cell transplant recipient. Pediatr Infect Dis J 2007;26(8): 760–2.
18. Horwitz MA. Cell-mediated immunity in Legionnaire's disease. J Clin Invest 1983; 71(6):1686–97.
19. McHugh SL, Newton CA, Yamamoto Y, et al. Tumor necrosis factor induces resistance of macrophages to *Legionella pneumophila* infection. Proc Soc Exp Biol Med 2000;224(3):191–6.
20. Tubach F, Ravaud P, Salmon-Céron D, et al. Emergence of *Legionella pneumophila* pneumonia in patients receiving tumor necrosis factor-alpha antagonists. Clin Infect Dis 2006;43(10):e95–100.
21. Lanternier F, Tubach F, Ravaud P, et al. Incidence and risk factors of *Legionella pneumophila* pneumonia during anti-tumor necrosis factor therapy: a prospective French study. Chest 2013;144(3):990–8.
22. Wondergem MJ, Voskuyl AE, van Agtmael MA. A case of legionellosis during treatment with a TNFalpha antagonist. Scand J Infect Dis 2004;36(4):310–1.
23. Jinno S, Pulido S, Pien BC. First reported United States case of *Legionella pneumophila* serogroup 1 pneumonia in a patient receiving anti-tumor necrosis factor-alpha therapy. Hawaii Med J 2009;68(5):109–12.
24. Mancini G, Erario L, Gianfreda R, et al. Tuberculosis and *Legionella pneumophila* pneumonia in a patient receiving anti-tumour necrosis factor-alpha (anti-TNF-alpha) treatment. Clin Microbiol Infect 2007;13(10):1036–7.
25. Hofmann A, Beaulieu Y, Bernard F, et al. Fulminant legionellosis in two patients treated with infliximab for Crohn's disease: case series and literature review. Can J Gastroenterol 2009;23(12):829–33.
26. Epping G, van der Valk PD, Hendrix R. *Legionella pneumophila* pneumonia in a pregnant woman treated with anti-TNF-α antibodies for Crohn's disease: a case report. J Crohns Colitis 2010;4(6):687–9.
27. Beigel F, Jürgens M, Filik L, et al. Severe *Legionella pneumophila* pneumonia following infliximab therapy in a patient with Crohn's disease. Inflamm Bowel Dis 2009;15(8):1240–4.
28. Eisendle K, Fritsch P. Fatal fulminant legionnaire's disease in a patient with severe erythodermic psoriasis treated with infliximab after long-term steroid therapy. Br J Dermatol 2005;152(3):585–6.
29. Kaku N, Yanagihara K, Morinaga Y, et al. Detection of *Legionella pneumophila* serogroup 1 in blood cultures from a patient treated with tumor necrosis factor-alpha inhibitor. J Infect Chemother 2013;19(1):166–70.
30. Wuerz TC, Mooney O, Keynan Y. *Legionella pneumophila* serotype 1 pneumonia in patient receiving adalimumab. Emerg Infect Dis 2012;18(11):1872–4.
31. Boivin S, Lacombe MC, Lalancette L, et al. Environmental factors associated with nosocomial legionellosis after anti-tumor necrosis factor therapy: case study. Am J Infect Control 2012;40(5):470–3.
32. Jacobson KL, Miceli MH, Tarrand JJ, et al. Legionella pneumonia in cancer patients. Medicine (Baltimore) 2008;87(3):152–9.

33. Nunnink JC, Gallagher JG, Yates JW. Legionnaire's disease in patients with cancer. Med Pediatr Oncol 1986;14(2):81–5.
34. Cordonnier C, Farcet JP, Desforges L, et al. Legionnaire's disease and hairy-cell leukemia. An unfortuitous association? Arch Intern Med 1984;144(12):2373–5.
35. Cunha BA, Munoz-Gomez S, Gran A, et al. Persistent Legionnaire's disease in an adult with hairy cell leukemia successfully treated with prolonged levofloxacin therapy. Heart Lung 2015;44(4):360–2.
36. Radaelli F, Langer M, Chiorboli O, et al. Severe *Legionella pneumophila* infection in a patient with hairy cell leukemia in partial remission after alpha interferon treatment. Hematol Oncol 1991;9(3):125–8.
37. Gutzeit MF, Lauer SJ, Dunne WM Jr, et al. Fatal *Legionella* pneumonitis in a neutropenic leukemic child. Pediatr Infect Dis J 1987;6(1):68–9.
38. Watts JC, Hicklin MD, Thomason BM, et al. Fatal pneumonia caused by *Legionella pneumophila*, serogroup 3: demonstration of the bacilli in extrathoracic organs. Ann Intern Med 1980;92(2 Pt 1):186–8.
39. Hendrick A. Fatal legionella pneumonia after fludarabine treatment in chronic lymphocytic leukaemia. J Clin Pathol 2001;54(5):412–3.
40. Sheldon PA, Tight RR, Renner ED. Fatal Legionnaire's disease coincident with initiation of immunosuppressive therapy. Arch Intern Med 1985;145(6):1138–9.
41. Del Castillo M, Lucca A, Plodkowski A, et al. Atypical presentation of *Legionella* pneumonia among patients with underlying cancer: A fifteen-year review. J Infect 2016;72(1):45–51.
42. Han XY, Lhegword A, Evans SE, et al. Microbiological and clinical studies of legionellosis in 33 patients with cancer. J Clin Microbiol 2015;53(7):2180–7.
43. Dworzack DL, Ferry JJ, Clark RB. Co-infection with *Legionella pneumophila* and *Pneumocystis carinii* in a patient with chronic lymphocytic leukemia. Nebr Med J 1989;74(4):73–5.
44. Arakaki N, Higa F, Tateyama M, et al. Concurrent infection with *Legionella pneumophila* and *Pneumocystis carinii* in a patient with adult T cell leukemia. Intern Med 1999;38(2):160–3.
45. Korvick J, Yu VL. Simultaneous infection with *Cryptococcus neoformans* and *Legionella pneumophila* in vivo expression of common defects in cell-mediated immunity. Respiration 1988;53(2):132–6.
46. Tkatch LS, Kusne S, Irish WD, et al. Epidemiology of legionella pneumonia and factors associated with legionella-related mortality at a tertiary care center. Clin Infect Dis 1998;27(6):1479–86.
47. Frenkel JK, Baker LH, Chonko AM. Autopsy diagnosis of Legionnaire's disease in immunosuppressed patients. A paleodiagnosis using Giemsa stain (Wohlbach modification). Ann Intern Med 1979;90(4):559–62.
48. Gump DW, Frank RO, Winn WC Jr, et al. Legionnaire's disease in patients with associated serious disease. Ann Intern Med 1979;90(4):538–42.
49. Gombert ME, Josephson A, Goldstein EJ, et al. Cavitary Legionnaire's pneumonia: nosocomial infection in renal transplant recipients. Am J Surg 1984; 147(3):402–5.
50. Bowie DM, Marrie TJ, Janigan DT, et al. Pneumonia in renal transplant patients. Can Med Assoc J 1983;128(12):1411–4.
51. Wilczek H, Kallings I, Nyström B, et al. Nosocomial Legionnaire's disease following renal transplantation. Transplantation 1987;43(6):847–51.
52. Campins M, Ferrer A, Callís L, et al. Nosocomial Legionnaire's disease in a children's hospital. Pediatr Infect Dis J 2000;19(3):228–34.

53. Lück PC, Schneider T, Wagner J, et al. Community-acquired Legionnaire's disease caused by *Legionella pneumophila* serogroup 10 linked to the private home. J Med Microbiol 2008;57(Pt 2):240–3.
54. Wewalka G, Schmid D, Harrison TG, et al. Dual infections with different *Legionella* strains. Clin Microbiol Infect 2014;20(1):O13–9.
55. Palmore TN, Stock F, White M, et al. A cluster of cases of nosocomial legionnaires disease linked to a contaminated hospital decorative water fountain. Infect Control Hosp Epidemiol 2009;30(8):764–8.
56. Copeland J, Wieden M, Feinberg W, et al. Legionnaire's disease following cardiac transplantation. Chest 1981;79(6):669–71.
57. Horbach I, Fehrenbach FJ. Legionellosis in heart transplant recipients. Infection 1990;18(6):361–3.
58. Bangsborg JM, Uldum S, Jensen JS, et al. Nosocomial legionellosis in three heart-lung transplant patients: case reports and environmental observations. Eur J Clin Microbiol Infect Dis 1995;14(2):99–104.
59. Guyot S, Goy JJ, Gersbach P, et al. *Legionella pneumophila* aortitis in a heart transplant recipient. Transpl Infect Dis 2007;9(1):58–9.
60. Mathys W, Deng MC, Meyer J, et al. Fatal nosocomial Legionnaire's disease after heart transplantation: clinical course, epidemiology and prevention strategies for the highly immunocompromized host. J Hosp Infect 1999;43(3):242–6.
61. Nichols L, Strollo DC, Kusne S. Legionellosis in a lung transplant recipient obscured by cytomegalovirus infection and *Clostridium difficile* colitis. Transpl Infect Dis 2002;4(1):41–5.
62. del Pozo JL. Update and actual trends on bacterial infections following liver transplantation. World J Gastroenterol 2008;14(32):4977–83.
63. Fraser TG, Zembower TR, Lynch P, et al. Cavitary *Legionella* pneumonia in a liver transplant recipient. Transpl Infect Dis 2004;6(2):77–80.
64. Singh N, Gayowski T, Wagener MM, et al. Predictors and outcome of early- versus late-onset major bacterial infections in liver transplant recipients receiving tacrolimus (FK506) as primary immunosuppression. Eur J Clin Microbiol Infect Dis 1997;16(11):821–6.
65. Halkic N, Ksontini R, Scholl B, et al. Recurrent cytomegalovirus disease, visceral leishmaniosis, and *Legionella* pneumonia after liver transplantation: a case report. Can J Anaesth 2004;51(1):84–7.
66. Singh N, Gayowski T, Wagener M, et al. Pulmonary infections in liver transplant recipients receiving tacrolimus. Changing pattern of microbial etiologies. Transplantation 1996;61(3):396–401.
67. Neumann UP, Langrehr JM, Kaisers U, et al. Simultaneous splenectomy increases risk for opportunistic pneumonia in patients after liver transplantation. Transpl Int 2002;15(5):226–32.
68. Harrington RD, Woolfrey AE, Bowden R, et al. Legionellosis in a bone marrow transplant center. Bone Marrow Transplant 1996;18(2):361–8.
69. Schindel C, Siepmann U, Han S, et al. Persistent *Legionella* infection in a patient after bone marrow transplantation. J Clin Microbiol 2000;38(11):4294–5.

Thoracic Imaging Features of Legionnaire's Disease

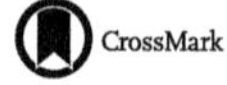

Sameer Mittal, MD, MS[a,*], Ayushi P. Singh, DO[b], Menachem Gold, MD[c], Ann N. Leung, MD[d], Linda B. Haramati, MD, MS[e,f], Douglas S. Katz, MD[a]

KEYWORDS

- Legionnaire's • Legionella • Pneumonia • Radiology • CT • Radiography • Imaging

KEY POINTS

- On chest radiography, legionella pneumonia usually presents as a patchy unilobar process that can progress to confluent opacities.
- Imaging findings in legionella pneumonia often lag behind clinical improvement.
- The most common thoracic computed tomography (CT) finding of legionella pneumonia is multilobar or multisegmental well-circumscribed air-space disease intermingled with ground-glass opacities.
- Although uncommonly identified on chest radiographs, small pleural effusions and lymphadenopathy are occasionally identified on thoracic CT in patients with legionella infection.

INTRODUCTION

Legionnaire's disease was first described following an outbreak of a respiratory illness that occurred during a 1976 convention of the American Legion in Philadelphia, with more than 200 reported cases and 34 deaths.[1,2] After extensive microbiologic and epidemiologic investigation, *Legionella pneumophila* was determined to be the causative organism 6 months after the outbreak occurred.[3] *L pneumophila* is a flagellated gram-negative bacterium that colonizes aquatic environments and enters the respiratory tract via inhalation of aerosols.[4]

Disclosure Statement. The authors have nothing to disclose.
[a] Department of Radiology, Winthrop-University Hospital, 259 First Street, Mineola, NY 11501, USA; [b] Department of Medicine, Maimonides Hospital, Fort Hamilton Parkway, Brooklyn, NY 11219, USA; [c] Department of Radiology, Lincoln Hospital, 234 East 149th Street, Suite 2C3, Bronx, NY 10461, USA; [d] Department of Radiology, Stanford University Medical Center, 300 Pasteur Drive, Room S078, MC5105, Stanford, CA 94305, USA; [e] Department of Radiology, Montefiore Medical Center, Albert Einstein College of Medicine, 200 East Gun Hill Road, Bronx, NY 10467, USA; [f] Department of Medicine, Montefiore Medical Center, Albert Einstein College of Medicine, 200 East Gun Hill Road, Bronx, NY 10467, USA
* Corresponding author.
E-mail address: smittal@winthrop.org

Infect Dis Clin N Am 31 (2017) 43–54
http://dx.doi.org/10.1016/j.idc.2016.10.004 id.theclinics.com

Risk factors for acquiring legionella pneumonia are advanced age, a smoking or substance abuse history, underlying lung disorders, and conditions leading to a compromised immune system.[5] A higher incidence in men, in the elderly, and during the summer months has been reported, the latter because of the association with inhaled aerosolization of contaminated water, commonly produced by air conditioning systems.

Clinical presentations of legionella pneumonia include cough, dyspnea, pleuritic chest pain, and nausea, as well as generalized malaise, weakness, and fatigue. Compromised renal function, microscopic hematuria, hyponatremia, and rhabdomyolysis also can be found on further workup of some affected patients.[6] Beta-lactams, which are commonly used as empiric antibiotics for pneumonia, are ineffective for the treatment of *L pneumophila* pneumonia.[7] Therefore, a high degree of clinical and radiologic suspicion is required, and a presumptive diagnosis should prompt specific testing and anti-legionella therapy to prevent intensive care unit (ICU) admission and substantial morbidity as well as potential mortality.

Establishing or suggesting the diagnosis of legionella infection rests on the identification of legionella antigen in the urine, immunofluorescent antibody, and enzyme-linked immunosorbent assay tests, or isolation of the organism by culture from sputum specimens. Treatment with macrolide or fluoroquinolone antibiotics has been shown to be effective, and portends a good prognosis if started early in the disease course.[6]

The literature to date has documented that the imaging findings in Legionnaire's disease are unfortunately relatively nonspecific, and it is therefore difficult to prospectively differentiate legionella pneumonia from other forms of pneumonia and from other noninfectious thoracic processes.[8] Through a selection of recent clinical cases at our institutions and a brief review of the literature, we aim to overview the thoracic imaging manifestations of legionella pneumonia.

DISCUSSION

Review of Thoracic Radiographic Features

Legionnaire's disease is classified as an "atypical pneumonia," which is usually defined as a bacterial pneumonia caused by organisms including mycoplasma, chlamydia, and legionella. These organisms are more difficult to identify and frequently have less severe clinical manifestations than classic causes of bacterial pneumonia, such as pneumococcus, streptococcus, and klebsiella.[9] Legionnaire's disease on chest radiography is often rapidly progressive, and asymmetric in pattern.[8] Several series have noted that the initial chest radiographic presentation of legionella pneumonia is frequently unilobar, with patchy air-space disease, although these findings are not specific for the diagnosis of legionella.[9–13] Tan and colleagues[9] studied the chest radiographs of 43 patients hospitalized with legionella pneumonia in Ohio. Forty of the patients had pulmonary findings on the initial chest radiographs. Seventy-seven percent of the 43 patients had patchy air-space disease, and 16% had confluent or lobar findings. More than two-thirds of the 77% of patients with patchy pulmonary findings had unilobar involvement.[9] Kroboth and colleagues noted that 76% of 34 patients with Legionnaire's disease had initial patchy air-space disease, and more than three-fourths of their patients had single-lobe disease at presentation.[11] Similarly, Kirby and colleagues[12] found that in a group of 65 nosocomially acquired Legionnaire's disease cases, almost all presented with unilobar patchy air-space disease on their initial chest radiographs. As the disease progressed, the most common pattern was progression to consolidation in the area of the initial air-space disease (**Figs. 1** and **2**). The abnormalities remained unilateral in 64% of cases.[12] Dietrich

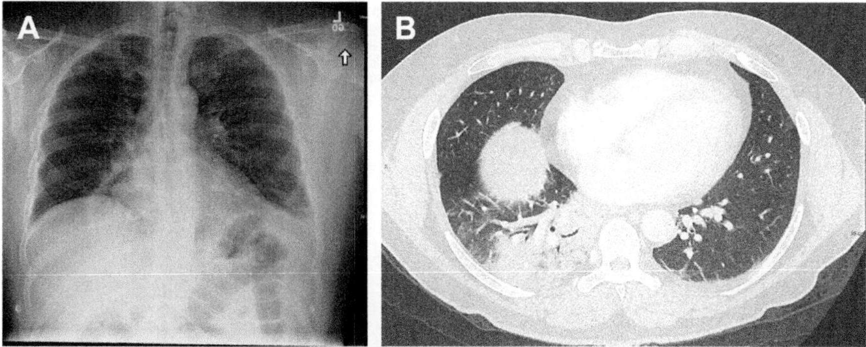

Fig. 1. A 42-year-old man presenting with nonproductive cough, fever, chills, and malaise for 4 days, with legionella pneumonia. (*A*) Initial chest radiograph demonstrates right medial lower lobe consolidation with air bronchograms. (*B*) Subsequent CT demonstrates right lower lobe consolidation.

and colleagues[14] found that 68% of patients with Legionnaire's disease had unilateral left lung air-space disease initially. The most common lung findings on radiographs were poorly marginated round opacities (46%), and diffuse patchy (25%) and peripheral opacities (21%).[14] Necrotizing pneumonia with cavitation was an occasional radiographic finding noted during the 2015 Bronx, NY outbreak (**Fig. 3**).

Immunocompromised patients may have different and variable chest radiographic manifestations compared with immunocompetent patients. Circumscribed peripheral opacities and cavitations are more common in immunocompromised patients, and may develop up to 14 days after presentation, despite the initiation of appropriate antibiotic therapy[8,15] (**Fig. 4**). Pedro-Botet and colleagues[13] studied 78 patients with legionella pneumonia: 28 with chronic disease who had received immunosuppressive treatment (group 1), 24 with chronic disease without immunosuppressive treatment (group 2), and 26 "controls". Unilateral involvement was observed in approximately 70% of patients in all 3 groups. A greater frequency of bilateral involvement was

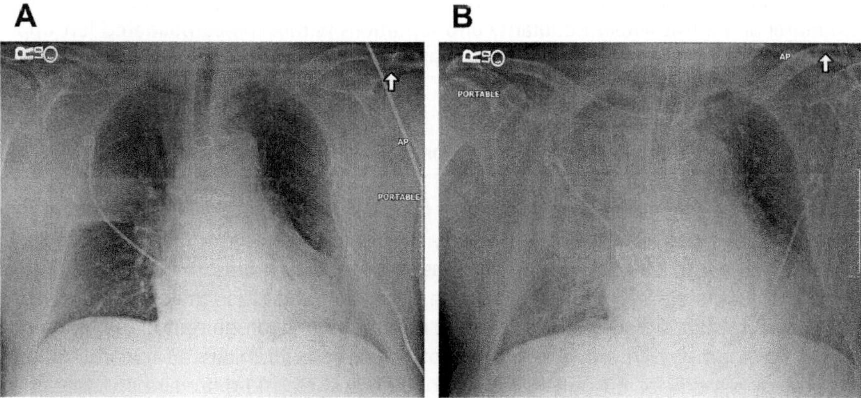

Fig. 2. A 73-year-old man on chronic high-dose prednisone presents with fevers and nonproductive cough. (*A*) Initial chest radiograph shows right upper lobe consolidation. (*B*) Subsequent chest radiograph demonstrates a worsening lobar pattern.

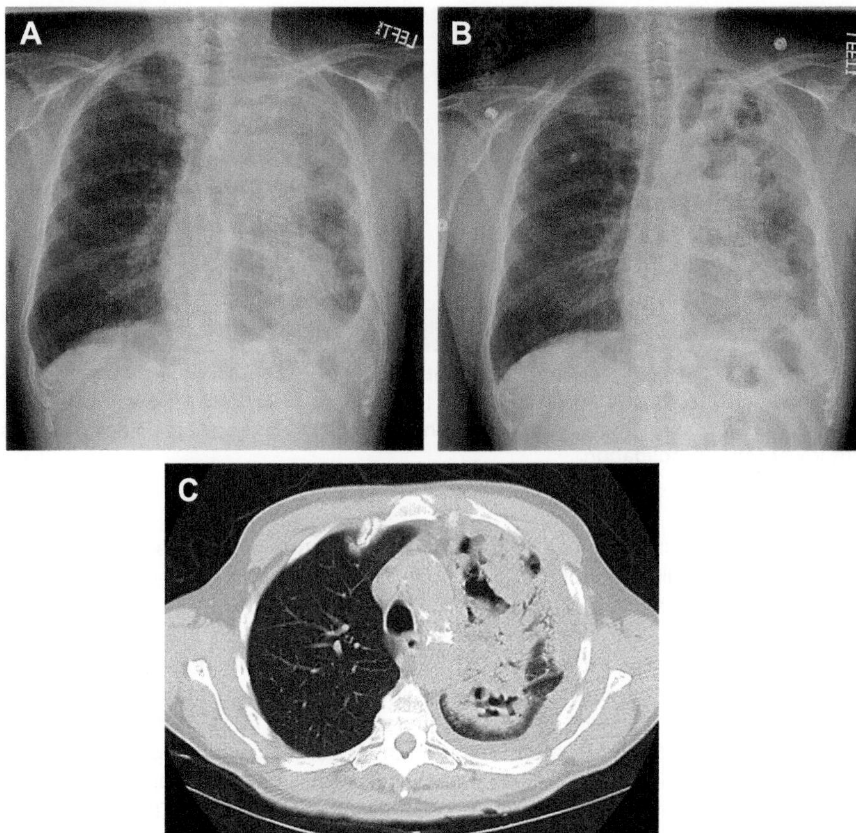

Fig. 3. A 58-year-old previously healthy man developed shortness of breath and cough productive of greenish sputum related to legionella infection. (*A*) Chest radiograph at presentation demonstrates dense consolidation within the left lung, predominantly in the upper lobe, with a small left pleural effusion. (*B*) Chest radiograph 5 days later demonstrates new cavitation within the consolidated left lung, and a persistent small left pleural effusion. (*C*) Chest CT on the same day as the follow-up radiograph demonstrates complex cavitation with mural and intracavitary nodularity and septations within the consolidated left upper lobe. There is a small left pleural effusion that tracks laterally, indicating that it is at least partially loculated.

observed in those who received immunosuppressive treatment (29%) than in the "controls" group (15%).[13]

Resolution of the thoracic radiographic findings in Legionnaire's disease may lag behind clinical improvement. This tendency for radiographic abnormalities to progress while the patient is clinically improving has been widely noted.[14,16,17] In a study of community-acquired Legionnaire's disease, 24 of 37 patients with serial radiographs during hospitalization had worsening chest radiographic findings during the first week (**Fig. 5**). Radiographic improvement was not observed until 6 days of hospitalization.[9] Similarly, in a study of 58 patients with hospital-acquired Legionnaire's disease, 11 showed progression of unilateral air-space disease in the same lung, and 6 showed progression to the opposite lung at days 8 to 10, despite receiving erythromycin[18] (**Fig. 6**). This tendency for radiographic progression despite clinical improvement should be

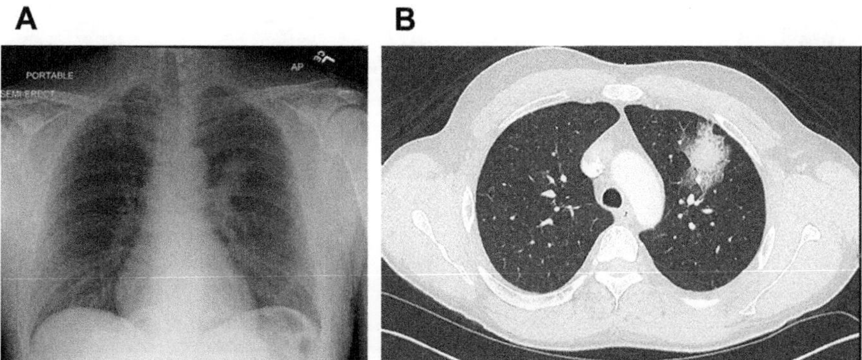

Fig. 4. A 43-year-old immunocompromised man presenting with sudden onset of fever, chills, malaise, nonproductive cough, and palpitations. (*A*) Initial chest radiograph demonstrates a circumscribed opacity in the left upper lung. (*B*) CT demonstrates a 2.9-cm left upper lobe circumscribed opacity with air bronchograms and surrounding ground-glass opacification, which proved to be legionella pneumonia.

considered before initiating further invasive diagnostic investigation or altering a patient's treatment plan. Also, the presence of several specific imaging findings argues strongly against the diagnosis of legionella pneumonia; these include rapid cavitation within 72 hours, hilar adenopathy, and massive or hemorrhagic pleural effusion(s).[19]

Review of Computed Tomography Features

Although otherwise nonspecific, typical computed tomography (CT) features of legionella pneumonia include multilobar or multisegmental well-circumscribed air-space opacities intermingled with ground-glass opacities.[18–21] In a review of the CT findings of 38 patients with Legionnaire's disease, Sarkai and colleagues[21] found that the opacities were scattered segmentally or subsegmentally within areas of nonsegmental ground-glass opacities in 24 patients. The segmental/subsegmental consolidations were predominantly in the perihilar region and had relatively sharp margins. The distribution was bilateral in 23 cases, and there was no preponderance for the upper or lower lungs. A less common presentation of legionella pneumonia in this study was bilateral diffuse ground-glass opacities mixed with foci of consolidation along the bronchovascular bundles, mimicking acute pulmonary edema. The presence of only consolidation or of only ground-glass opacities was distinctly unusual, and was present in 2 and 1 patients, respectively. The CT appearance did not correlate with clinical severity, time after onset of symptoms, patient age, or patient sex.[21]

In a review of the thoracic CT findings in 16 patients with Legionnaire's disease, Kim and colleagues[18] found multilobar or multisegmental parenchymal air-space disease in at least 2 lobes in all 12 patients. The average number of affected lobes in this study was 3.4, and there was no upper or lower lobar predominance (**Fig. 7**). All 12 patients had ground-glass opacities, and 10 of 12 also had air-space consolidation. Most of the lobar and segmental consolidations were associated with surrounding ground-glass opacities. Four patients in this study developed cavitation during their hospital course, which was evident on CT. All 4 of these patients were on high-dose steroid therapy.[18]

A review by Yu and colleagues[20] of 23 patients with sporadic legionella pneumonia found that air-space consolidation mixed with ground-glass opacities was the predominant pattern on CT. In 22 of the patients, air bronchograms were observed within the areas of air-space disease. Pleural effusions were observed in most patients. In

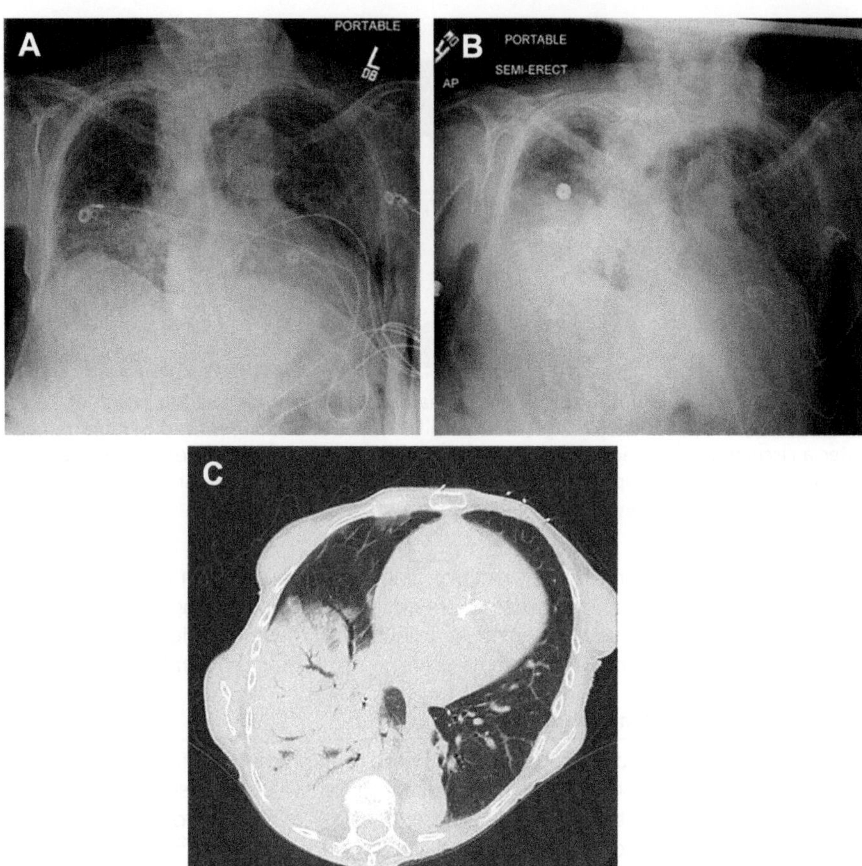

Fig. 5. An 81-year-old woman presenting with fevers, myalgias, generalized weakness, and decreased appetite for 3 days. (*A*) Chest radiograph demonstrates patchy opacity in the right middle to lower lung. (*B*) Radiograph 2 days later demonstrates worsening air-space disease, despite clinical improvement and a decreasing white blood cell count. (*C*) CT better demonstrates the right lower lobe consolidation with air bronchograms, which proved to be legionella pneumonia.

this series, a nonsegmental distribution was substantially more common than a segmental distribution. Twelve patients had multilobar involvement; the right lower lobe was most frequently involved (31%)[20] (**Fig. 8**).

Occasionally, CT may reveal a "reversed halo sign," which is characterized by a central ground-glass opacity surrounded by denser air-space consolidation in the shape of a crescent or a ring[22] (**Fig. 9**). However, this is a somewhat nonspecific finding, as it has been reported in association with a relatively wide range of pulmonary disorders, including invasive pulmonary fungal infections, pneumocystis pneumonia, tuberculosis, community-acquired pneumonia, lymphomatoid granulomatosis, Wegener granulomatosis, lipoid pneumonia, and sarcoidosis.[22] A "bulging fissure sign" also may be present if there is an increase in lobar volume. This sign is classically seen with *Klebsiella pneumoniae* and with *Streptococcus pneumoniae* thoracic infection.[19]

Small pleural effusions on CT are common in legionella pneumonia. Sarkai and colleagues[21] found effusions in 23 of 38 cases; 11 were bilateral (**Fig. 10**). Kim and

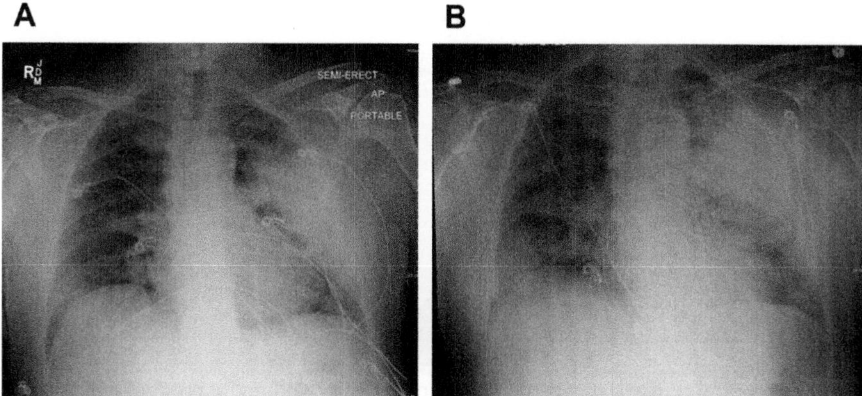

Fig. 6. A 65-year-old man presenting with shortness of breath, lethargy, and fever. (*A*) Chest radiograph demonstrates left mid-lung consolidation and patchy opacity in the right lower lobe laterally. (*B*) Radiograph 3 days later shows worsening of the left mid-lung consolidation and right lower lobe air-space disease, despite clinical improvement, which is very typical for thoracic legionella infection.

colleagues[18] found effusions in 6 of 12 patients on CT. In both series, pleural effusions were predominantly ipsilateral to the consolidations. Although lymphadenopathy is uncommonly recognized in Legionnaire's disease on chest radiographs, it was found on CT in 20 of 38 cases reported by Sarkai and colleagues,[21] and in 5 of 12 patients reported by Kim and colleagues[18] (**Fig. 11**).

Differential Diagnosis

Legionella may resemble typical bacterial community-acquired pneumonias on radiographs and on CT, including those due to pneumococcus, klebsiella, and staphylococcus. More often, it presents on imaging similarly to other atypical pneumonias, particularly mycoplasma pneumonia and viral pneumonias.[23] Pneumococcal pneumonia usually presents as a consolidation limited to a single lobe. However, it can be multifocal or bilateral in some patients. It almost always abuts a visceral pleural surface. Air bronchograms are usually present.[24] Pleural effusions are seen in up to 50%

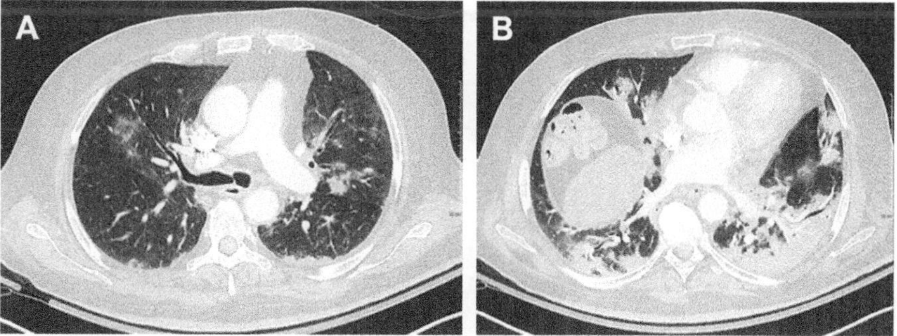

Fig. 7. A 70-year-old man with B-cell lymphoma, on chemotherapy, presenting with weakness, nonproductive cough, and shortness of breath for 1 week. (*A*) CT shows multiple small nodular patchy opacities in the upper lobes. (*B*) CT also demonstrates bibasilar consolidations.

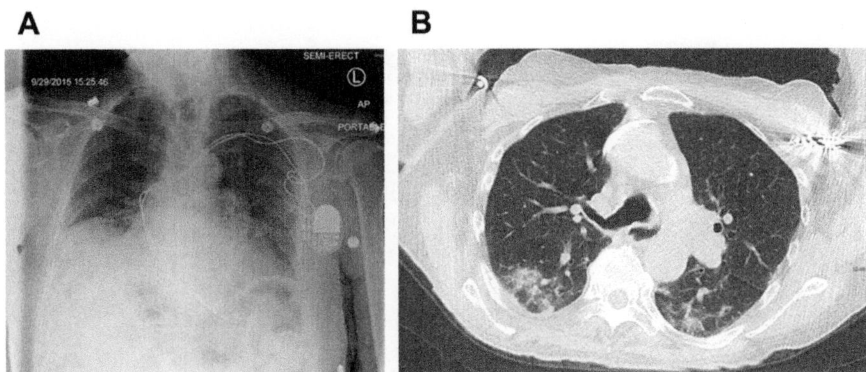

Fig. 8. A 92-year-old man with worsening shortness of breath and a productive cough for 2 weeks, with legionella pneumonia. (*A*) Chest radiograph demonstrates multilobar involvement, with patchy bibasilar opacities. (*B*) Subsequent CT demonstrates irregular patchy opacities in the superior segment of the right lower lobe and in the left lower lobe.

of cases. On CT, the consolidation is frequently more extensive than expected based on the radiographs, with ground-glass opacities surrounding the consolidation. Although both *S pneumoniae* community-acquired pneumonia (CAP) and Legionnaire's disease can present as "ground-glass" opacification, the ground-glass attenuation in *S pneumoniae* usually occurs only in the peripheral portions of the consolidation. In addition, the consolidation with *S pneumoniae* is usually not as sharply demarcated as the consolidation in Legionnaire's disease. Unlike Legionnaire's disease, *S pneumoniae* usually does not progress with appropriate therapy.[19,22] Lymphadenopathy is seen in 50% of cases of *S pneumoniae*. Cavitations and abscesses are rare. A bronchopneumonia pattern with reticular or nodular opacities also can be seen on radiographs or on CT.[25]

Klebsiella pneumonia is usually a nosocomial infection, which typically presents radiographically as lobar consolidation. As noted, a bulging interlobar fissure can be seen in up to 30% of cases.[24] Cavitation can be seen in 30% to 50% of cases, and can be multiple and chronic, potentially mimicking tuberculosis. Pleural effusions are also commonly seen.[26] CT shows consolidation, which is initially nonsegmental,

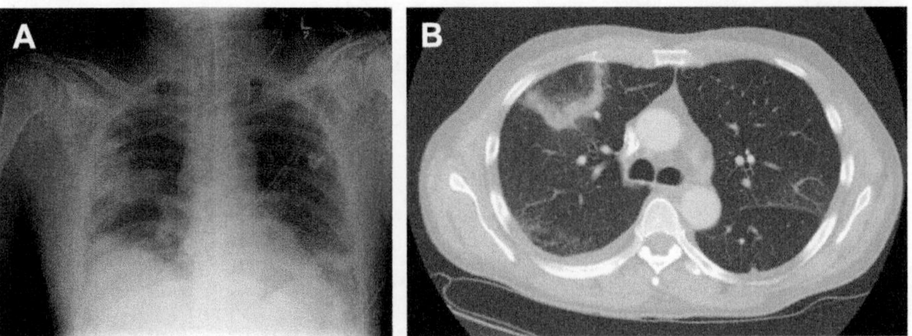

Fig. 9. A 62-year-old man presenting with diarrhea, weakness, and fever. (*A*). Initial chest radiograph shows a right upper lobe opacity. (*B*) CT demonstrates a central ground-glass opacity surrounded by denser air-space consolidation in the shape of a crescent or a ring, the "reverse halo sign", which was due to legionella.

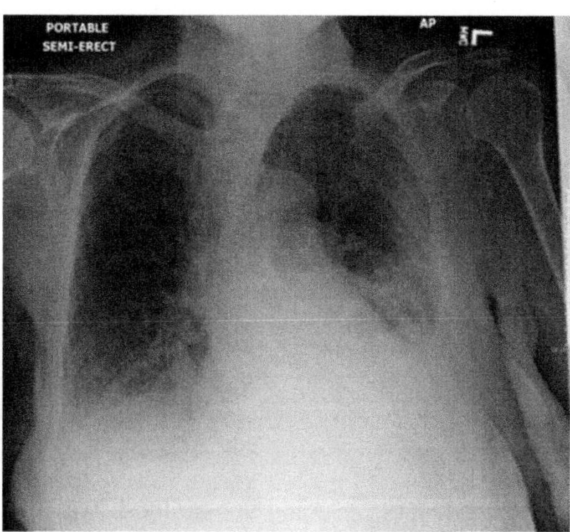

Fig. 10. An 82-year-old woman with a history of CLL, presenting with productive cough and fever for 5 days. Chest radiograph demonstrates air-space disease in the middle and lower lungs bilaterally, and small bilateral effusions, left larger than right. CLL, chronic lymphocytic leukemia.

but which quickly becomes lobar. There is expansion of the consolidated lobe. There may be necrosis, which shows an enhancing consolidation with low-density areas and small air cavities. Lung abscesses can be seen on CT in 16% to 50% of cases.[26,27] Lymphadenopathy is uncommon. Additional CT findings include interlobular septal thickening, bronchial wall thickening, pleural effusion, fibrosis, and bronchiectasis.[27]

Staphylococcal pneumonia is often nosocomial, especially in ICU patients. Typical radiographic findings are consolidation, which can range from a patchy nonsegmental to a bilateral multilobar distribution. Rapid progression of the disease is typically seen on serial radiographs. Unlike legionella and pneumococcal pneumonia, in which abscesses are rare, abscesses are present in 15% to 30% of cases with staphylococcal pneumonia. On CT, similar to pneumococcal pneumonia, consolidations are often

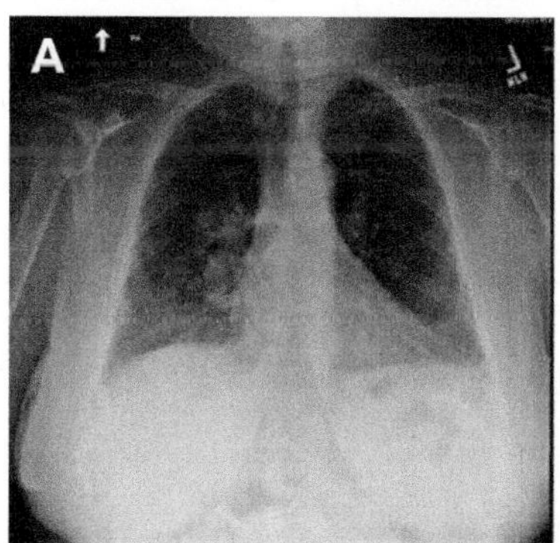

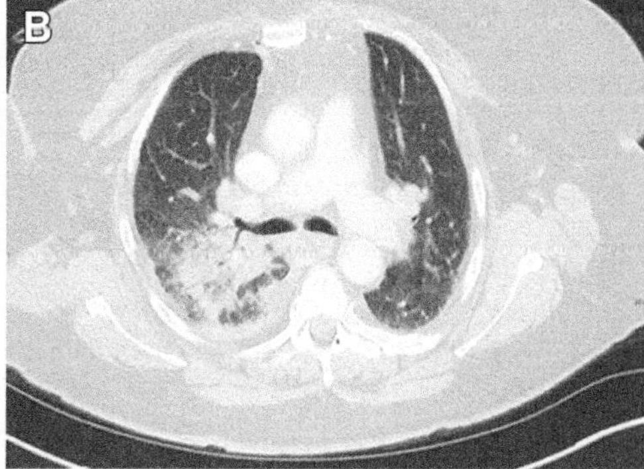

Fig. 11. A 64-year-old woman with a history of asplenia presenting with a 1-week history of generalized weakness, headache, and nonproductive cough. (*A*) Chest radiograph demonstrates patchy opacities in the right lower lobe, with a rounded density in the right hilum. (*B*) Subsequent CT shows patchy consolidation in the right lower lobe and right hilar adenopathy, due to legionella.

more extensive than are expected from the radiographs. CT better depicts the cavitations/abscesses, which may heal with pneumatocele formation. Abscesses can take weeks to months to heal. Additional CT findings can range from small centrilobular lung nodules to large parenchymal masses. Septal thickening is occasionally seen. Pleural effusions are common and can be loculated.[28,29]

Mycoplasma pneumonia is often included in the differential diagnosis of legionella CAP due to the similarity in their clinical presentation. On radiographs, mycoplasma pneumonia and legionella pneumonia may be difficult to differentiate, as they can both present with bilateral patchy air-space disease. CT, however, can be helpful for suggesting the diagnosis of mycoplasma pneumonia, because nearly all patients will have diffuse bronchial wall thickening.[19] Additional CT findings in mycoplasma pneumonia include centrilobular nodules with tree-in-bud opacities and regional lymphadenopathy.[30] Another atypical pneumonia, *Chlamydophila pneumoniae*, also presents on CT with diffuse bronchial wall thickening, but peripheral airway dilatation also will be present.[31]

Viral pneumonias have a variable imaging appearance. Typical radiographic findings are of a bronchiolitis pattern with hyperinflation, and vague small nodular opacities. Bronchial wall thickening and consolidations that present as hazy or dense air-space opacities also can be seen. Unlike legionella pneumonia, lobar consolidation is uncommon in patients with viral pneumonia.[32,33]

SUMMARY

Although the imaging findings of Legionnaire's disease (or legionella pneumonia) are nonspecific, there are patterns on both radiographs and on CT, which, in concert with the clinical presentation, can be used to suggest legionella pneumonia in the differential diagnosis. On radiographs, Legionnaire's disease usually presents as patchy unilobar air-space disease, which can progress to a confluent opacity over several days. Worsening of radiographic findings in the setting of clinical improvement is common and should not alter therapy. The most common CT findings are multilobar or multisegmental well-circumscribed air-space consolidations intermingled with ground-glass opacities. Cavitation is usually not present at disease onset, but may occasionally develop during the disease course, especially in immunocompromised patients. Although uncommonly identified on radiographs, pleural effusions and adenopathy may be identified on CT.

REFERENCES

1. Fraser DW, Tsai TR, Orenstein W, et al. Legionnaire's disease: description of an epidemic of pneumonia. N Engl J Med 1977;297:1189–97.
2. Washington CW. Legionnaire's disease: historical perspective. Clin Microbiol Rev 1988;1:60–81.
3. McDade JE, Shepard CC, Fraser DW, et al. Legionnaire's disease: isolation of a bacterium and demonstration of its role in other respiratory disease. N Engl J Med 1977;297(22):1197–203.
4. Farnham A, Alleyne L, Cimini D, et al. Legionnaire's disease incidence and risk factors. Emerg Infect Dis 2014;20(11):1795–802.
5. Atlas RM. Legionella: from environmental habitats to disease pathology, detection and control. Environ Microbiol 1999;1(4):283–93.
6. Phin N, Parry-Ford F, Harrison T, et al. Epidemiology and clinical management of Legionnaire's disease. Lancet Infect Dis 2014;14(10):1011–21.

7. Nguyen MH, Stout JE, Yu VL. Legionellosis. Infect Dis Clin North Am 1991;5: 561–84.
8. Coletta FS, Fein AM. Radiological manifestations of Legionella/Legionella-like organisms. Semin Respir Infect 1998;13(2):109–15.
9. Tan MJ, Tan JS, Hamor RH, et al. The radiological manifestations of Legionnaire's disease. Chest 2000;117(2):398–403.
10. Zhigang Z, Xinmin L, Luzeng C, et al. Chest radiographic characteristics of community-acquired Legionella pneumonia in the elderly. Chin Med J 2014; 127(12):2270–4.
11. Kroboth FJ, Yu VL, Reddy SC, et al. Clinicoradiographic correlation with the extent of Legionnaire's disease. Am J Roentgenol 1983;141:263–8.
12. Kirby BD, Snyder KM, Meyer RD, et al. Legionnaire's disease: report of sixty-five nosocomially acquired cases and review of the literature. Medicine 1980;59: 188–205.
13. Pedro-Botet ML, Sabria-Leal M, Sopena N, et al. Role of immunosuppression in the evolution of Legionnaire's disease. Clin Infect Dis 1998;26:14–9.
14. Dietrich PA, Johnson RD, Fairbanks JT, et al. The chest radiograph in Legionnaire's disease. Radiology 1978;127:577–82.
15. Kumpers P, Tiede A, Kirschner P, et al. Legionnaire's disease in immunocompromised patients: a case report of Legionella longbeachae pneumonia and review of the literature. J Med Microbiol 2008;57:384–7.
16. Mulazimoglu L, Yu VL. Can Legionnaire's disease be diagnosed by clinical criteria? A critical review. Chest 2001;120(4):1049–53.
17. Domingo C, Roig J, Planas F, et al. Radiographic appearance of nosocomial Legionnaire's disease after erythromycin treatment. Thorax 1991;46:663–6.
18. Kim KW, Goo JM, Lee HJ, et al. Chest computed tomographic findings and clinical features of legionella pneumonia. J Comput Assist Tomogr 2007;31(6):950–5.
19. Cunha BA. Legionnaire's disease: clinical differentiation from typical and other atypical pneumonias. Infect Dis Clin North Am 2010;24(1):73–105.
20. Yu H, Higa F, Hibiya K, et al. Computed tomographic features of 23 sporadic cases with *Legionella pneumophila* pneumonia. Eur J Radiol 2010;74:73–8.
21. Sarkai F, Tokuda H, Goto H, et al. Computed tomographic features of *Legionella pneumophila* pneumonia in 38 cases. J Comput Assist Tomogr 2007;31(1): 125–31.
22. Godoy MCB, Vishwanathan C, Marchioro E, et al. The reverse halo sign: update and differential diagnosis. Br J Radiol 2012;85(1017):1226–35.
23. Watkins RR, Lemonovich TL. Diagnosis and management of community-acquired pneumonia in adults. Am Fam Physician 2011;83(11):1299–306.
24. Reynolds JH, McDonald G, Alton H, et al. Pneumonia in the immunocompetent patient. Br J Radiol 2010;83(996):998–1009.
25. Yagihashi K, Kurihara Y, Fujikawa A, et al. Correlations between computed tomography findings and clinical manifestations of *Streptococcus pneumoniae* pneumonia. Jpn J Radiol 2011;29(6):423–8.
26. Okada F, Ando Y, Honda K, et al. Clinical and pulmonary thin-section CT findings in acute *Klebsiella pneumoniae* pneumonia. Eur Radiol 2009;19(4):809–15.
27. Okada F, Ando Y, Honda K, et al. Acute *Klebsiella pneumoniae* pneumonia alone and with concurrent infection: comparison of clinical and thin-section CT findings. Br J Radiol 2010;83(994):854–60.
28. Hayden GE, Wrenn KW. Chest radiograph vs. computed tomography scan in the evaluation for pneumonia. J Emerg Med 2009;36(3):266–70.

29. Nguyen ET, Kanne JP, Hoang LM, et al. Community-acquired methicillin-resistant *Staphylococcus aureus* pneumonia: radiographic and computed tomography findings. J Thorac Imaging 2008;23(1):13–9.
30. Lee I, Kim TS, Yoon HK. *Mycoplasma pneumoniae* pneumonia: CT features in 16 patients. Eur Radiol 2006;16(3):719–25.
31. Okada F, Andy Y, Wakisaka M, et al. *Chlamydia pneumoniae* pneumonia and *Mycoplasma pneumoniae* pneumonia: comparison of clinical findings and CT findings. J Comput Assist Tomogr 2005;29:626–32.
32. Franquet T. Imaging of pulmonary viral pneumonia. Radiology 2011;260(1):18–33.
33. Kim EA, Lee KS, Primack SL, et al. Viral pneumonias in adults: radiologic and pathologic findings. Radiographics 2002;22(Spec No):S137–49.

Nervous System Abnormalities and Legionnaire's Disease

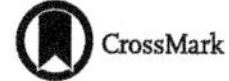

John J. Halperin, MD[a,b,*]

KEYWORDS

- Legionnaire's disease • Nervous system abnormalities • Parainfectious
- Encephalopathy • Critical illness polyneuropathy

KEY POINTS

- Although patients with Legionnaire's disease frequently develop alterations of consciousness, this is no more frequent than in patients hospitalized with other, equally severe forms of bacterial pneumonia.
- Legionella meningitis occurs rarely, if ever.
- Patients with Legionnaire's are susceptible to critical illness polyneuropathy/myopathy, as are other critically ill patients.
- Legionnaire's patients may develop MRI hyperdensities in the splenium of the corpus callosum, as may other patients with severe infections.
- Patients with Legionnaire's may be at increased risk of, and rarely develop, immune-mediated multifocal brain (acute disseminated encephalomyelitis) or peripheral nerve disease (Guillain-Barré syndrome).

In 1977, the American Legion's name became inextricably linked to both the severe respiratory infection, Legionnaire's disease (LD), and the responsible pathogen, *Legionella pneumophila*. The initial report provided a brief description of the clinical syndrome.[1] Patients' "earliest symptoms (included) malaise, muscle aches and a slight headache"; patients then developed high fever and respiratory symptoms. The description continued to add that "one fifth of the patients became obtunded." Subsequent reports attributed changes to nervous system involvement in up to 50% or more of patients with Legionnaire's.[2,3] Today, however, the Centers for Disease Control and Prevention does not even consider nervous system involvement

[a] Sidney Kimmel Medical College of Thomas Jefferson University, 99 Beauvoir Avenue, Summit, NJ 07902, USA; [b] Department of Neurosciences, Overlook Medical Center, 99 Beauvoir Avenue, Summit, NJ 07902, USA
* Sidney Kimmel Medical College of Thomas Jefferson University, 99 Beauvoir Avenue, Summit, NJ 07902.
E-mail address: John.halperin@atlantichealth.org

Infect Dis Clin N Am 31 (2017) 55–68
http://dx.doi.org/10.1016/j.idc.2016.10.005
id.theclinics.com
0891-5520/17/

sufficiently notable to track it separately.[4] This evolution is strikingly illustrative—not just of the maturing understanding of LD, aided by improving laboratory techniques for diagnosing it, but also about the pitfalls of anchoring biases, framing errors, and perhaps most importantly, widespread misunderstanding about what does and does not constitute neurologic disease.

BACKGROUND

Nervous System Infections

Context is critical in considering early thinking about nervous system involvement in Legionnaire's. In patients with the most common bacterial pneumonia, that due to *Streptococcus pneumoniae*, altered mental status commonly reflects the presence of pneumococcal meningitis, a potentially fatal complication. Hence, it was certainly reasonable for clinicians first confronting this novel bacterial pneumonia to have a high level of concern about possible central nervous system (CNS) infection in individuals with altered mental status. Second, definitive diagnosis at the time relied on early serologic tests using an immunofluorescence assay (IFA), with limited data on test cross-reactivity, specificity, and sensitivity. Organism-based testing was several years off in the future. Third, in the late 1970s, neuroimaging was primitive: CT scanning was in its infancy; clinical MRI had not yet been introduced. Physicians investigating outbreaks used the best tools they had available to study a novel disease with high mortality. Now, with years of accumulated data, there is more clarity, although there are still some intriguing and yet to be answered questions.

Understanding this changing perspective requires, first, appreciating what does and does not constitute neurologic disease, and second, differentiating between causality and association. Earliest series, in which neurologic abnormalities were described frequently, emphasized 2 conditions: altered consciousness including delirium, visual hallucinations and stupor, and cerebellar ataxia.[5–7] Nevertheless, just a few years later, a large series of 65 patients, in which the authors combined their observations with 332 published cases,[8] concluded that the most common neurologic abnormalities were confusion, disorientation, and lethargy, and only rarely cerebellar ataxia, hallucinations, or focal neurologic findings, and, in 1 patient, generalized seizures. Occasional small series described a variety of rare disorders: postinfectious myelopathy, an axonal peripheral neuropathy, and then, with the advent of MRI, rare events including areas of abnormal signal in the splenium of the corpus callosum.

Using this framework, it is convenient to divide the disorders of nervous system function attributed to Legionnaire's into 2 broad groups—those described in many patients, and almost certainly not attributable to nervous system infection, and those that are rare, in which causality is suggested but not proven. Pathophysiologically, if there is a causal relationship, for the latter, it is probably immunologic rather than directly infectious.

OBSERVED NEUROLOGIC ABNORMALITIES

Altered Consciousness, Hallucinations

On any general inpatient neurology consultation service, alterations of consciousness are probably the most common reason for consultations. Patients with systemic illness: sepsis, high fever, hyponatremia, hypoglycemia, to name just a few, frequently develop what is variably referred to as a delirium or encephalopathy, an acute confusional state, often accompanied by an altered level of consciousness, up to and including coma. Although patients may develop transient focal neurologic signs, clinical findings suggestive of localized damage to the CNS, these are rarely constant over time. It may at first seem paradoxic that such a state, reflecting global dysfunction of the nervous system, is rarely caused by neurologic disease. However, this relates to a fundamental premise of clinical neurology: that neurologic disorders involve structural damage to the nervous system. The degree of nervous system damage required to cause such global nervous system dysfunction is almost always accompanied by persistent and focal findings, reflected in abnormal and localizing brainstem or cortical dysfunction. In the absence of any such localizing clinical findings, it is highly unlikely that such an encephalopathy is due to nervous system damage. Rather, these global disorders of consciousness are likely related to the effect of cytokines or other systemic factors impairing nervous system function, typically without causing irreversible damage to the affected structures.

Infectious meningitis occupies an intermediate position in the spectrum of nervous system–involving disorders. Inflammation of the meninges, in and of itself, causes severe headaches, often accompanied by systemic symptoms of infection. However, as exemplified by viral meningitis, unless the brain parenchyma becomes involved (which by definition is an encephalitis or meningoencephalitis, not meningitis), there is typically minimal effect on consciousness or other neurologic function. Bacterial meningitis can be quite different, in large part because the inflammation can damage brain blood vessels (as well as the cranial nerves) and invade the surrounding brain, causing substantial parenchymal CNS swelling and damage.

In this context, the fact that 20% of patients in the initial series became obtunded (**Table 1**) certainly made it reasonable to suspect that this organism, like *S pneumoniae*, directly invaded the CNS. However, as patients were systematically evaluated, cerebrospinal fluid (CSF) was virtually universally normal, and recovery from the acute illness rarely left residual CNS dysfunction, essentially excluding a bacterial meningeal infection. Moreover, when advanced imaging became available, the brain usually looked normal. Then, in 1982, a prospective study of 142 patients with pneumonia,[9] in whom serologic testing suggested Legionnaire's in 32, found that abnormalities of neurobehavioral function were no more common in patients with Legionnaire's than in those with pneumonia of other causes, occurring in 50% to 55% of both groups. The following year, a systematic study of autopsied brains from 40 patients with Legionnaire's,[10] 37 of whom had mental status changes and 16 that were thought to be CNS signs, found no evidence of related brain infection or damage in any. Then, a 1991 prospective study of 55 patients with nosocomial pneumonia[11] found no meaningful clinical differences between the 27 with Legionnaire's and the remainder, attributed to other pathogens. Perhaps most informative was a patient diagnosed based on urine antigen testing and positive culture from bronchoalveolar lavage, who presented with fever and mental status changes.[12] CSF demonstrated a mild pleocytosis, elevated protein, and increased immunoglobulin G (IgG) index, but negative CSF Legionella culture and polymerase chain reaction–based testing (PCR), leading the investigators to postulate an immune mechanism.

Given the high prevalence of altered consciousness in the Legionnaire's patients, the virtually universally negative CSF in affected LD patients, the absence of any findings on neuropathologic examination, and the typically normal neurologic recovery of these patients, it seems fair to conclude that altered consciousness is not caused by brain infection with Legionella. Similarly, the finding that altered cognition is no more common than in patients with bacterial pneumonia of other causes argues strongly that this is not attributable to some unique mechanism related to this bacterium, such as an exotoxin, as was suggested in the early literature.

Table 1
Patients with delirium, cerebellar ataxia

Author	Cases	Diagnosed by	# Cerebellar	Altered Mental Status	Imaging	CSF	Confounders
Fraser et al,[1] 1977	182	IFA	Not stated	20%	—	—	—
Terranova et al,[7] 1977	11	IFA	1	1	—	1 Normal	Minimal information
Friedman,[5] 1978	5	IFA	4	Visual hallucinations	1 Normal brain scan	1/4 increased protein	At least 2 probably Wernicke
Gregory et al,[14] 1979	7	IFA	1	4; visual hallucinations in 3; $^1/_4$ also unsteady gait	Normal brain scan	Normal	ETOH denied
Kirby et al,[8] 1980	65 & lit review 332	IFA	Rare	Most common; rare visual hallucinations	—	Normal	ETOH as risk factor for LD
Shetty et al,[15] 1980	1	IFA	1	—	CT -	Normal	"10 ounces wine per day"
Baker et al,[16] 1981	1	IFA	1	Bipolar	CT -	Normal	High-dose neuroleptic, high fever; ?NLM
Bone et al,[18] 1981	27	—	"50%"	—	—	—	Minimal information
Kennedy et al,[17] 1981	16		8/16	14/16			
Harris,[30] 1981	1	IFA 4× to 1:128	—	Delirium	—	Protein 101: WBC 160 (90% M)	Low IFA; ?spurious
Yu et al,[9] 1982	32	IFA 4 1:128 or increased	—	Same as other pneumonias	—	—	Prospective, all in-patient pneumonia

Pendlebury et al,[10] 1983	40	IFA, pathology	—	37	CT -Nuclear med-	Normal × 1 protein 66	Autopsy: alternate explanations in 5; no pathologic evidence of LD in brain
Johnson et al,[2] 1984	21	IFA	—	9	CT, nuc -	2/9 pleocytosis; 1 w/ protein 72	—
Johnson, Lit review	912	IFA	3.6%	29.6%	CT, nuc -	21/78 pleocytosis	—
Granados et al,[39] 1989	32	IFA, culture	—	14%	ND	ND	Prospective vs 37 *S pneumoniae*; no difference in neurologic findings
Roig et al,[11] 1991	27	IFA, culture	0	0	—	—	Prospective vs 28 other bacterial nosocomial pneumonia; no difference
Hasegawa et al,[12] 2013	1	Ur Ag, culture	—	1	—	Mild pleocytosis, increased protein	Meningeal signs, confusion; antibiotic responsive. Postulated immune mechanism as CSF culture/PCR -

Abbreviations: Ag, antigen-based test; CT-, brain computerized tomography scan normal; ETOH, ethyl alcohol; ND, not done; NLM, neuroleptic malignant syndrome; nuc-, nuclear medicine brain scan normal.

Cerebellar Ataxia, Brainstem Abnormalities

The other alteration of neurologic function emphasized in the early literature[5] was cerebellar dysfunction (see **Table 1**). Of a series of 5 non-Legionnaires with sporadic LD, all diagnosed based on having pneumonia and a positive IFA serology, all were thought to have some form of neurologic involvement. Four had cerebellar signs: 1 of these also had visual hallucinations and peripheral neuropathy. At least 2 of these 4 provided histories of heavy alcohol intake; an additional one admitted to "1 pint of beer daily," and the other denied alcohol consumption. The provided clinical descriptions actually sound quite typical of Wernicke encephalopathy, which, given the subsequent description of a strong association between LD and excessive alcohol intake,[8] may provide a better explanation. The fifth patient in this initial series presented with an acute thoracic transverse myelitis, with severe persisting but improved myelopathy after treatment. Given the unavailability of advanced imaging at the time, the fact that this was the only patient of the 5 with a significant CSF pleocytosis, that he had a cough but apparently not pneumonia, that diagnosis was based on a serum IFA of 256, and that there have been few[13] additional similar cases described, it is entirely possible this patient's illness was not directly caused by Legionnaire's.

For comparison, another series,[7] also published in 1978, described 30 patients with pneumonia and serologic evidence of Legionnaire's, who attended a convention of the Independent Order of Odd Fellows at the same Philadelphia hotel as the Legionnaire's, but in 1974, 2 years earlier. Of these 30, 1 became obtunded but had normal CSF, and 1 developed persistent ataxia, but no other information was provided. No others had evidence of neurologic compromise. In a report of a pair of patients with pneumonia and IFA-based diagnosis,[6] 1 became comatose and developed a left extensor plantar; CSF showed "only a slight leukocytosis." Brain CT was unrevealing, and IFA increased from 64 to 256. The patient recovered but was left with aphasia and ataxia. The other patient, who also presented with pneumonia and coma, had an IFA that increased from 64 to 1028 and was similarly left with expressive language difficulty; however, that patient presented in atrial fibrillation. No imaging was available to determine the cause of the neurologic residua, but it seems likely this was due to a thromboembolic stroke related to the atrial fibrillation. In another series of 7 cases,[14] 4 had CNS changes but normal CSF. All had altered mental status; 3 had visual hallucinations and 1 had a seizure. Nevertheless, another case report[15] described a patient with pneumonia, positive serology, cerebellar signs, and normal CSF. Not unlike most other such cases, the patient admitted to significant alcohol consumption, in her case "10 ounces of wine per day." An additional case report[16] described a psychiatric patient with pneumonia, high fever, on high-dose haloperidol, who developed ataxia and brainstem dysfunction, with normal CSF, quite possibly as a consequence of hyperthermia due either to his pneumonia or to neuroleptic malignant syndrome. Finally, a 1981[17] report described 16 patients, in whom diagnosis was again based on serology. Seven were evaluated by a neurologist; the remainder were reviewed retrospectively. Fourteen had a confusional state; 8 had hallucinations, and 8 had ataxia as well as a variety of other CNS signs. In a subsequent letter to the editor,[18] the same group of authors expanded their series to 27 and reported that half developed confusion, cerebellar ataxia (in 1 this persisted for at least 5 years). No CSF or imaging findings were provided. In neither paper did the authors comment on alcohol consumption.

In sum, although cerebellar abnormalities were described frequently in early reports of patients with LD, this is now described rarely if ever; a causal relation seems unlikely. In light of the consistently negative CSF in affected patients, the negative autopsy data cited above,[10] and the fact that these clinical findings were often self-limited, an early hypothesis was that this might be due to a toxin produced by the bacterium. It seems that in many patients, there were other, more plausible explanations for the cerebellar findings (eg, Wernickes from alcohol; hyperthermia).

Given the studies comparing Legionnaire's to other pneumonias, it would appear that there is no large-scale increase in the frequency of neurologic changes in this pneumonia compared with others; in particular, Legionnaire's-related meningitis seems strikingly infrequent. However, it is entirely possible that there are infrequently occurring forms of associated nervous system involvement, notwithstanding the rarity of such reports in the modern imaging era. These less frequent associations form the focus of the remainder of this discussion.

Peripheral Nervous System Abnormalities

Infectious diseases can cause peripheral nervous system (PNS) disease (**Table 2**) by at least 3 different mechanisms: direct microorganism invasion of nerves, immune-mediated damage to myelin or axons, and what has been termed critical illness polyneuropathy.[19–21] Leprosy directly invades the peripheral nerve. Spirochetal infections can attack nerve roots (syphilis) or possibly dorsal root ganglia (Lyme); there is little evidence this mechanism plays a role in other infections, with none suggesting this occurs in LD.

Some infections (best understood with Campylobacter[22]), by virtue of presumptive antigenic cross-reactivity between bacterial and peripheral nerve antigens, cause an immune-mediated acute, typically reversible, polyneuropathy: Guillain-Barré syndrome, also known as acute inflammatory demyelinating polyneuropathy (AIDP). A 1981 case report[23] from England described a patient who, at the time of admission for an acute pneumonia (subsequently attributed to Legionnaire's based on a 4-fold increase in IFA titer), presented with diffuse hyporeflexia and extensor plantars; by day 5, he developed bulbar and subsequently severe limb weakness, all of which resolved over 2 months. CSF was initially normal; on repeat, it was acellular, but protein was at the upper limit of normal. Median motor conduction velocity was in the demyelinating range, but there was no description of conduction block or other findings typical of AIDP. The onset of this neuropathy early in the course of the presumed precipitating infection, the normal CSF protein, and the neurophysiologic findings would all be highly unusual for Guillain-Barré. A second report described a 13-year-old Turkish child[24] with weakness associated with respiratory failure with Legionnaire's. In this case, nerve conduction studies demonstrated both slowing consistent with demyelination and conduction block. Of 3 other case reports, 1 patient from Turkey[13] had both transverse myelitis and an axonal neuropathy, and 1 from the United States showed conduction block but also changes of an axonal neuropathy.[25] One from Italy, with diabetes and markedly elevated creatine kinase (CK), had mixed demyelinating and axonal changes.[26] Although several of these patients had rather atypical features, the close temporal relationship between syndrome onset and apparent Legionnaire's does suggest a causal relationship. However, the fact that there is just 1 US case report, in the face of a current estimated annual incidence of approximately 1/100,000 in the United States[4] (or 3000 cases/yr) suggests this is a quite rare event that might have occurred by chance.

Perhaps of greater relevance is the fact that severe infections can be associated with critical illness polyneuropathy and myopathy,[19,20,27] a disorder thought to be related to cytokine changes occurring in sepsis. This variably severe axonal neuropathy can cause profound weakness in intensive care unit (ICU) patients, particularly those with sepsis and multiorgan compromise, and probably occurs more

Table 2
Patients with peripheral nervous system disorders

Author	Cases	Diagnosed by	No. of PNS	EMG	CSF	Detail
Kennedy et al,[17] 1981	15	IFA	5	Axonal	—	Subclinical in 4; persisting motor neuropathy in 1
Morgan et al,[23] 1981	1	IFA	1	Mixed; demyelinating features	Protein 40 mg% early; 60 f/u	Areflexic but Babinski; bulbar × week 1–2; left w/ distal weakness, facial diplegia; weakness resolved but areflexic
Ellie et al,[28] 1949	1	(in French)	—	—	—	Severe persistent polyneuropathy
Madsen et al,[29] 1998	1	(in Danish)	—	—	—	Severe persistent polyneuropathy in both legs
Akyildiz et al,[24] 2008	1	Serology; Ag in bronchoalveolar lavage; serology	1	Demyelinating	No cells; protein 181 mg%	Bulbar, then BLE weakness; responded to IVIg
Canpolat et al,[13] 2013	1	LD Ag, lung	1	Axonal	No cells, protein 112 mg%	Acute motor/sensory neuropathy + Transverse myelitis
Lui et al,[25] 2014	1	Urine Ag	1	Mixed axonal & demyelinating	ND	71 y, primarily GI disease. confused
Vigneri et al,[26] 2014	1	Urine Ag	1	Mixed axonal & demyelinating; motor > sensory	No cells, protein 54	DM; CK >2000. Respiratory failure; modest response to pheresis

Abbreviations: BLE, bilateral lower extremities; DM, diabetes mellitus; f/u, follow-up; GI, gastrointestinal; IVIg, intravenous immunoglobulin.

frequently than is generally understood, both in ICU patients in general and in Legionnaire's patients in particular.[28,29] Such a process is suggested by the frequently elevated CK described in LD,[26] including in 1 of the cases described above. In such patients, particularly those in whom the electrophysiologic evidence of acquired demyelination is ambiguous, critical illness polyneuropathy/myopathy might be a better fit. Interestingly, having identified a single patient with severe persistent motor neuropathy following LD, that may well have been attributable to this disorder,[17,18] LD patients at 1 center underwent neurophysiologic testing, which identified an acute but subclinical axonal polyneuropathy in 5, reversible in 4. Whether this represents a milder "forme frusta" of a critical illness polyneuropathy remains to be determined.

Focal Central Nervous Changes

Several case reports have described patients with Legionnaire's and focal CNS changes (**Table 3**). As already mentioned, at least 2 patients have developed transverse myelitis.[5,13] The first, reported before MRI, had a neutrophil-predominant CSF pleocytosis (910 white blood cells [WBC]/mm^3) and normal myelogram. In the second, CSF was acellular with modestly elevated protein (112 mg%); brain MRI was normal, whereas spine demonstrated a slightly enhancing area of abnormal signal at C6. In both instances, both the mechanism and the potential causal relationship to Legionnaire's are unclear. Although it is tempting to consider them instances of parainfectious acute demyelinating encephalomyelitis (ADEM), the noninflammatory CSF in the second would be quite atypical for this immune-mediated disorder. Whether the first was a patient with multiple sclerosis and a first event, perhaps precipitated by a significant infection, cannot be ascertained. However, the observation that both occurred in close temporal relationship to LD at least raises the possibility of a causal relationship, regardless of pathophysiologic mechanism.

Several additional reports have suggested an association between ADEM and Legionnaire's—in most, the LD diagnosis has similarly been made based on evolving serologies—an approach that may be problematic in patients with active systemic inflammatory states of other causes, which can trigger increases in production of a broad array of antibodies, causing deceptively positive-appearing serologic results.

The early case cited above,[6] of a woman who seroconverted and developed persisting but improving aphasia and a transient left Babinski sign, with a mild CSF lymphocytic pleocytosis, might have had LD-related CNS disease. A 1981 case report[30] described a febrile 26-year-old man with delirium, a mononuclear-predominant CSF pleocytosis (160 WBC/mm^3), protein 101 mg%, and, like all other reported cases, normal CSF glucose. He subsequently developed pulmonary infiltrates and right arm paralysis. He was diagnosed with ADEM and recovered completely after antimicrobial therapy. In the series reported by Van Arsdall and colleagues,[31] 5 of 12 patients diagnosed serologically were thought to have CNS involvement. In 1, nuclear medicine brain scan demonstrated multifocal brain defects; CSF had 5 WBC/mm^3. At autopsy, this patient was thought to have necrotizing hemorrhagic leukoencephalitis, a variant of ADEM. Two others in this series had 20 and 28 WBC/mm^3, respectively. One developed status epilepticus. Other than the 1 autopsied patient, apparently outcome was favorable. A separate report described 3 patients, who recovered completely, who presented with apparent encephalitis[32] and positive LD serologies. One patient[33] diagnosed with ADEM based on widespread nonenhancing white matter changes on brain MRI, mildly inflammatory CSF (19 WBC/mm^3) and protein 70 mg% was diagnosed with Legionnaire's based on a 4-fold decrease in IFA; he recovered after corticosteroid treatment. Surprisingly few cases have been described in the past few

Table 3
Patients with focal central nervous system abnormalities

Author	Cases	Diagnosed by	Imaging	CSF	Details
Friedman,[5] 1978	1	IFA	Myelogram -	910 WBC, 96% n	T5 transverse myelitis; persistent paraplegia
Lees & Tyrrell,[6] 1978	2	IFA	CT -	"Slight increase lymphs"	Multifocal, residual aphasia, ataxia
	—	IFA	—	—	Focal; residual aphasia, hemisensory; new onset atrial fibrillation
Harris,[30] 1981	—	IFA 128	ND	WBC 160, 90% m; protein 101	Delirium + myelitis
Bamford & Hakin,[40] 1982	1	IFA 256 1 y later	Nuclear scan -	nl	Ataxic, dysarthric, Babinski; residual chorea, dysphonia, persisted; 2 y later PD but subsequently resolved
van Arsdall et al,[31] 1983; Johnson et al,[2] 1984	1	IFA	Nuclear scan+	nl	Autopsy: necrotizing hemorrhagic leukoencephalitis; direct fluorescence of brain negative
	1	IFA	ND	nl	Status epilepticus
Andersen & Sogaard,[41] 1987	1	IFA neg>512 wk 2	CT: 1 ring enhancing	23 WBC, 602 RBC, protein 70, nl glucose	Seizure as 1st symptom; developed aphasia, R hemiparesis; over months symptoms resolved except memory difficulty
Potasman et al,[32] 1990	3	IFA	n/a	n/a	"Viral encephalitis-like picture"
Sommer et al,[33] 2000	1	IFA 256	MRI extensive Gd-, WM disease	19 L, protein 70; no OCB	3 wk p treated pneumonia; brainstem signs; CT, SPECT neg; better p steroids w/ CSF nl, IFA 64; ADEM

Morgan et al,[34] 2004	1	Sputum + DFA; + urine Ag	MRI + SCC; DWI+; Gd- resolved 13 d later	nl	Transient splenium corpus callosum; presented dysarthric, dysmetric, difficult standing; declining mental status
de Lau et al,[42] 2010	2	Adm 1024; 1, 2, & 3 wk later all 265	MRI multifocal WM, Gd+	7 WBC; else nl	1 mo p pneumonia; behavioral change, unsteady gait; apractic, chorea; afebrile; recovered w/o steroids; dx ADEM
Hasegawa et al,[12] 2013	—	LD Urine Ag+	MRI: ext WM, Gd-; including CC	no WBC; protein mildly increased IgG index 0.7	3 wk p admission, seizures; multifocal, decreased LOC; treated steroids pheresis; gradual recovery; ADEM
Robbins et al,[35] 2012	—	LD Urine Ag+	MRI SCC DWI, Gd-	nl	HIV, <20 viral load; headache, delirium; SCC; better w/ antibiotics
Kilic et al,[36] 2013	—	LD Urine Ag+	MRI SCC, +DWI FLAIR	ND	SCC, coma
Canpolat et al,[13] 2013	1	LD Ag, lung	MRI T2 at C6; Gd+	No cells; protein 112	Also axonal polyneuropathy; response to steroids, IVIg
Tomizawa et al,[37] 2015	1	Seroconvert	MRI T2, DWI	No cells, protein 22, nl IgG index	Reversible, splenium of corpus callosum

Abbreviations: Adm, on admission; CC, corpus callosum; DFA, direct fluorescent antibody; DWI, diffusion-weighted image; FLAIR, fluid-attenuated inversion recovery; Gd + or –, enhancing or not with gadolinium; HIV, human immunodeficiency virus; LOC, level of consciousness; n/a, not available; nl, normal; OCB, oligoclonal bands; RBC, red blood cells; SPECT, single-photon emission computed tomography; in differential n, neutrophils; m, monocytes; SCC, splenium of the corpus callosum; w/, with; w/o, without; WM, white matter.

decades when one would expect the increasing incidence (or recognition) of Legionnaire's, and widespread availability of improved diagnostic testing and MRI to have increased the frequency of this diagnosis.

Finally, 4 patients have been reported with reversible MRI abnormalities limited to the splenium of the corpus callosum.[34–37] This finding, reported in several other infectious and noninfectious disorders,[38] is of unclear cause but possibly cytokine mediated or pathophysiologically related to posterior reversible encephalopathy syndrome, is typically self-limited and ultimately benign.

SUMMARY

It appears, with the benefit of 4 decades of experience, that the abnormalities of nervous system function observed in patients with Legionnaire's are largely similar to those seen in patients with other infectious diseases of comparable severity. Altered consciousness, up to and including hallucinations and coma, occurs frequently but is not typically related to CNS infection; in fact, reports of inflammatory CSF are quite rare in LD. Rather, this appears to be the same "toxic metabolic encephalopathy" seen in myriad other patients with severe pneumonia and/or sepsis. The cerebellar abnormalities emphasized in early series are now described rarely and may well have been an artifact of a rather high prevalence of excessive alcohol intake in early populations. Somewhat underemphasized, there probably is a significant incidence of peripheral nerve involvement, primarily due to critical illness polyneuropathy, a disorder occurring quite frequently in patients with severe infections and sepsis.

On the other hand, there are scattered case reports of patients who appear to develop noninfectious, inflammatory peripheral or CNS disorders: Guillain-Barré–like neuropathies, focal inflammation of the spinal cord or brain, the latter perhaps contributing to seizures on rare occasions. In most cases, the temporal association between Legionnaire's and the neurologic disorder is suggestive of a causal link. However, in most of these cases, Legionnaire's was diagnosed simply on the basis of low titer antibody in serum, a test that can be deceptive in inflammatory states of many causes. With these disorders occurring so rarely, a pathophysiologic link must be considered possible but definitely not proven.

Finally, the peculiar MRI disorder in which transient abnormalities appear, and then disappear, in the splenium of the corpus callosum, may well be linked to Legionnaire's as it is to numerous other infections. All of these associations, as well as their pathophysiologic mechanisms, await further clarification.

REFERENCES

1. Fraser DW, Tsai TR, Orenstein W, et al. Legionnaire's disease: description of an epidemic of pneumonia. N Engl J Med 1977;297:1189–97.
2. Johnson JD, Raff MJ, Van Arsdall JA. Neurologic manifestations of Legionnaire's disease. Medicine (Baltimore) 1984;63:303–10.
3. Cunha BA, Burillo A, Bouza E. Legionnaire's disease. Lancet 2016;387:376–85.
4. Dooling KL, Toews KA, Hicks LA, et al. Active bacterial core surveillance for Legionellosis—United States, 2011-2013. MMWR Morb Mortal Wkly Rep 2015;64:1190–3.
5. Friedman HM. Legionnaire's disease in non-Legionnaires. A report of five cases. Ann Intern Med 1978;88:294–302.
6. Lees AW, Tyrrell WF. Severe cerebral disturbance in legionnaire's disease. Lancet 1978;2:1336–7.

7. Terranova W, Cohen ML, Fraser DW. 1974 outbreak of Legionnaire's disease diagnosed in 1977. Clinical and epidemiological features. Lancet 1978;2:122–4.
8. Kirby BD, Snyder KM, Meyer RD, et al. Legionnaire's disease: report of sixty-five nosocomially acquired cases of review of the literature. Medicine (Baltimore) 1980;59:188–205.
9. Yu VL, Kroboth FJ, Shonnard J, et al. Legionnaire's disease: new clinical perspective from a prospective pneumonia study. Am J Med 1982;73:357–61.
10. Pendlebury WW, Perl DP, Winn WC Jr, et al. Neuropathologic evaluation of 40 confirmed cases of Legionella pneumonia. Neurology 1983;33:1340–4.
11. Roig J, Aguilar X, Ruiz J, et al. Comparative study of Legionella pneumophila and other nosocomial-acquired pneumonias. Chest 1991;99:344–50.
12. Hasegawa J, Horikawa T, Endo K. [A case of Legionnaire's infection with meningeal irritation and abnormal cerebrospinal fluid]. Rinsho Shinkeigaku 2013;53: 526–30.
13. Canpolat M, Kumandas S, Yikilmaz A, et al. Transverse myelitis and acute motor sensory axonal neuropathy due to Legionella pneumophila: a case report. Pediatr Int 2013;55:778–82.
14. Gregory DW, Schaffner W, Alford RH, et al. Sporadic cases of Legionnaire's disease: the expanding clinical spectrum. Ann Intern Med 1979;90:518–21.
15. Shetty KR, Cilyo CL, Starr BD, et al. Legionnaire's disease with profound cerebellar involvement. Arch Neurol 1980;37:379–80.
16. Baker PC, Price TR, Allen CD. Brain stem and cerebellar dysfunction with Legionnaire's disease. J Neurol Neurosurg Psychiatry 1981;44:1054–6.
17. Kennedy DH, Bone I, Weir AI. Early diagnosis of Legionnaire's disease: distinctive neurological findings. Lancet 1981;1:940–1.
18. Bone I, Weir AI, Kennedy D. Pronounced cerebellar features in legionnaire's disease. Br Med J (Clin Res Ed) 1981;283:730.
19. Guarneri B, Bertolini G, Latronico N. Long-term outcome in patients with critical illness myopathy or neuropathy: the Italian multicentre CRIMYNE study. J Neurol Neurosurg Psychiatry 2008;79:838–41.
20. Khan J, Harrison TB, Rich MM, et al. Early development of critical illness myopathy and neuropathy in patients with severe sepsis. Neurology 2006;67:1421–5.
21. Latronico N, Bolton CF. Critical illness polyneuropathy and myopathy: a major cause of muscle weakness and paralysis. Lancet Neurol 2011;10:931–41.
22. Nachamkin I, Ung H, Moran AP, et al. Ganglioside GM1 mimicry in Campylobacter strains from sporadic infections in the United States. J Infect Dis 1999; 179:1183–9.
23. Morgan DJ, Gawler J. Severe peripheral neuropathy complicating legionnaire's disease. Br Med J (Clin Res Ed) 1981;283:1577–8.
24. Akyildiz B, Gumus H, Kumandas S, et al. Guillain-Barre syndrome associated with Legionnella infection. J Trop Pediatr 2008;54:275–7.
25. Lui JK, Touray S, Tosches WA, et al. Acute inflammatory demyelinating polyradiculopathy in Legionella pneumonia. Muscle Nerve 2014;50:868–9.
26. Vigneri S, Spadaro S, Farinelli I, et al. Acute respiratory failure onset in a patient with Guillain-Barre syndrome after Legionella-associated pneumonia: a case report. J Clin Neuromuscul Dis 2014;16:74–8.
27. Hermans G, De Jonghe B, Bruyninckx F, et al. Interventions for preventing critical illness polyneuropathy and critical illness myopathy. Cochrane Database Syst Rev 2014;(1):CD006832.
28. Ellie E, Wiart L, Vital A, et al. Severe polyneuropathy in Legionnaire's disease. Presse Med 1991;20:1949 [in French].

29. Madsen KH. Peripheral polyneuropathy in legionellosis. Ugeskr Laeger 1998; 160:288–9 [in Danish].
30. Harris LF. Legionnaire's disease associated with acute encephalomyelitis. Arch Neurol 1981;38:462–3.
31. Van Arsdall JA 2nd, Wunderlich HF, Melo JC, et al. The protean manifestations of Legionnaire's disease. J Infect 1983;7:51–62.
32. Potasman I, Liberson A, Schwartz M, et al. [Encephalitis without pneumonia caused by Legionella bozemanii]. Harefuah 1990;118:198–201 [in Hebrew].
33. Sommer JB, Erbguth FJ, Neundorfer B. Acute disseminated encephalomyelitis following Legionella pneumophila infection. Eur Neurol 2000;44:182–4.
34. Morgan JC, Cavaliere R, Juel VC. Reversible corpus callosum lesion in legionnaire's disease. J Neurol Neurosurg Psychiatry 2004;75:651–4.
35. Robbins NM, Kumar A, Blair BM. Legionella pneumophila infection presenting as headache, confusion and dysarthria in a human immunodeficiency virus-1 (HIV-1) positive patient: case report. BMC Infect Dis 2012;12:225.
36. Kilic EC, Aksoy S, Sahin AR, et al. The presentation of a transient hyperintense lesion with Legionnaires disease in a patient–is it a coincidence or an incidental finding? Ideggyogy Sz 2013;66:63–6.
37. Tomizawa Y, Hoshino Y, Sasaki F, et al. Diagnostic utility of splenial lesions in a case of Legionnaire's disease due to Legionella pneumophila serogroup 2. Intern Med 2015;54:3079–82.
38. Zhang S, Ma Y, Feng J. Clinicoradiological spectrum of reversible splenial lesion syndrome (RESLES) in adults: a retrospective study of a rare entity. Medicine (Baltimore) 2015;94:e512.
39. Granados A, Podzamczer D, Gudiol F, et al. Pneumonia due to Legionella pneumophila and pneumococcal pneumonia: similarities and differences on presentation. Eur Respir J 1989;2:130–4.
40. Bamford JM, Hakin RN. Chorea after Legionnaire's disease. Br Med J (Clin Res Ed) 1982;284:1232–3.
41. Andersen BB, Sogaard I. Legionnaire's disease and brain abscess. Neurology 1987;37:333–4.
42. de Lau LM, Siepman DA, Remmers MJ, et al. Acute disseminating encephalomyelitis following legionnaires disease. Arch Neurol 2010;67:623–6.

Legionnaire's Disease

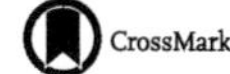

Cardiac Manifestations

John L. Brusch, BS, MD[a,b,c,d,*]

KEYWORDS

• Legionnaire's • Legionella • Endocarditis • Cardiac infections

KEY POINTS

- Most cardiac infections with *Legionella* are secondary to bacteremias arising from a pulmonary focus. Other possible sites of origin are infected sternotomy wounds or equipment such as transesophageal echocardiography probes contaminated by *Legionella* spp.
- Legionella endocarditis is truly a "stealth" infection, with almost no hallmarks of bacterial endocarditis. Echocardiography fails to detect any vegetations in most cases. There are no classic peripheral stigmata of endocarditis. Fever if present is quite low-grade. Standard blood cultures are negative.
- The key step in making the diagnosis of *Legionella* endocarditis is for the physician be aware of the clinical causes of culture-negative infective endocarditis (CNIE) and to include in *Legionella* cardiac involvement in this differential. It is the onset of congestive heart failure that his the usual stimulus to look for unusual causes of valvular infection. The most common infectious causes of CNIE in this country are *Bartonella* and the organism of Whipple disease.
- The most frequent profile of *Legionella* valvular infection is an individual with prosthetic valve in place that was implanted in an institution in which there have been outbreaks of Legionnaire's disease. Many times these individuals will have postoperative pneumonia.
- The initial diagnostic approach should be urinary antigen testing for *Legionella*. This is the most available test with the caveat that it will consistently detect only *Legionella* pneumobilia type I. Blood endocarditis cultures should then be redrawn and subcultured on special media. Many times the issue of endocarditis arises only on examination of resected valvular material.

OVERVIEW

Legionella organisms currently are considered to cause fewer than 1% of all types of bacterial cardiac infections. The incidence of *Legionella* endocarditis, myocarditis, and pericarditis may be underestimated simply because they are not thought of as

[a] Medical Department, Cambridge Health Alliance, 1493 Cambridge Street, Cambridge, MA 02139, USA; [b] Division of Infectious Diseases, Cambridge Health Alliance, 1493 Cambridge Street, Cambridge, MA 02139, USA; [c] Ambulatory Medicine, Cambridge Health Alliance, 1493 Cambridge Street, Cambridge, MA 02139, USA; [d] Medicine, Harvard Medical School, 25 Shattuck Street, Boston, MA 02155, USA

* Cambridge Hospital, Primary Care Center, 1493 Cambridge Street, Cambridge, MA 02139.
E-mail address: jbrusch@challiance.org

Infect Dis Clin N Am 31 (2017) 69–80
http://dx.doi.org/10.1016/j.idc.2016.10.006 id.theclinics.com
0891-5520/17/

part of the differential of an extremely ill patient who is not responding to empiric treatment and for whom no definitive diagnosis has been established. Clinicians are often unfamiliar with the various manifestations of extrapulmonary *Legionella* infection and may not be aware of which diagnostic tests should be ordered and when. *Legionella* valvular infection is often stumbled on during the workup for more common causes of culture-negative infective endocarditis (CNIE) or when the patient fails to respond to appropriate therapy of *Legionella* pneumonia.[1] Legionella endocarditis is truly a "stealth" type of valvular infection. It is not recoverable from the usual types of blood cultures. Echocardiographically fails to demonstrate any valvular vegetations. It is without peripheral stigmata of endocarditis. This review is timely because of the recent recognition of the rapid rise of Legionnaire's disease, a primary source of *Legionella* cardiac infection, in the United States. It has increased almost fourfold from 2000 to 2014. The mortality rate is approximately 10%.[2]

THE ORGANISM

Legionellae are quite tiny gram-negative bacteria that are found in a variety of watery sites. Individuals are infected by breathing organisms that have been aerosolized from sites of potable hot water or air conditioning systems. Most cases of cardiac *Legionella* infection are caused by *Legionella pneumophilia*. Other species of *Legionella*, such as *Legionella dumoffii* and *Legionella longbeachae*, have been involved.[3]

L pneumophila serves as a model of the effectiveness of the multiple virulence factors that are possessed by the intracellular pathogens. *L pneumophila* is resistant to chlorination of various water reservoirs. This may be because of their ability to produce biofilms within hot water and air conditioning systems. Biofilm production also promotes their ability infect prosthetic heart valves. Their intracellular status within various protozoans, including amebae, allows them both to multiply and meet their nutritional needs.[4]

The organism's uptake by macrophages is promoted by opsonization with complement C3. Binding to C1 and CR3 receptors enhances its intracellular survival by dampening the macrophage's oxidative burst. After entering the cell, it lives within its phagosomes. This organelle protects it from being killed by vacuolar acidification and by lysosomal enzymes. The organism continues to multiply within an enlarging phagosome but eventually their luxuriant growth ruptures the macrophage. The pathogens then are free to infect the adjacent tissue.[5]

It appears that iron is essential for intracellular and extracellular replication. Low levels of thiamine and thymidine trigger expression of various virulence genes.

Despite being excised by monocytes and polymorphonuclear leukocytes, *Legionella* spp are resistant to being killed by these cells.[6] Some of the important pathogenic properties of *Legionella* spp are displayed in **Table 1**.

CLINICAL *LEGIONELLA* CARDIAC INVOLVEMENT

Legionella spp have been documented to cause valvular infection, pericarditis, and myocarditis, with endocarditis being the most common.[7]

Legionella valvular infection was first described in a 60-year-old woman who had undergone replacement of the mitral and aortic valve with porcine prosthetic valves. Postoperatively, she developed a fever but there was no evidence of pneumonia. She received multiple courses of antibiotics. Seven months later, an echocardiogram was repeated when she developed a new aortic regurgitation murmur. On echocardiography, there was some suggestion of valvular vegetations on the aortic valve. Both valves were removed. *Legionella pneumophilia* serotype was documented by culture

Table 1
Some of the pathogenic properties of *Legionella* species

Property	Results
Production of biofilm	a. Survival in the watery collections of health care facilities despite the presence of usual disinfectants b. Promotes their ability to infect prosthetic material c. Provides a safe haven from the effect of antibiotics
Able to penetrate macrophages	Protection from a variety of host extracellular defenses
Establishment of a replicative phagosome within the macrophage	Allows the pathogen to replicate while being protected from the effect of the macrophages' intracellular endosomal and lysosomal bactericidal actions
Causes death of the macrophage	It uses the macrophage as a vehicle to circulate throughout the body; on its death, the organisms are deposited in various organs

and direct fluorescent antibody staining.[8] No route of infection was determined in this first-described case of cardiac Legionellosis.

Initially, it was speculated that local infection of sternal wounds was the primary cause of *Legionella* prosthetic valve endocarditis (PVE). Intuitively, it would seem most likely that the infection would start during the actual surgery; however, *Legionella* spp are infrequently recovered from the operating room environment. One of the first large series of nosocomial extrapulmonary infections occurred in cardiac surgical patients of the Stanford University Medical Center. There were 7 patients with PVE; 1 of whom also had a sternotomy infection. There were 2 separate strains of *L pneumophilia* serogroup 1 and 1 strain of *L dumoffii*. The same strains were retrieved from the hospital water supply as well as other reservoirs of water, such as nebulizers. Early on, it was documented that the sternal wound could become contaminated during its irrigation with tap water to remove the povidone iodine solution that was applied before surgery. These wounds are characteristically described as being nonpurulent with serosanguineous drainage and delayed healing.[9] The presence of a localized wound infection does not rule out disseminated *Legionella*. Eighty percent of those with such infections had evidence of disseminated *Legionella* on autopsy.[10]

It appears that *Legionella* can infect the heart and other extrapulmonary sites via hematogenous spread that originates in the infected pulmonary tissue. Autopsy studies of *Legionella* pneumonia have documented the presence of this pathogen in the myocardium, bone marrow, intrathoracic lymph nodes, pericardial effusions, kidneys, and prosthetic valves. Interestingly, there did not seem to be any inflammatory response to the embedded *Legionella* in these extrapulmonary sites. The organisms may arise from a primary pneumonia with *Legionella*. There may be an interval of several weeks before the extrapulmonary infection becomes clinically apparent. Ironically, a nosocomial outbreak of *L pneumophila* pneumonia was associated with contaminated transesophageal echocardiography probes.[11]

Although there was no proof of any cases of endocarditis, this outbreak highlighted the ubiquity of the organism throughout the hospital environment. Infections of cardiac prosthetic material also may occur outside of health care institutions.[12] This occurs usually following an attack of *Legionella* pneumonia. The clinical presentation of the valvular infection may be concurrent with the pulmonary infection or delayed by several weeks. The characteristic size of the vegetation in *Legionella* endocarditis, if present at all, is quite small.[13]

Most identified cases of *Legionella* endocarditis result from *L pneumophila* infection of prosthetic valves. Other *Legionella* spp also have been implicated. These include *Legionella micdadei* and *L dumoffii*.[14]

More recently, native valve endocarditis, due to *Legionella* spp has been described.[15,16]

The major risk factors for development of *L pneumophila* respiratory infection are older age (older than 58 years) and male sex (75%). In 55.6% of patients, there is at least one comorbid condition. These include heart disease, diabetes mellitus, and chronic lung disease due to smoking.[17]

It is not clear whether the risk factors for developing the complication of valvular infection are any different from those of *Legionella* pneumonia. Very likely, this is because of the small number of the studies available due to the low degree of recognition of *Legionella* cardiac infections. A distinctive exception is the presence of prosthetic heart valves. Twenty percent of patients are immunosuppressed, especially heart transplant recipients.[18] In addition, the presence of a post cardiotomy syndrome greatly increases the chance of developing *Legionella* valvular infection.

Legionella PVE and native valve endocarditis are characteristically incredibly chronic infections that can extend for 3 to 19 months after surgery. They are characterized by low-grade fever, weight loss, malaise, and fatigue. If undiagnosed, the slowly progressive valvular destruction will lead to congestive failure. Leukocytosis is quite unusual. Thrombocytopenia can occur. The degree of the anemia is associated with the chronicity of the infection. The peripheral stigmata and other complications of acute and subacute endocarditis, such as Osler nodes and Janeway lesions are absent. This is because there does not appear to be any significant degree of septic emboli or immune complex disease. Echocardiograms often are unremarkable. *Legionella* endocarditis has been described as fibrinous without prominent vegetations. **Box 1** presents this lack of clinical clues that make its diagnosis so difficult.[19,20]

DIFFERENTIAL DIAGNOSES

Legionella endocarditis is classified as CNIE. This term describes valvular infections that are diagnosed on the basis of the Duke Criteria, in which at least 3 sets of standard blood cultures have remained negative after 5 to 7 days of incubation and subculturing. The more common causes of CNIE are listed in **Box 2**.

CNIE, due to poor blood culture techniques can be divided into individuals previously given antibiotics and those in whom an insufficient amount of blood was cultured. In the case of the fastidious, intracellular organisms that we are discussing, proper blood culture techniques are aimed at avoiding unnecessary diagnostic delays when 3 sets of properly drawn blood cultures would have retrieved the usual pathogens of endocarditis.

Box 1
Challenges to diagnosing *Legionella* endocarditis

Negative standard blood cultures.

Although infection may be related to *Legionella* pneumonia, manifestation of the valvular infection may be separated by weeks from this event.

Little clinical evidence that valvular infection exists: rare embolic or immune complex manifestations of endocarditis. Often normal echocardiogram. No spiking temperatures.

Effects may mimic those of noninfectious diseases.

Box 2
Causes of culture-negative endocarditis

Prior antibiotic therapy: most common cause in the United States

Difficult to culture organisms

Right-sided endocarditis: weakly pathogenic organism such as *Streptococcal viridans* species that are filtered out in the pulmonary circulation

Infected pacemaker wires and prosthetic valves: probably due to biofilm laid down by coagulase-negative staphylococci

Because the concentration of organisms in the blood in endocarditis is fewer than 100 colony-forming units per milliliter, it is not the number of blood cultures that are obtained, but the volume of blood placed in each bottle. It appears that 10 mL of blood injected into each bottle is the optimum volume. Three sets of such prepared blood cultures will retrieve approximately 99% of the usual pathogens.[21]

The blood cultures should be obtained from a peripheral venipuncture. If at all possible, they should not be collected from central venous catheters because of the risk of contamination.[22]

Antibiotics that are administered before obtaining blood cultures certainly can sterilize those samples. It is the streptococci, especially viridans streptococci, whose growth is most susceptible. *Staphylococcus aureus* and enterococci are markedly less so.[23,24]

State-of-the-art blood culture techniques have reduced the percentage of CNIE cases from 30% to 5%. Infective endocarditis due to members of the HACEK (*Haemophilus*, *Aggregatibacter*, *Cardiobacterium*, *Eikenella*, *Kingella*) group, *Brucella* spp, and *Abiotrophia* spp are no longer classified as CNIE. Current blood culture techniques detect pathogens within 1 week. HACEK organisms usually grow out within 5 days. *Brucella* spp and *Abiotrophia* spp will often require longer than 1 week to retrieve.[25]

Resins or charcoal may be added to the media to neutralize the suppressive effects of antibiotics. There is a wide variation in their effectiveness. They themselves may inhibit bacterial growth as advised "As far as possible," blood cultures should be obtained before initiating antibiotic therapy.

The organisms that cause CNIE have strong associations with specific geographic areas. However, with globalization of infections, the clinician must have a worldwide awareness of those pathogens that have been associated with valvular infections. For example, among 348 cases of CNIE collected in southern France, 48% were attributed to *Coxiella burnetii*, and 28% to *Bartonella* spp. Approximately 1% were caused by a combination of organisms, including *Tropheryma whipplei*, *Legionella pneumophila*, *Abiotrophia* spp, and *Mycoplasma hominis*; 28% of patients had been given antibiotics before culturing of their blood.[1] In the United States, *Bartonella* spp appear to be the most common cause of CNIE.

It is important for the clinician to be aware of the epidemiology of clinical presentations when empirically choosing an initial antibiotic regimen that would need to cover 1 or more of these fastidious intracellular organisms. **Boxes 2** and **3** and **Tables 2–6** present helpful clinical characteristics of the most common causes of true CNIE.

MIMICS OF ENDOCARDITIS

The diseases that most commonly mimic CNIE are forms of vasculitis, marantic endocarditis, and atrial myxomas (**Table 7**).

Box 3
Mimics of culture-negative endocarditis

Marantic endocarditis

Rheumatologic diseases such as lupus

Atrial myxomas

Myocarditis and pericarditis also may complicate *Legionella* infection. They most likely are a consequence of bacteremia, originating from a pulmonary focus of *Legionella* infection. Clinical signs of pneumonia may or may not be present. Cardiac tamponade and constrictive pericarditis are fairly frequent complications. There are no distinctive symptoms or signs of *Legionella* pericarditis. Fever, chest pains, and myalgias are often present. Because it may respond temporarily to nonsteroidal anti-inflammatory drugs, it may be misdiagnosed as a viral process.

Myocarditis, due to *Legionella*, may be asymptomatic or present as flagrant congestive heart failure. Cases may be mistaken as viral myocarditis. However, most cases occur in the setting of clinical pneumonia. Usually, they respond to appropriate antibiotic treatment of the primary *Legionella* infection.[9,26,27]

DIAGNOSTIC APPROACHES

The most important step making the diagnosis of *Legionella* is for the clinician to suspect the possibility of such. Then, laboratory testing for *Legionella* cardiac infection should be based on a reasonable pretest probability that the patient has this disease: "Don't order a test just because you can."[28] This diagnosis should be considered in patients with prosthetic valves, no matter how long after their implantation and in whom blood cultures that have been properly obtained and negative. Under these conditions, if the patient has had *Legionella* pneumonia within the past few years or any other pneumonia without an etiologic diagnosis should further raise concern. The history of having been an inpatient in a facility that has had nosocomial outbreaks of Legionellosis is another point favoring the diagnosis. Certainly the lack of echocardiographic findings actually strengthens the likelihood that a given patient has *Legionella* endocarditis.

Legionella spp will grow out in standard blood culture media, but the concentration of the organisms is below that detectable by subculturing on routine media. However,

Table 2
Leading bacterial causes of culture-negative endocarditis

Organism	Comments
Bartonella spp	Most common cause of CNIE in the United States. Fever, acute heart failure, murmur with vegetation on echocardiogram. *Bartonella quintana* associated with homelessness. *Bartonella henselae* associated with cats.
Coxiella burnetii	Occurs in immunosuppressed individuals and in those with prosthetic valves. Usually no vegetation on echocardiogram.
Tropheryma whipplei	Multiorgan involvement especially gastrointestinal neurologic and musculoskeletal systems. Vegetation on echocardiogram. Acute cardiac failure.
Legionella spp	Highly associated with prosthetic valves, mechanical or bioprosthetic. Mild heart failure. Negative for vegetations on echocardiogram.

Table 3
Distinguishing clinical characteristics of chronic Q fever CNIE

1. Epidemiology	Typical patient is 60-year-old man who is exposed to farm animals and parturient cats. 10% of patients drink raw milk. 9% have various immunosuppression states. Currently remains an unusual cause of CNIE in the United States.
2. Clinical course	This chronic type of endocarditis can be present for up to a decade before the diagnosis is made.
3. Heart disease	90% have underlying valvular disease with prosthetic valves in >50% of patients. 39% of cases of chronic Q fever develop valvular infection. Valvular vegetations are really identified on either TTE or TEE. 20% develop arterial embolization, especially to the CNS. 67% develop CHF.
4. Peripheral stigmata	Splenomegaly is present in 50% of cases. There is a high rate of clubbing and purpuric rashes of the mucosa and of the extremities. These are secondary to the deposition of immune complexes. Immune complex disease can lead to glomerulonephritis with microscopic hematuria and renal insufficiency.
5. Mortality rate is approximately 30%	Comment: Q fever is the CNIE that most resembles Legionnaire's disease, especially with regard to the lack of valvular vegetations.[37]

Abbreviations: CHF, congestive heart failure; CNIE, culture-negative infective endocarditis; CNS, central nervous system; TEE, transesophageal echocardiography; TTE, transthoracic echocardiography.

Data from Refs.[24,36,37]

Table 4
Distinguishing clinical features of *Bartonella* CNIE

1. Epidemiology	Essentially all cases are caused by *Bartonella quintana* and *Bartonella henselae*. Patients with *B henselae* are infected from close contact with chronically bacteremic cats. The organism is transmitted by bites of cat fleas or by cat scratches. Typical patients with *B quintana* are homeless alcoholic men (70% of cases) who live in shelters. They are infected by body lice.
2. Clinical course	The course of *Bartonella* CNIE is typical of subacute endocarditis. The symptoms are nonspecific of low-grade fever and weight loss.
3. Heart disease	There is underlying heart disease present in 88% of individuals with *B henselae* and in 30% of those with *B quintana*. 96% of infected valves exhibit large and often calcified vegetations. There is a high rate of prior cardiac surgery in patients with *B henselae* infection.
4. Peripheral stigmata	These may be due to antineutrophil cytoplasmic antibody–positive pauci-immune necrotizing vasculitis that can lead to glomerulonephritis and other manifestations of immune complex disease.
5. Mortality rate	<20%

Abbreviation: CNIE, culture-negative infective endocarditis.

Data from Refs.[24,38,39]

Table 5
Distinguishing clinical features of *Chlamydophila psittaci* CNIE

1. Epidemiology	90% of patients have history of exposure to domestic or wild psittacine birds. Although unusual, human-human transmission has been documented in the hospital setting. Patients are usually younger than those suffering from Q fever or *Bartonella* CNIE.
2. Clinical course	It is usually subacute in nature.
3. Heart disease	Underlying aortic valve disease is common.
4. Peripheral stigmata	There does not seem to be any increased incidence of vasculitic type of rashes.
5. Mortality rate	Remains high at approximately 40% despite the combined use of surgery and antibiotics.

Abbreviation: CNIE, culture-negative infective endocarditis.

Comment: In the past, with the use of the polyclonal antibody test, which cross-reacts between *Chlamydia* and *Bartonella*, there had been a high rate of *Bartonella* valvular infection being ascribed to *C psittaci*.

Data from Refs.[24,36,40,41]

periodic subculturing on buffered, charcoal yeast extract (BCYE) will recover the organism in approximately 40% of patients. Full identification of the organism on this media requires special staining and use of a dissecting microscope. Retrieval and identification of the organism may take up to 3 to 5 days.[8,13]

The most commonly used test for diagnosing Legionellosis is the urinary antigen test. Results are available within a few hours. It is reliable only for diagnosis of

Table 6
Distinguishing characteristics of *Tropheryma whipplei* CNIE

1. Epidemiology	The typical patient with this form of CNIE is a 50-year-old male white of European descent. Valvular infection may be part of the classic presentation of Whipple disease with polyarthritis, central nervous system involvement, fever or weight loss, diarrhea and abdominal pain, or it may be an isolated event. Endocarditis may occur in up to 55% individuals with *T whipplei* infection. This organism may be the third most common cause of CNIE.
2. Clinical course	Those with isolated Whipple disease suffer from minimal systemic symptoms of malaise and anorexia. It may well be discovered on examination of the valve that was resected due to significant incompetence. Often there is no fever. In those with Whipple disease, clinical course may range from seronegative migratory polyarthritis to full-blown Whipple disease.
3. Heart disease	There may be associated myocarditis and pericarditis.
4. Peripheral stigmata	There does not seem to be any significant rash associated with valvular involvement.
5. Mortality rate	There are no reliable figures for mortality due to valvular infection because of the difficulty in separating the effect of localized valvular infection from the consequences of systemic infection.

Abbreviation: CNIE, culture-negative infective endocarditis.

Data from Refs.[25,36,42,43]

Table 7
Mimics of CNIE

Disease	Comments
1. Marantic endocarditis	Because cases have cardiac murmur cardiac vegetation and negative blood cultures, this entity is an almost perfect mimic of CNIE. This entity is associated with a host of chronic conditions. These include solid tumors, vasculitis, malnutrition. An important point of difference is that patients with marantic endocarditis are usually afebrile. Most types of CNIE will have some degree of fever.
2. Viral myocarditis	Patients will have fever, murmur, and peripheral emboli. Viral myocarditis is a disease of young adults. There are no valvular vegetations in viral myocarditis.
3. Systemic lupus erythematosus	Verrucous valvular vegetations (Libman–Sacks) may be seen uncommonly in systemic lupus erythematosus.
4. Atrial myxomas	Patients are often febrile with emboli, as well as positive rheumatoid factors. Because of fever and the presence of significant vegetations, these cases may be easily diagnosed as CNIE.

Abbreviation: CNIE, culture-negative infective endocarditis.

Adapted from Cunha BA. Mimics of endocarditis. In: Brusch JL, editor. Endocarditis essentials. Sudbury (MA): Jones and Bartlett; 2011. p. 157–9.

L pneumophilia primarily serotype 1. It does appear to also detect other *Legionella* spp; however, its sensitivity and specificity in doing so has not been established.[29,30]

In a recent study, the Binax urine antigen test was up to 96% sensitive for detecting *L pneumophila*. The Binax NOW Legionella Urinary Antigen Kit has been useful in detecting *Legionella pneumophila* 6.[26] The investigators emphasized the challenges of assessing the utility of a specific testing modality in the case of an extremely low prevalence disease such as *Legionella* cardiac infections.[31,32]

On resected valvular tissue, broad-range polymerase chain reaction (16 S rRNA) for CNIE is more sensitive (66.1%).[25] There does not seem to be a great deal of experience in using this technique for detection of *Legionella* spp in such tissue (**Box 4**). These diagnostic modalities are applicable for use in all 3 types of *Legionella* cardiac involvement.

TREATMENT

In the 1980s and 1990s, therapy for *Legionella* endocarditis consisted mainly of erythromycin 2 g intravenously with rifampin 600 to 1200 mg per day orally as a standard

Box 4
Suggested diagnostic approach to diagnosis of *Legionella* CNIE in the United States

1. Obtain urinary antigen
2. If available, any sputum and wound discharge for culture on buffered, charcoal yeast extract (BCYE) media
3. Direct fluorescent antibody testing of sputum *Legionella* if available
4. Obtain serologic testing for *Bartonella* spp and *Tropheryma whipplei*
5. Use appropriate staining, culture, and broad-range polymerase chain reaction testing of excised valvular tissue.

Box 5
Antibiotic treatment of *Legionella* endocarditis

Ciprofloxacin 400 mg intravenously (IV) every 12 hours + 500 mg azithromycin IV every 24 hours for 3 to 6 months[a]
or

Doxycycline 200 mg IV every 12 hours for 3 days and 100 mg IV every 12 hours for 3 to 6 months[a]
or

Doxycycline 200 mg every 12 hours by mouth (PO) for 3 days, then 100 mg PO every 12 hours for 3 to 6 months[a]

[a] In the presence of a prosthetic valve, consider addition of rifampin 300 mg PO every 8 hours.

regimen. Ciprofloxacin alone had been used as well as doxycycline. These antibiotics were administered for 5 months. Sixty-seven percent of patients required removal of the prosthetic valve.[13]

It is well recognized that the effectiveness of an antibiotic in treating Legionellosis is dependent on the degree of its intracellular penetration.

Based on clinical experience, primarily in treating *Legionella* pneumonia, the use of a quinolone combined with azithromycin has been advocated.[33]

In vitro techniques, such as high-throughput intracellular antimicrobial susceptibility testing of *L pneumophila*, indicate that combining ciprofloxacin with azithromycin or rifampin or minocycline resulted in significant synergism. However, these combinations with levofloxacin instead of ciprofloxacin did not do as well. In all probability, one could substitute doxycycline for minocycline (**Box 5**).[34,35] Overall, mortality rate approximates 10% for endocarditis.

Antibiotic regimens for *Legionella* peritonitis and myocarditis are identical to those used for treating Legionella endocarditis. What is in question is the duration of antibiotic therapy. Most likely it should be at least 2 to 3 months in duration. Pericardiectomy is usually required in cases of constrictive pericarditis.[5]

REFERENCES

1. Houpikian P, Raoult D. Blood culture negative endocarditis in a reference center. Medicine 2005;84:162–73.
2. CDC Vital Signs. Legionnaire's disease. Available at: cdc.gov/vitalsigns/. Accessed July 7, 2016.
3. Brusch JL. Gram-negatives and other organisms. In: Brusch JL, editor. Infective endocarditis: management in the era of intravascular devices. New York: Informa Healthcare; 2007. p. 51–99.
4. Cianciotto NP. Pathogenicity of *Legionella pneumophilia*. Int J Med Microbiol 2001;291:331–43.
5. Vezza PR, Lack EE, Chandler FW. Legionellosis chapter. In: Connor DH, Chandler FW, Manz HJ, et al, editors. Pathology of infectious diseases. Stamford (CT): Appleton and Lange; 1997. p. 597–604.
6. Miyake M. Intracellular survival and replication of *Legionella pneumophilia* within host cells. YakugakZasshi 2008;128:1763–70.
7. Nelson DP, Rensimer ER, Burke CM, et al. Cardiac Legionellosis. Chest 1984;86: 807–8.
8. McCabe RS, Baldwin JC, McGregor CA, et al. Prosthetic valve endocarditis by *Legionella pneumophilia*. Ann Intern Med 1984;100:525–7.

9. Lowry PW, Tompkins LS. Nosocomial legionellosis: A review of pulmonary and extrapulmonary syndromes. Am J Infect Control 1993;21:21–7.
10. Braybender W, Hinthorn DR, Asher M, et al. *Legionella pneumophilia* wound infection. JAMA 1983;250:3091–2.
11. Levy PY, Teysseire N, Etiene J, et al. Nosocomial outbreak of *Legionella pneumophilia* caused by contaminated transesophageal echocardiographic probes. Infect Control Hosp Epidemiol 2003;24:619–22.
12. Massey R, Kumar P, Pepper JP. Innocent victim of a localized outbreak: *Legionella* endocarditis. Heart 2003;89:e16. Available at: http://www.heartjnl.com/cgi/content/full.89/5/e16.
13. Tompkins LS, Rossler BJ, Redd SC, et al. Legionella prosthetic valve endocarditis. N Engl J Med 1988;318:530–5.
14. Park D, Puglisi A, Cunha AB. *Legionella micdadei* prosthetic valve endocarditis. Infection 1994;22:213–5.
15. Samuel V, Bajwa AA, Curry JD. First case of *Legionella pneumophilia* native valve endocarditis. Int J Infect Dis 2011;15:e576–7.
16. Compain F, Bruneval P, Jarraud S, et al. Chronic endocarditis due to *Legionella anisa*: the first case difficult to diagnose. New Microbes New Infect 2015;8:113–5.
17. Viasus D, DiYacovo S, Garcia-Vidal C, et al. Community-acquired *Legionella pneumophilia* pneumonia: a single center experience with 214 hospitalized sporadic cases over 15 years. Medicine 2013;92:51–60.
18. Guyot S, Goy P, Gersbach K, et al. *Legionella* pneumonia aortitis in a heart transplant recipient. Transpl Infect Dis 2007;9:58–9.
19. Hernandez K, Kirby BD, Stanley TM, et al. Legionnaire's disease. Postmortem pathologic findings of 20 cases. Am J Clin Pathol 1980;73(4):488–95.
20. Fukuta Y, Yildiz-Aktas IZ, Pascuille W, et al. *Legionella micdadei* prosthetic valve endocarditis complicated by brain abscess: case reported and review of the literature. Scand J Infect Dis 2012;44:414–8.
21. Towns ML, Reller LB. Diagnostic methods: current best practices and guidelines for isolation of bacteria and fungi in infective endocarditis. Infect Dis Clin North Am 2002;16:363–76.
22. Lamy B, Dargere S, Arendrup MC, et al. How to optimize the use of blood cultures with a diagnosis of blood stream infections? A state of the art. Front Microbiol 2016;7:697–7010.
23. Tattevin P, Watt G, Revest M, et al. Update and blood culture negative endocarditis. Med Mal Infect 2015;45:1–9.
24. Brouqu IP, Raoult D. Endocarditis due to rare and fastidious bacteria. Clin Microbiol Rev 2001;14:177–207.
25. Fournier PE, Thuny F, Richet H, et al. Comprehensive diagnosis strategy for blood culture-negative endocarditis: a prospective study of 819 cases. Clin Infect Dis 2010;51:131–40.
26. Antonarakis ES, Wung PK, Durand DJ, et al. An atypical complication of atypical pneumonia. Am J Med 2006;119:824–7.
27. Ishimuru N, Suzuki H, Tokuda Y, et al. Severe *Legionella* disease with pneumonia and biopsy confirmed myocarditis most likely caused by *Legionella pneumophilia* serogroup 6. Intern Med 2012;51:3207–12.
28. Cunha BA. Characteristic predictors that increase the pretest probability of Legionnaire's disease: "Don't order a test just because you can" revisited. South Med J 2015;108:761.

29. Benson RF, Tang PW, Fields BS. Evaluation of Binax and Biotest test urinary antigen kits for detection of Legionnaire's disease due to multiple serogroups and species of *Legionella*. J Clin Microbiol 2000;38:2763–6.
30. Chen DJ, Procop GW, Vogel S, et al. Utility of PCR, culture and antigen detection methods the diagnosis of Legionellosis. J Clin Microbiol 2015;53:3474–7.
31. Lepid H, Coulibaly B, Casalta JP, et al. Autoimmunohistochemistry: a method for the histologic diagnosis of infective endocarditis. J Infect Dis 2006;193:1711–7.
32. Bruneval P, Choucair J, Paraf F, et al. Detection of fastidious bacteria and cardiac valves in cases of blood culture-negative endocarditis. J Clin Pathol 2001;54:238–40.
33. Pedro-Botet ML, Yu VL. Treatment strategies for *Legionella* infection. Expert Opin Pharmacother 2009;10:1109–21.
34. Chiaraviglio L, Kirby JE. High-throughput intracellular antimicrobial susceptibility testing of *Legionella pneumophilia*. Antimicrob Agents Chemother 2015;59:7517–29.
35. Cunha BA, Brusch JL, Nichols RL, et al. Empiric therapy based on clinical syndrome. In: Cunha BA, Cunha C, editors. Antibiotic essentials. 14th edition. New Delhi: Jaypee Brothers Medical Publishers; 2015. p. 17–184.
36. Brusch JL. Microbiology of infective endocarditis and clinical correlates: gram-negatives and other organisms. In: Brusch JL, editor. Infective endocarditis: management in the era of intravascular devices. New York: Informa Healthcare USA Incorporated; 2007. p. 51–99.
37. Cunha B, Nausheen S, Busch L. Severe Q fever community-acquired pneumonia (CAP) mimicking Legionnaire's disease: clinical significance of cold agglutinins, anti-smooth muscle antibodies and thrombocytosis. Heart Lung 2009;38:354–62.
38. Shah SH, Grahame-Clarke C, Ross CN. Touch not the cat bot a glove: ANCA positive pauci-immune necrotizing glomerulonephritis secondary to *Bartonella henselae*. Clin Kidney J 2014;7:179–81.
39. Raoult D, Fournier PE, Drancourt M, et al. Diagnosis of 22 new cases of *Bartonella* endocarditis. Ann Intern Med 1996;125:646–52.
40. Yung AP, Grayson ML. Psittacosis—a review of 135 cases. Med J Aust 1988;148:228.
41. Jones RB, Priest JB, Kuo CC. Subacute chlamydial endocarditis. JAMA 1982;247:655.
42. Weisman A, Rebick G, Morris A, et al. Whipple's endocarditis: An enigmatic cause of culture-negative bacterial endocarditis. Can J Infect Dis Med Microbiol 2013;24:e29–30.
43. Alozie A, Zimpfer A, Koller K, et al. Arthralgia and blood culture negative endocarditis in middle-aged men suggest Tropheryma whipplei infection. BMC Infect Dis 2015;15:339–47.

Legionnaire's Disease

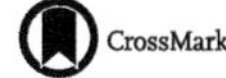

A Clinical Diagnostic Approach

Burke A. Cunha, MD, MACP[a,b,*], Cheston B. Cunha, MD[c]

KEYWORDS

- Relative bradycardia • Erythrocyte sedimentation rate • C-reactive protein • Ferritin
- Hypophosphatemia • Microscopic hematuria

KEY POINTS

- Legionnaire's disease is a atypical pneumonias with nonspecific radiographic and clinical findings.
- With pneumonia, low phosphorus or high ferritin suggest Legionnaire's disease.
- If key characteristic extrapulmonary features are present, Legionella is likely.
- Testing all pneumonias for Legionella is unwarranted.
- If several Legionella predictors are present, then testing should be done.
- If Legionella is suspected based on key findings, titers and urinary antigen should be ordered.

BACKGROUND

Since 1977, it has been appreciated that Legionnaire's disease is a nonzoonotic atypical pneumonia with several distinctive features.[1–4] With typical bacterial pneumonias, clinical findings are limited to the lungs, and atypical pneumonias differ from typical bacterial pneumonias by the presence of extrapulmonary findings.[5–7] Zoonotic and nonzoonotic atypical pneumonias are systemic infectious diseases with prominent extrapulmonary manifestations. Each atypical pneumonia has a characteristic pattern of organ involvement, which provides important clues in pneumonia differential diagnosis.

The diagnostic challenge for clinicians is to recognize the characteristic pattern of extrapulmonary organ involvement associated with each atypical pneumonia. Key

Conflict of Interest: The authors declare no conflict of interest.

[a] Infectious Disease Division, Winthrop-University Hospital, 222 Station Plaza North (#432), Mineola, NY 11501, USA; [b] School of Medicine, State University of New York, Stony Brook, NY, USA; [c] Division of Infectious Disease, Rhode Island Hospital, The Miriam Hospital, Brown University Alpert School of Medicine, Providence, RI, USA

* Corresponding author. Infectious Disease Division, Winthrop-University Hospital, 222 Station Plaza North (#432), Mineola, NY 11501.

E-mail address: bacunha@winthrop.org

Infect Dis Clin N Am 31 (2017) 81–93
http://dx.doi.org/10.1016/j.idc.2016.10.007
id.theclinics.com

clinical findings from the history, physical examination, and characteristic nonspecific laboratory tests determine the pattern of organ involvement.[8–11] The clinical problem is not which tests should be ordered to diagnose Legionnaire's disease. Rather, clinicians should try to identify which patients are likely to have Legionnaire's disease based on characteristic nonspecific findings that when considered together point to the diagnosis and should prompt specific *Legionella* sp testing.[12–18]

Clinically, Legionnaire's disease is readily differentiated from typical bacterial pneumonias by the presence of extrapulmonary findings.[12–16] Pneumococcal pneumonia, like Legionnaire's disease, is accompanied by fever and pulmonary symptoms, but not extrapulmonary findings, for example, relative bradycardia, mental confusion, loose stools/diarrhea, abdominal pain, which are often present with Legionnaire's disease.[7,13,16] After eliminating typical bacterial pneumonias from further diagnostic consideration, the next step in the clinical approach is to differentiate the zoonotic from non-zoonotic atypical pneumonias on the basis of zoonotic contact history. Zoonotic atypical pneumonias are not acquired from others but are acquired from zoonotic vectors. A negative recent zoonotic contact history, for example, psittacine birds for psittacosis, rabbit/deer contact for tularemia, or sheep or parturient cat exposure for Q fever, effectively rules out zoonotic atypical pneumonias from further diagnostic consideration.[13–15]

After eliminating zoonotic atypical pneumonias on the basis of a negative vector contact history, the clinician should try to differentiate the nonzoonotic atypical pneumonias, *Mycoplasma pneumoniae*, *Chlamydia pneumoniae*, and Legionnaire's disease. Because Legionnaire's disease is accompanied by its own set of characteristic and extrapulmonary findings, it is relatively straightforward clinically to differentiate Legionnaire's disease from *M pneumoniae* and *C pneumoniae*, for example, no relative bradycardia, sore throat, fevers less than 102°F, hoarseness (*C pneumoniae*).[15,16] Because neither chest film appearance or individual nonspecific findings are pathognomonic of Legionnaire's disease, an effective clinical approach involves recognizing the diagnostic significance of the combined presence of several characteristic Legionnaire's disease findings, for example, fever usually greater than 102°F, relative bradycardia, mental confusion, abdominal pain, loose stools/diarrhea, hypophosphatemia, highly elevated ferritin levels, elevated creatinine phosphokinase, microscopic hematuria (**Table 1**).[15–18]

Legionnaire's disease clinical syndromic diagnosis is based on recognizing the characteristic extrapulmonary abnormalities associated with Legionnaire's disease. The more characteristic findings present, the more likely the atypical pneumonia is due to Legionnaire's disease.[12,13,15,16] Not all abnormalities have equal diagnostic significance, for example, hyponatremia versus hypophosphatemia.[8,12,13,15,16] Hyponatremia, although common with Legionnaire's disease, alone is unhelpful diagnostically because hyponatremia due to the syndrome of inappropriate antidiuretic hormone may accompany any pneumonia as well as a variety of noninfectious pulmonary disorders.[15,16] In contrast, otherwise unexplained hypophosphatemia is associated only with Legionnaire's disease and not other typical, for example, *Streptococcus pneumoniae*, *Haemophilus influenzae*, *Moraxella catarrhalis* or other atypical pneumonias, for example, *M pneumoniae*, Q fever, tularemia, psittacosis.[15,16]

CLINICAL DIAGNOSTIC APPROACH

A clinical syndromic diagnosis of Legionnaire's disease is based on the relative diagnostic importance of several nonspecific clinical and laboratory findings.[17–19] A presumptive clinical syndromic diagnosis is useful in focusing the diagnostic workup to

Table 1
Community acquired pneumonia: a clinical diagnostic approach to Legionnaire's disease

1. Verify the diagnosis of community-acquired pneumonia
   - New patchy, segmental, or lobar infiltrates (with pulmonary symptoms suggestive of pneumonia, eg, cough, shortness of breath)
   - Viral community-acquired pneumonias (*excluding* adenovirus) do *not* have focal segmental/lobar infiltrates on chest radiograph
   - Rule out mimics of pneumonia by history, physical examination, nonspecific laboratory tests, and chest radiograph appearance
2. Determine if clinical findings are limited to the lungs or if there are extrapulmonary findings
   Typical community-acquired pneumonia
   - Community-acquired pneumonia *without* extrapulmonary findings is likely due to a typical bacterial pathogen (*S pneumoniae*, *H influenzae*, or *M catarrhalis*). Order sputum, blood cultures, and treat appropriately

   Atypical community-acquired pneumonia
   - Community-acquired pneumonia *with* extrapulmonary findings is likely due to an atypical pneumonia pathogen (either 1 of 3 zoonotic pathogens or 1 of 3 nonzoonotic pathogens)
3. If the community-acquired pneumonia has extrapulmonary manifestations (an atypical pneumonia), inquire regarding recent zoonotic exposure
   Differential diagnosis of zoonotic atypical community-acquired pneumonia (positive recent vector exposure or contact history)
   - Psittacine birds (psittacosis)
   - Parturient cats/sheep (Q fever)
   - Rabbits/deer (tularemia)

   Differential diagnosis of nonzoonotic atypical community-acquired pneumonia (negative recent vector exposure or contact history)
   - *M pneumoniae*
   - *C pneumoniae*
   - Legionnaire's disease
4. With a nonzoonotic atypical community-acquired pneumonia, determine if key Legionnaire's disease *characteristic* findings are present, that considered together, suggest Legionnaire's disease
   - If pattern of organ involvement is *not characteristic* of Legionnaire's disease, order tests for *M pneumoniae* (immunoglobulin M [IgM] and IgG titers are cold agglutinin titers) and *C pneumoniae* (IgM and IgG titers)
   - If pattern of organ involvement *is characteristic* of Legionnaire's disease, order Legionella titers, Legionella sputum culture, direct fluorescent antibody testing of sputum, and Legionella urinary antigen tests

Adapted from Cunha BA, editor. Pneumonia essentials. 3rd edition. Sudbury (MA): Jones & Bartlett; 2010.

limit *Legionella* sp testing to confirm or rule out the diagnosis.[15,20] Legionnaire's disease should also be considered in patients with otherwise unexplained severe pneumonia.[9,11,21,22] Nosocomial Legionnaire's disease has the same clinical features as community-acquired Legionnaire's disease, but nosocomial Legionnaire's disease occurs in clusters/outbreaks, not as isolated or sporadic cases because nosocomial Legionnaire's disease results from common *Legionella* sp containing aerosolized water exposure.[23–25]

The key characteristic clinical findings of Legionnaire's disease include otherwise unexplained fever greater than 102°F (with relative bradycardia), loose stools/watery diarrhea (±abdominal pain), headache/mental confusion, highly elevated erythrocyte sedimentation rate (ESR; >90 mm/h), highly elevated ferritin levels

(>2 × normal), mildly/transiently increased serum transaminases, hyponatremia, hypophosphatemia (early/transient), and microscopic hematuria (early/transient).[2,4,8,15,16] Clinically, the most important of these is relative bradycardia (if temperature > 102°F and patient does not have a pacemaker, heart block, or is on a ß-blocker, diltiazem, or verapamil).[13,26] In a patient with pneumonia, the most important nonspecific laboratory tests are an otherwise explained highly elevated ESR (>90 mm/h), hypophosphatemia, and elevated ferritin levels, which when considered in concert, are highly predictive of Legionnaire's disease.[27] Similarly, "diagnostic eliminators" are clinical features that argue strongly against the diagnosis of Legionnaire's disease. The lack of such findings argues strongly against the diagnosis of Legionnaire's disease and should suggest an alternate diagnosis, for example, no relative bradycardia (with temperature > 102°F).[13,14,27,28]

RADIOLOGIC ABNORMALITIES

Radiologic manifestations of Legionnaire's disease are varied and have no pathognomonic radiographic appearance.[9–11,16] The most common chest film findings are rapidly progressive patchy infiltrates that may occur, but all types of infiltrates have been reported. Consolidation or pleural effusions are not uncommon. Lung abscess is a rare complication of Legionnaire's disease. Round nodular opacities should suggest Legionnaire's disease. Cavitation may occur during the first 2 weeks of antibiotic therapy.[29,30]

Even with appropriate antibiotic therapy during the first week, rapid asymmetric progression of infiltrates is common. Generally, radiographic improvement lags behind clinical improvement, and complete resolution of infiltrates takes 1 to 4 months, sometimes longer.[29,30] Radiographs correlate well with CT findings. A variety of chest CT scan manifestations have been described, that is, "tree-in-bud" configuration, but none are pathognomonic for Legionnaire's disease.[31]

CLINICAL EXTRAPULMONARY MANIFESTATIONS

In addition to the lungs, Legionnaire's disease is a systemic infection that directly or indirectly affects multiple organs. The characteristic pattern of extrapulmonary organ involvement in Legionnaire's disease includes the central nervous system, heart, liver, gastrointestinal tract, and kidney.[2,4,8,11,14,20]

Central Nervous System Manifestations

Headache and mental confusion are the commonest central nervous system manifestations of Legionnaire's disease.[8,32] Some causes of pneumonia are accompanied by headache, but few with encephalopathy, for example, rarely with *M pneumoniae*.[15,16] Meningismus and meningitis are not features of Legionnaire's disease, but some patients have had lumbar puncture to rule out meningitis/encephalitis. Cerebrospinal fluid in Legionnaire's disease with mental confusion may demonstrate a mild lymphocyte pleocytosis but is otherwise unremarkable.[13,32]

Cardiac Manifestations

The most common cardiac manifestation of Legionnaire's disease is relative bradycardia.[2,4,5,13] Relative bradycardia may be considered present in adults with temperatures greater than 102°F, but not if the temperature is less than 102°F, or with a pacemaker, with a heart block, or if receiving drugs that affect pulse-temperature relationships, for example, β-blockers, diltiazem, or verapamil.[16,26] Besides Legionnaire's disease, relative bradycardia also may accompany psittacosis or Q fever

(**Fig. 1**, **Table 2**). Pericarditis, myocarditis, and endocarditis (native or prosthetic valve) are rare complications of Legionnaire's disease.[15,26]

Hepatic Manifestations

Hepatic involvement is commonly manifested by early mild/transient elevations of serum transaminases.[8–11] Alkaline phosphatase levels are usually not elevated. Very high serum transaminases or alkaline phosphatase levels should suggest an alternate diagnosis.[15,16] Elevated serum transaminases are not a feature of bacterial *M pneumoniae*, *C pneumoniae*, or tularemia pneumonias.[15,16] An atypical pneumonia with splenomegaly should suggest psittacosis or Q fever, rather than Legionnaire's disease.[15,16,33,34]

Pancreatic Manifestations

Although rare, *Legionella* sp involvement of the pancreas may manifest as acute pancreatitis. The only other pneumonias that may present with acute pancreatitis are adenovirus and *M pneumoniae* pneumonias.[35]

Gastrointestinal Manifestations

Loose stools and watery diarrhea are the commonest gastrointestinal manifestations of Legionnaire's disease.[8,15] Watery diarrhea is also common with *M pneumoniae* pneumonia. Abdominal pain may occur with or without diarrhea. Pneumonia presenting with otherwise unexplained abdominal pain should suggest Legionnaire's

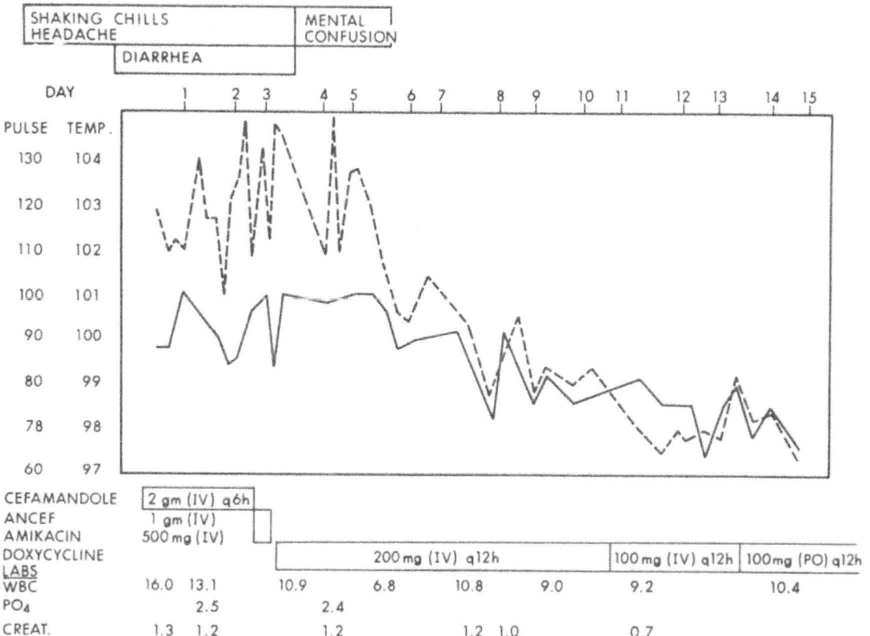

Fig. 1. Legionnaire's disease with relative bradycardia treated with doxycycline showing resolution of relative bradycardia in 5 to 7 days. CREAT, creatine; IV, intravenous; PO, orally; PO_4, phosphate; q6h, every 6 hours; q12h, every 12 hours; WBC, white blood cells. (*From* Cotton E, Strainpfer M, Cunha B. Legionella and Mpplarma piietrinoriiac-a community hospital experience with atypical pneumonias. Clin Chest Med 1987;8:441–53; with permission.)

Table 2
The diagnostic importance of relative bradycardia in Legionnaire's disease diagnosis

Diagnostic Criteria for Relative Bradycardia: Temperature-Pulse Relationships

Temperature, °F (°C)	Appropriate Pulse Response for Temperature/min	Relative Bradycardia Present if Pulse/min
106°F (41.1°C)	150/min	<140/min
105°F (40.6°C)	140/min	<130/min
104°F (40.7°C)	130/min	<120/min
103°F (39.4°C)	120/min	<110/min
102°F (38.9°C)	110/min	<100/min

The only pneumonias with relative bradycardia are psittacosis, Q fever, and Legionnaire's disease. Relative bradycardia is not a feature of other pneumonias, for example, tularemia, *C pneumoniae*, or *M pneumoniae*.

In a patient with pneumonia and otherwise unexplained relative bradycardia, if psittacosis and Q fever are unlikely, that is, negative recent appropriate zoonotic exposure/contact, *Legionnaire's disease is highly likely.*

Because relative bradycardia is a constant finding in Legionnaire's disease (in adults with temperatures ≥102°F), the absence of relative bradycardia *argues strongly against* the diagnosis of Legionnaire's disease.

Relative bradycardia refers to heart rates that are inappropriately slow relative to body temperature (pulse must be taken simultaneously with temperature elevation). Applies only to adults with temperature ≥102°F and does not apply to patients with second-/third-degree heart block, pacemaker-induced rhythms, or those taking β-blockers, diltiazem, or verapamil.

[a] Negative recent zoonotic exposure/contact history.

[b] If present, look for other causes.

Adapted from Cunha BA, editor. Pneumonia essentials. 3rd edition. Sudbury (MA): Jones & Bartlett; 2010.

disease.[13,15] As with central nervous system manifestations, gastrointestinal symptoms may overshadow pulmonary findings.[15]

Renal Manifestations

Acute renal failure is the primary renal manifestation of Legionnaire's disease.[8,15] Because critically ill pneumonia patients are often hypotensive, resulting in acute renal failure, it is often difficult to ascribe acute renal failure to Legionnaire's disease. However, with pneumonia, otherwise unexplained acute renal failure should suggest Legionnaire's disease.[9–11]

Musculoskeletal Manifestations

Myalgias, if present, are mild. Muscle involvement is not uncommon early in Legionnaire's disease and is manifested by elevated creatine phosphokinase. Rhabdomyolysis and myoglobinuria may complicate Legionnaire's disease.[12,13,15]

NONSPECIFIC LABORATORY FINDINGS

Hematologic Manifestations

Leukocytosis with a left shift is usual with Legionnaire's disease. Otherwise unexplained thrombocytopenia, thrombocytosis, lymphocytosis, or atypical lymphocytes (>5%) should suggest an alternate diagnosis.[15–17] The most characteristic white blood cell finding in Legionnaire's disease is otherwise unexplained relative lymphopenia.[8,15] Relative lymphopenia also has prognostic significance, that is, resolving relative lymphopenia is predictive of clinical improvement.

Erythrocyte Sedimentation Rate and C-Reactive Protein

Mild/moderate elevations of ESR and C-reactive protein (CRP) levels may occur with any pneumonia.[16] However, an otherwise unexplained highly elevated ESR (>90 mm/h) or CRP levels (>35 mg/L) should suggest Legionnaire's disease.[36] *S pneumoniae* pneumonia may also be associated with a high ESR, but *S pneumoniae* pneumonia is easily differentiated from Legionnaire's disease by the absence of characteristic extrapulmonary findings, for example, relative bradycardia.[16]

Hypophosphatemia and Hyponatremia

Hyponatremia and hypophosphatemia are common in Legionnaire's disease.[8–11] Hyponatremia occurs most often with Legionnaire's disease, but may accompany other pneumonias or noninfectious pulmonary disorders.[16] Severe hyponatremia is more common with Legionnaire's disease versus other pneumonias. However, pneumonia with otherwise unexplained hypophosphatemia points to Legionnaire's disease.[8,13,37] Because decreased serum phosphorus levels occur early and rapidly return to normal, transient hypophosphatemia is easily missed (**Fig. 2**).[37] Importantly, unlike hyponatremia, hypophosphatemia, if present, is uniquely associated with Legionnaire's disease.[15,37]

Highly Elevated Ferritin Levels

Ferritin levels may be mildly elevated acutely as part of the acute phase response, but acute phase elevations are mild/transient.[16] However, with pneumonia otherwise unexplained, high/persistent serum ferritin level is characteristic of Legionnaire's disease.[38] If pneumonia is accompanied by otherwise unexplained highly/persistently elevated serum ferritin levels, Legionnaire's disease is highly likely (**Fig. 3**).[16,38]

Highly Elevated Creatinine Phosphokinase Levels

Elevated creatinine phosphokinase levels occur with Legionnaire's disease. Very high creatinine phosphokinase levels may be accompanied by rhabdomyolysis and related renal failure.[8] The only other pneumonia commonly associated with highly/elevated creatinine phosphokinase levels is influenza (**Fig. 4**).[16,17]

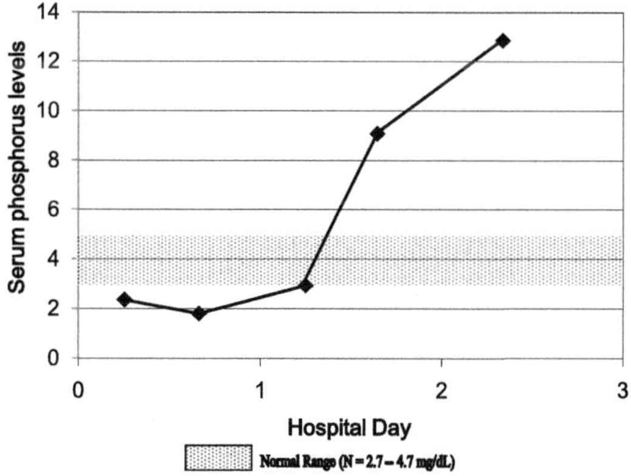

Fig. 2. Legionnaire's disease with typical early transient hypophosphatemia. (*Reproduced from* Cunha BA. Hypophosphatemia: diagnostic significance in Legionnaire's disease. Am J Med 2006;119:e5–6; with permission.)

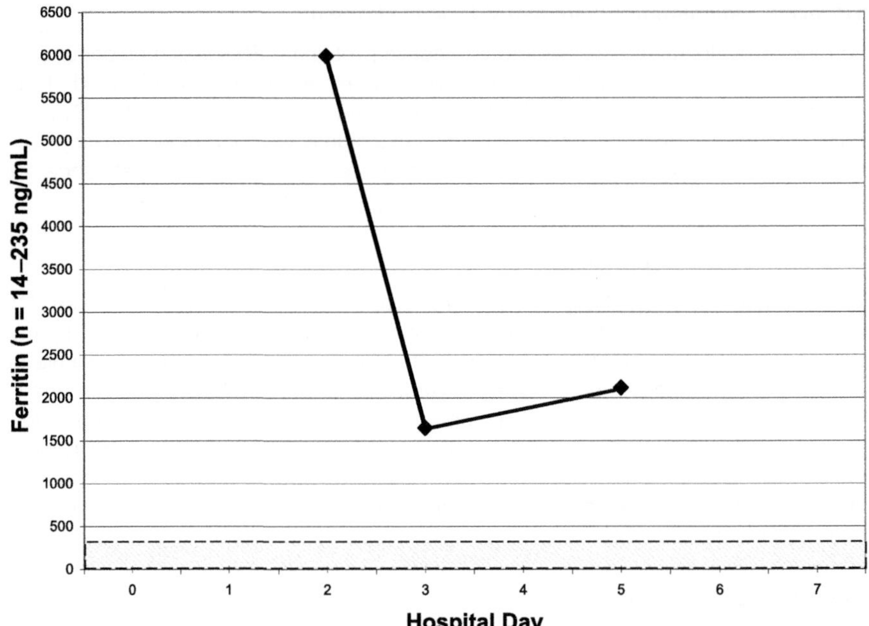

Fig. 3. Serial ferritin levels with Legionnaire's disease. (*From* Cunha BA, Klein NC, Strollo S, et al. Legionnaires disease mimicking swine influenza (H1N1) pneumonia during the "herald wave" of the pandemic. Heart Lung 2010;39:242–8; with permission.)

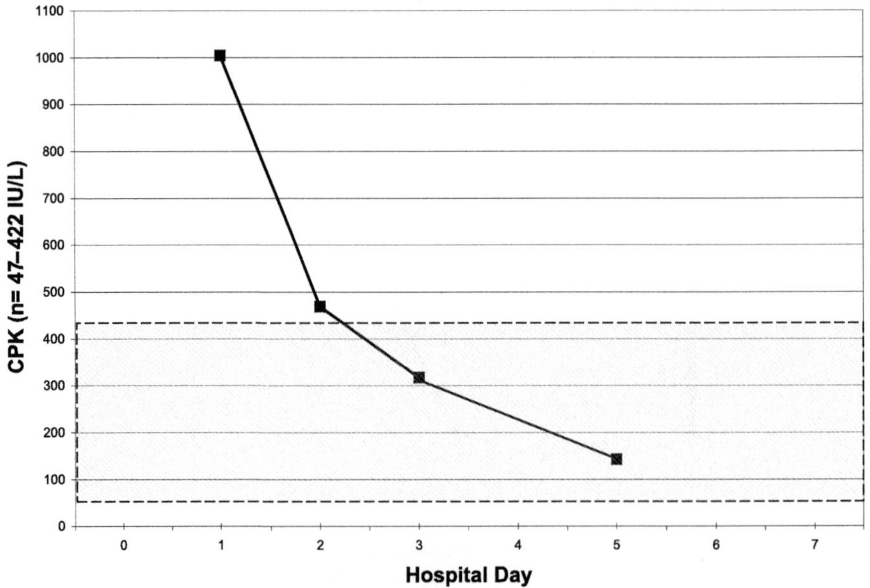

Fig. 4. Serial CK levels with Legionnaire's disease. CPK, creatine kinase. (*From* Cunha BA, Klein NC, Strollo S, et al. Legionnaires disease mimicking swine influenza (H1N1) pneumonia during the "herald wave" of the pandemic. Heart Lung 2010;39:242–8; with permission.)

Microscopic Hematuria

Microscopic hematuria occurs early/transiently in Legionnaire's disease and is an important clue. Other pneumonias are not associated with microscopic hematuria. With pneumonia, an otherwise unexplained microscopic hematuria should suggest Legionnaire's disease.[13,15,39]

LEGIONNAIRE'S DISEASE MIMICS

Because Legionnaire's disease is a multisystem infection with several extrapulmonary manifestations, it is not surprising that some other pneumonias may mimic some radiologic or clinical features of Legionnaire's disease.[16]

Influenza and Influenzalike Illnesses

Influenza and influenzalike illnesses (ILIs), due to other respiratory viruses, may mimic the clinical presentation of Legionnaire's disease with fever, headache, and shortness of breath. However, sore throat, myalgias, and fatigue are typical of influenza but are not the predominant findings in Legionnaire's disease. The chest film appearance of influenza and influenzalike illnesses is negative for infiltrates early, and later often has bilateral interstitial, but not asymmetric or localized infiltrates as does Legionnaire's disease. In hospitalized adults with influenza, leukopenia, relative lymphopenia, and thrombocytopenia are common. Although relative lymphopenia is a feature of Legionnaire's disease, leukopenia and thrombocytopenia argue against a diagnosis of Legionnaire's disease.[13,17] A cardinal finding in Legionnaire's disease is a pulse temperature deficient, that is, relative bradycardia. In hospitalized adults, relative bradycardia is not a feature of influenza or any viral pneumonia.[16] Mildly elevated serum transaminases or elevated creatine kinase (CK) levels also often present with Legionnaire's disease, but a highly elevated ferritin level effectively rules out influenza.[15–17]

Adenovirus

Adenovirus pneumonia on chest radiograph may mimic a bacterial pneumonia. Unlike other respiratory viral pneumonias with either negative infiltrates (early) or bilateral interstitial infiltrates (late), adenoviral pneumonia often presents with a localized segmental/lobar infiltrate.[16] Adenoviral pneumonia, as with other viral pneumonias, may be distinguished from Legionnaire's disease by the absence of relative bradycardia and elevated ferritin levels. If present, in a hospitalized adult with pneumonia, conjunctival suffusion and/or sore throat suggests the possibility of adenoviral pneumonia.[16,40]

Psittacosis and Q Fever

Psittacosis and Q fever may resemble Legionnaire's disease, that is, both may be accompanied by relative bradycardia. Hyponatremia may be present, but hypophosphatemia, elevated CK levels, and elevated serum ferritin levels are not features of either psittacosis or Q fever pneumonia.[16] Facial Horder spots point to psittacosis. Splenomegaly, if present, effectively rules out Legionnaire's disease. Psittacosis and Q fever are the only pneumonias often accompanied by an enlarged spleen.[16] Epidemiologically, the possibility of psittacosis or Q fever, both zoonotic atypical pneumonias, is suggested by recent psittacine bird (psittacosis) exposure or cat or sheep exposure (Q fever).[33,34]

Streptococcus pneumoniae

Pneumococcal pneumonia is a typical bacterial pneumonia that may resemble Legionnaire's disease in a few aspects. Headache may be present and mental confusion may be secondary to high fevers, particularly in the elderly.[16] However, unlike Legionnaire's disease, *S pneumoniae* fevers are not accompanied by relative bradycardia (unless the patient is on a β-blocker, diltiazem, or verapamil, which will slow the pulse). Pneumococcal pneumonia, like Legionnaire's disease, may be accompanied by a very high ESR, that is, greater than 90 mm/h (D. Schlossberg, MD, personal communication, 1998). Hyponatremia may be present in *S pneumoniae* but is not accompanied by hypophosphatemia, highly elevated ferritin levels, or microscopic hematuria.[16]

LEGIONNAIRE'S DISEASE DIAGNOSIS

Selective Testing

The clinical dilemma is choosing which pneumonias should be tested for Legionnaire's disease. Some physicians test all pneumonias for Legionnaire's disease. Because Legionnaire's disease is relatively uncommon (low pretest probability), this approach results in overtesting.[18] Legionnaire's disease should be considered in those with severe pneumonia or impaired cellular immunity.[21,22] Furthermore, Legionnaire's disease incidence is highest in the summer and fall and during periods of increased precipitation.

The preferred clinical approach is to identify pneumonias likely due to Legionnaire's disease based on the presence of several key characteristic findings.[28] When present, these clinical predictors of Legionnaire's disease increase the pretest probability of *Legionella* sp.[18]

Definitive Testing

Following infection, not all infectious diseases are accompanied by specific titer elevations. *Legionella* sp titers may be blunted, delayed, or eliminated by early anti-Legionella therapy, and a negative titer does not rule out the diagnosis. *Legionella* sp titers may be elevated early, but titers often become elevated in 4 to 6 weeks, and in some cases, 10 weeks later. If Legionnaire's disease is likely, then serial testing over 4 to 6 weeks should be done.[9–11] *Legionella* sp urinary antigen testing is helpful if positive, but if negative may be a function of timing. Alternately, in Legionnaire's disease, negative urinary *Legionella* sp antigen testing may be due to non-*Legionella pneumophila* (serotypes 1–6). *Legionella* sp urinary antigen test may be negative early, but if positive, remains persistently positive for weeks. *Legionella* sp antigenuria is most useful in patients with *Legionella* sp titers that are not elevated that may subsequently test positive for *Legionella* sp by urinary antigen.[15,16] Always order both *Legionella* sp titers and urinary antigen tests because titers may be elevated, when *Legionella* sp urinary antigen tests are negative.[12,15,20]

SUMMARY

Clinical diagnostic reasoning is used to narrow diagnostic possibilities to direct the workup and focus testing based on the most likely diagnostic probabilities. Clinical syndromic diagnosis is based on recognizing and combining characteristic clinical findings. The diagnostic importance of grouped characteristic findings is based on increased specificity derived from the simultaneous presence of multiple key (characteristic) clinical clues. This approach is not based on possibilities or findings "consistent with the diagnosis." Rather, characteristic findings when grouped are the basis of a probability based syndromic diagnosis. Clinically, when applied to patients presenting with pneumonia, the task for clinicians is first to verify the patient has pneumonia versus the mimics of pneumonia. Second, the next step in the diagnosis sequence is to differentiate typical from atypical pneumonia. Third, eliminate zoonotic atypical pneumonias, by obtaining a recent negative zoonotic vector exposure. Remaining are the 3 common nonzoonotic atypical pneumonias, that is, *M pneumoniae*, *C pneumoniae*, or Legionnaire's disease. The last step is to look for characteristic clinical findings or diagnostic eliminators that alone or together will increase or decrease the diagnostic probability of Legionnaire's disease.

It is relatively straightforward among admitted adults with pneumonia to identify characteristic clinical and nonspecific laboratory findings of Legionnaire's disease. Alternately, it is equally useful to eliminate Legionnaire's disease from further consideration if diagnostic eliminators are present. If fever is >102°F and accompanied by relative bradycardia (not due to a pacemaker, heart block, β-blocker, diltiazem, or verapamil), Legionnaire's disease is effectively ruled out.

The most common characteristic nonspecific early laboratory abnormalities in Legionnaire's disease are otherwise unexplained hypophosphatemia and microscopic hematuria (on admission/early). Mild serum transaminases elevations are common. Elevated creatine phosphokinase levels (excluding viral pneumonias, eg, influenza) are not infrequent. Aside from hypophosphatemia, the most diagnostically important nonspecific laboratory abnormality is a highly elevated serum ferritin level (>2 × normal). Importantly, otherwise unexplained highly elevated ferritin levels are not associated with any other typical or atypical pneumonia. In a hospitalized adult with pneumonia and an otherwise unexplained highly elevated ESR (>90 mm/h), diagnostic possibilities are limited to *S pneumoniae* and Legionnaire's disease. However, with Legionnaire's disease, other characteristic findings will be present, for example, relative bradycardia, hypophosphatemia, elevated ferritin, microscopic hematuria, which are not present in *S pneumoniae* and readily eliminate *S pneumoniae* from further diagnostic consideration (**Table 3**).

The more otherwise unexplained *Legionella* sp characteristic findings present, that is, hypophosphatemia, highly elevated ESR, highly elevated serum ferritin level,

Table 3
Legionnaire's disease: clinical predictors and diagnostic eliminators in admitted adults with pneumonia[a]

Diagnostic Predictors	Diagnostic Eliminators
Clinical predictors	Clinical eliminators
• Fever (>102°F) with relative bradycardia	• Fever (>102°F) without relative bradycardia
Laboratory predictors[b]	• Severe myalgias
• Highly elevated ESR (>90 mm/h) or highly elevated CRP (>35 mg/L)	Laboratory eliminators
• Highly elevated serum ferritin levels (>2 × normal)	• Negative chest radiograph (no infiltrates)
• Hypophosphatemia (on admission/early) or hyponatremia	• No relative lymphopenia
• Elevated CK (>2 × normal)	• Leukopenia
• Microscopic hematuria (on admission)	• Thrombocytopenia
	• Levels of ferritin minimal or not elevated
Legionnaire's disease *very likely if >3 predictors present*	Legionnaire's disease *very unlikely if <3 predictors or any diagnostic eliminators present*

[a] Pulmonary symptoms: shortness of breath, cough, and so forth, with fever and a new focal/segmental infiltrate on chest film.

[b] Otherwise unexplained. If finding is due to an existing disorder, it should not be used as a clinical predictor.

Adapted from Cunha BA, editor. Pneumonia essentials. 3rd edition. Sudbury (MA): Jones & Bartlett; 2010; Cunha BA, Wu G, Raza M. Clinical diagnosis of Legionnaire's disease: six characteristic criteria. Am J Med 2015;128:e21–2.

microscopic hematuria, the more probable is Legionnaire's disease. The presence of several characteristic extrapulmonary findings increases the diagnostic pretest probability of Legionnaire's disease, permitting selective *Legionella* sp testing with serum titers and urinary antigen.

REFERENCES

1. Fraser DW, Tsai TR, Orenstein W, et al. Legionnaire's disease: description of an epidemic of pneumonia. N Engl J Med 1977;297:1189–97.
2. Lattimer GL, Rhodes LV 3rd. Legionnaire's disease. Clinical findings and one-year follow-up. JAMA 1978;240:1169–71.
3. Sharrar RG, Friedman HM, Miller WT, et al. Summertime pneumonias in Philadelphia in 1976. An epidemiologic study. Ann Intern Med 1979;90:577–80.
4. Meyer RD, Edelstein PH, Kirby BD, et al. Legionnaire's disease: unusual clinical and laboratory features. Ann Intern Med 1980;93:240–3.
5. Cunha BA, Quintiliani R. The atypical pneumonias: a diagnostic and therapeutic approach. Postgrad Med 1979;66:95–102.
6. Johnson DH, Cunha BA. Atypical pneumonias. Clinical and extrapulmonary features of Chlamydia, Mycoplasma, and Legionella infections. Postgrad Med 1993; 93:69–72.
7. Musher DM, Thorner AR. Community acquired pneumonia. N Engl J Med 2014; 371:1619–28.
8. Strampfer MJ, Cunha BA. Legionnaire's disease. Semin Respir Infect 1987;2: 228–34.
9. Bouza Santiago E, Rodriguez Creixems M. Legionnaire's disease. Review. Med Clin 1981;77:298–310.
10. Diederen BM. Legionella sp. and Legionnaire's disease. J Infect 2008;56:1–12.
11. Cunha BA, Burillo A, Bouza E. Legionnaire's disease. Lancet 2016;387:376–85.
12. Cunha BA. The atypical pneumonias: clinical diagnosis and importance. Clin Microbiol Infect 2006;3:12–24.
13. Cunha BA. Legionnaire's disease: clinical differentiation from typical and other atypical pneumonias. Infect Dis Clin North Am 2010;24:73–105.
14. Basarab M, Macrae MB, Curtis CM. Atypical pneumonia. Curr Opin Pulm Med 2014;20:247–51.
15. Cunha BA. Atypical pneumonias: current clinical concepts focusing on Legionnaire's disease. Curr Opin Pulm Med 2008;14:183–4.
16. Cunha BA, editor. Pneumonia essentials. 3rd edition. Sudbury (MA): Jones & Bartlett; 2010.
17. Cunha BA, Klein NC, Strollo S, et al. Legionnaires disease mimicking swine influenza (H1N1) pneumonia during the "herald wave" of the pandemic. Heart Lung 2010;39:242–8.
18. Cunha BA. Characteristic predictors that increase the pretest probability of Legionnaire's disease: "don't order a test just because you can" revisited. South Med J 2015;108:761.
19. Viasus D, Di Yacovo S, Garcia-Vidal C, et al. Community-acquired Legionella pneumophila pneumonia: a single-center experience with 214 hospitalized sporadic cases over 15 years. Medicine 2013;92:51–60.
20. Phin N, Parry-Ford F, Harrison T, et al. Epidemiology and clinical management of Legionnaire's disease. Lancet 2014;14:1011–21.
21. Gump DW, Frank RO, Winn WC, et al. Legionnaire's disease in patients with associated serious disease. Ann Intern Med 1979;90:538–42.

22. Vergis EN, Akbas E, Yu VL. Legionella as a cause of severe pneumonia. Semin Respir Crit Care Med 2000;21:295–304.
23. Lowry PW, Tompkins LS. Nosocomial legionellosis: a review of pulmonary and extrapulmonary syndromes. Am J Infect Control 1993;21:21–7.
24. Roig J, Sabria M, Pedro-Botet ML. Legionella sp.: community acquired and nosocomial infections. Curr Opin Infect Dis 2003;16:145–51.
25. Cunha BA, Thekkel V, Schoch PE. Community-acquired versus nosocomial Legionella pneumonia: lessons learned from an epidemiologic investigation. Am J Infect Control 2011;39:901–3.
26. Cunha BA. The diagnostic significance of relative bradycardia in infectious disease. Clin Microbiol Infect 2000;6:633–4.
27. Cunha BA. The clinical diagnosis of Legionnaire's disease: the diagnostic value of combining non-specific laboratory tests. Infection 2008;56:395–7.
28. Cunha BA, Wu G, Raza M. Clinical diagnosis of Legionnaire's disease: six characteristic criteria. Am J Med 2015;128:e21–2.
29. Lo CD, MacKeen AD, Campbell DR, et al. Radiographic analysis of the course of Legionella pneumonia. J Can Assoc Radiol 1983;34:116–9.
30. Coletta FS, Fein AM. Radiological manifestations of Legionella/Legionella-like organisms. Semin Respir Infect 1998;13:109–15.
31. Yu H, Higa F, Hibiya K, et al. Computed tomographic features of 23 sporadic cases with Legionella pneumophila pneumonia. Eur J Radiol 2010;74:e73–8.
32. Johnson JD, Raff MJ, Van Arsdall JA. Neurologic manifestations of Legionnaire's disease. Medicine 1984;63:303–10.
33. Marrie TJ. Q fever pneumonia. Infect Dis Clin North Am 2010;24:27–41.
34. Cunha BA, Nausheen S, Cusch L. Severe Q fever community acquired pneumonia mimicking Legionnaires disease: clinical significance of cold agglutinins, anti-smooth muscle antibodies and thrombocytosis. Heart Lung 2009;38:354–62.
35. Franchini S, Marinosci A, Ferrante L, et al. Pancreatic involvement in Legionella pneumonia. Infection 2015;43:367–70.
36. Cunha BA, Strollo S, Schoch P. Extremely elevated erythrocyte sedimentation rates (ESR) in Legionnaire's disease. Eur J Clin Microbiol Infect Dis 2010;30: 1567–9.
37. Cunha BA. Hypophosphatemia: diagnostic significance in Legionnaire's disease. Am J Med 2006;119:e5–6.
38. Cunha BA. Serum ferritin levels in legionella community-acquired pneumonia. Clin Infect Dis 2008;46:1789–91.
39. Cunha BA, Strollo S, Schoch P. Legionnaire's disease. Incidence and intensity of microscopic hematuria. Infection 2010;61:275–6.
40. Lynch JR 3rd, Fishbein M, Echavarria M. Adenovirus. Semin Respir Crit Care Med 2011;32:494–511.

Legionnaire's Disease and its Mimics: A Clinical Perspective

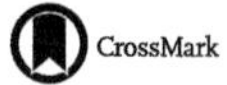

Burke A. Cunha, MD, MACP[a,b,*], Cheston B. Cunha, MD[c]

KEYWORDS

• Q fever • Psittacosis • Influenza like illnesses (ILIs) • Mimics • Adenovirus • HPIV-3

KEY POINTS

- Legionnaire's disease most often manifests as community acquired pneumonia (CAP) with characteristic extrapulmonary features that serve as diagnostic clues.
- Radiologically, legionnaire's disease presents as a rapidly progressive asymmetric multifocal pneumonia.
- For hospitalized adults with fever greater than 38.9°C (102°F), relative bradycardia is an important diagnostic finding in legionnaire's disease. Relative bradycardia also occurs with psittacosis and Q fever, but not with typical bacterial causes of CAP, such as *Streptococcus pneumoniae*, or nonzoonotic atypical pneumonias, such as *Mycoplasma pneumoniae* and *Chlamydophila pneumoniae*.
- Legionnaire's disease mimics are those CAPs that have otherwise unexplained clinical and or laboratory test findings in common with legionnaire's disease; for example, mental confusion, watery diarrhea, acute renal failure, highly increased C-reactive protein (CRP) level or erythrocyte sedimentation rate (ESR), microscopic hematuria, highly otherwise unexplained increased ferritin levels, mildly elevated serum transaminase levels, hypophosphatemia, or hyponatremia.
- Mycoplasma CAP is not usually considered a legionnaire's disease mimic. Except for watery diarrhea, mycoplasma pneumonia does not resemble legionnaire's disease radiographically. Furthermore, with *Mycoplasma* CAP, fevers are usually less than 38.9°C (102°F) (without relative bradycardia), and ESR, CRP, and ferritin levels are not highly increased. Serum transaminase levels are not increased and hypophosphatemia/hyponatremia are also not present. The presence of highly elevated cold agglutinin titers (>1:64) in hospitalized adults with CAP should suggest mycoplasma pneumonia and argues strongly against a diagnosis of legionnaire's disease.

Continued

[a] Infectious Disease Division, Winthrop-University Hospital, 222 Station Plaza North, #432, Mineola, NY 11501, USA; [b] School of Medicine, State University of New York, Stony Brook, NY, USA; [c] Division of Infectious Disease, Rhode Island Hospital, The Miriam Hospital, Brown University Alpert School of Medicine, Providence, RI, USA

* Corresponding author. Infectious Disease Division, Winthrop-University Hospital, 222 Station Plaza North, #432, Mineola, NY 11501.

E-mail address: bacunha@winthrop.org

Infect Dis Clin N Am 31 (2017) 95–109
http://dx.doi.org/10.1016/j.idc.2016.10.008 id.theclinics.com

Continued

- The most common bacterial mimics of legionnaire's disease are *S pneumoniae*, psittacosis, and Q fever.
- In hospitalized adults the most common viral mimics of legionnaire's disease are influenza, and viral pneumonias caused by influenzalike illness; for example, respiratory syncytial virus (RSV), rhinovirus/enterovirus (R/E), human metapneumovirus (hMPV), human parainfluenza virus type 3 (HPIV-3), and adenovirus.

CLINICAL DIAGNOSTIC APPROACH

If a disorder resembles another in one or more clinically important aspects, the potential for one disease masquerading or mimicking another is present. Unlike typical bacterial pneumonias, with clinical findings confined to the lungs, legionnaire's disease, a nonzoonotic atypical pneumonia, has several characteristic extrapulmonary findings. Pneumonias with one or more characteristic features of legionnaire's disease may mimic legionnaire's disease.[1–5] The more characteristics findings there are in common with legionnaire's disease, the more closely a pneumonia mimics legionnaire's disease (**Box 1**).

The characteristic clinical features of legionnaire's disease are not present in all cases.[1,3–5] Furthermore, individually, characteristic findings of legionnaire's disease are not diagnostic of legionnaire's disease. However, when characteristic findings of legionnaire's disease are otherwise unexplained and considered together, the probability of legionnaire's disease is greatly increased.[6] In contrast, clinical findings that are only

Box 1
Legionnaire's disease: characteristic clinical findings that increase pretest probability in hospitalized adults with pneumonia

Clinical findings[a]

- New onset of pneumonia symptoms
- Fever greater than 38.9°C (102°F) (with relative bradycardia)

Chest film features[a]

- New rapidly progressive unilateral or bilateral interstitial/nodular infiltrates
- New rapidly progressive bilateral multifocal infiltrates

Laboratory test abnormalities[a]

- Leukocytosis
- Relative lymphopenia
- Highly increased erythrocyte sedimentation rate (>90 mm/h) or highly increased C-reactive protein level (>180 mg/L)
- Highly increased ferritin levels (>2 × normal)
- Hypophosphatemia (on admission/early)
- Highly increased creatine phosphokinase level (>2 × normal)
- Microscopic hematuria (on admission)

[a] Otherwise unexplained.

Adapted from Cunha BA, Wu G, Raza M. Clinical diagnosis of legionnaire's disease: six characteristic criteria. Am J Med 2015;128:e21–2.

consistent with the diagnosis of legionnaire's disease are not useful diagnostically because they may be present with many other pneumonias; for example, fever, myalgias, headache, pleuritic chest pain, shortness of breath, cough. Similarly, nonspecific laboratory tests consistent with legionnaire's disease may be present in many other community-acquired pneumonias (CAPs); for example, leukocytosis with a left shift and hyponatremia are not useful in narrowing diagnostic possibilities.[7] Disorders that mimic others should have cardinal or characteristic findings in common with the mimicked disorder, but consistent findings are unhelpful diagnostically and should not be considered as legionnaire's disease mimics. Clinicians should be familiar with the characteristic findings of legionnaire's disease as the basis for clinical syndromic diagnosis as well as having the potential for mimicking legionnaire's disease[1–5] (**Table 1**).

With a CAP with extrapulmonary findings and a negative zoonotic contact history, a cardinal finding in legionnaire's disease in hospitalized adults with fever greater than 38.9°C (102°F) is relative bradycardia.[1–4] To be diagnostically meaningful, relative bradycardia must be otherwise unexplained; that is, not a pneumonia with fever if the patient is taking β-blockers, verapamil, or diltiazem (or has a permanent pacemaker or heart block). If a hospitalized adult pneumonia patient has otherwise unexplained relative bradycardia, then the diagnosis is narrowed to Q fever, psittacosis, or legionnaire's disease.[7–10] A negative recent zoonotic contact vector history with cats, sheep, and so forth (Q fever) and psittacine birds (psittacosis) effectively limits the diagnosis of CAP to legionnaire's disease[7] (**Table 2**).

RADIOLOGIC MIMICS OF LEGIONNAIRE'S DISEASE

The main value of the chest film is not in identifying a specific pneumonia pathogen but in eliminating nonpneumonia diagnoses that may resemble pneumonia; for example, congestive heart failure (CHF) or systemic lupus erythematosus (SLE) pneumonitis.[7] Excluding adenoviral pneumonia, a focal segmental/lobar infiltrate on chest radiograph, effectively rules out viral pneumonia.[7,11–13] Following influenza pneumonia, *Streptococcus pneumoniae* or *Haemophilus influenzae* may present as bacterial coinfection, which is not the case with the other respiratory viral influenzalike illnesses (ILIs).[7,14–16] Therefore, with the exception of adenovirus, a focal segmental/lobar chest film infiltrate effectively is a diagnostic eliminator for nearly all viral pneumonias.[13,17] Because legionnaire's disease has no characteristic radiologic appearance either on the chest film or chest computed tomography (CT) scan, many disorders may radiographically resemble legionnaire's disease.[18,19] Chest CT findings are usually reported as having ground-glass opacities or as having a tree-in-bud appearance, but these patterns have a large differential diagnosis and are not specific for legionnaire's disease.[20–22] As mentioned previously, the main value of the chest film in pneumonia differential diagnosis is in eliminating nonpneumonia diagnoses; for example, CHF, SLE, or bronchogenic carcinomas.[7] The presence of focal/segmental infiltrates confined to a lobar distribution argues strongly against legionnaire's disease as the cause of pneumonia.[1–3] If the chest film infiltrates are round or nodular in appearance, this finding is helpful in narrowing the differential diagnosis.[7] There are many causes of round or nodular infiltrates associated with a variety of noninfectious pulmonary disorders, but there are relatively few causes of pneumonia with round or nodular infiltrates.[7,23] Pneumonia with otherwise unexplained new round or nodular infiltrates suggests *S pneumoniae* or Q fever as likely diagnostic possibilities.[23] New bilateral round or nodular infiltrates not only point to legionnaire's disease but particularly suggest *Legionella micdadei* as the most likely *Legionella* species with round or nodular infiltrates.[7,18,24]

Table 1
Legionnaire's disease: clinical mimics in hospitalized adults

	Relative Bradycardia (with Fever >38.9°C [102°F])	Dry Cough	Headache and or Mental Confusion	Loose Stools or Watery Diarrhea
Bacterial LD Clinical Mimics	• Q fever • Psittacosis • Leptospirosis • Any typical bacterial CAP (with drug fever)	• *Mycoplasma pneumoniae* • *Chlamydophila pneumoniae* • Pertussis	• Psittacosis • Q fever • Tularemia • Leptospirosis • *M pneumoniae*[a]	• *M pneumoniae* • Any pneumonia (on stool softeners or laxatives)

Viral LD Clinical Mimics	• Any viral CAP (with drug fever)
	• hMPV (rare)
		• Influenza
		• Respiratory noninfluenza ILI viruses
		  ○ RSV
		  ○ HPIV-3
		  ○ hMPV
		• Adenovirus
			• Influenza
			• Respiratory noninfluenza ILI viruses
			  ○ RSV
			  ○ HPIV-3
			  ○ hMPV
			• Adenovirus
				• Influenza
				• Respiratory noninfluenza ILI viruses
				  ○ RSV
				  ○ HPIV-3
				  ○ hMPV
				• Adenovirus

Noninfectious LD Clinical Mimics	• Hypersensitivity pneumonitis[b] • SLE pneumonitis[b] • Pulmonary hemorrhage[b] • Lymphoma (with pulmonary involvement) • Any pulmonary disorder (with drug fever)	• Bronchogenic carcinomas • CHF	• Bronchogenic carcinomas (with CNS metastases) • SLE cerebritis • Pulmonary sarcoidosis (with basilar meningitis)	• Any pulmonary disorder (on stool softeners or laxatives)

Abbreviations: CHF, congestive heart failure; CNS, central nervous system; hMPV, human metapneumovirus; HPIV-3, human parainfluenza virus-3; ILI, influenzalike illnesses; LD, legionnaire's disease; RSV, respiratory syncytial virus; SLE, systemic lupus erythematosus.

[a] With meningoencephalitis (cold agglutinin titers >1:512).

[b] On β-blockers, verapamil, diltiazem, heart block, or pacemaker rhythm.

Table 2
Relative bradycardia

Temperature, °F (°C)	Appropriate Pulse Response For Temperature, /min	Relative Bradycardia Present If Pulse, /min
106°F (41.1°C)	150/min	<140/min
105°F (40.6°C)	140/min	<130/min
104°F (40.7°C)	130/min	<120/min
103°F (89.4°C)	120/min	<110/min
102°F (38.9°C)	110/min	<100/min

Diagnostic Criteria for Relative Bradycardia: Temperature-Pulse Relationships

Relative bradycardia refers to heart rates that are inappropriately slow relative to body temperature (pulse must be taken simultaneously with temperature increase). Applies to adult patients with temperature greater than or equal to 38.9°C (102°F); does not apply to patients with second-degree/third-degree heart block, pacemaker-induced rhythms, or those on β-blockers, diltiazem, or verapamil.

Adapted from Cunha CB, Cunha BA. Antibiotic Essentials. 15th edition. New Delhi: Jay Pee Medical Publishers; 2016.

In hospitalized adults admitted with CAP, the lack of characteristic radiologic findings by chest radiograph means that chest film findings in viral pneumonias often resemble legionnaire's disease.[14–16] During the 2009 to 1010 swine influenza (H1N1) pandemic, influenza was most often confused with legionnaire's disease.[25–29] With the widespread use of viral respiratory polymerase chain reaction (PCR) in adults, the clinical features of the respiratory noninfluenza viral ILI have become clear.[30] With a specific ILI viral pneumonia diagnosis with viral PCR of respiratory specimens, it has been shown that respiratory syncytial virus (RSV), human parainfluenza virus type 3 (HPIV-3), and human metapneumovirus (hMPV) are the most likely ILI viral pneumonias to have chest film features in common with legionnaire's disease.[31–40]

CHARACTERISTIC CLINICAL FINDINGS IN LEGIONNAIRE'S DISEASE

Clinicians should be aware of the nonspecific characteristic clinical findings in legionnaire's disease and its mimics.[1–5,9,41–45] In admitted adults with CAP and with otherwise unexplained mental confusion, the differential diagnosis is essentially limited and points to legionnaire's disease or *Mycoplasma pneumoniae* meningoencephalitis.[7,41–49] In the setting of CAP, otherwise unexplained loose watery stools suggest legionnaire's disease or *M pneumoniae*.[40,46] With CAPs, excluding influenza with appendicitis, otherwise unexplained abdominal pain occurs only with legionnaire's disease.[2–4,46,50–52]

The diagnostic importance of combining nonspecific but characteristic findings cannot be overemphasized.[6,7] For example, hospitalized adults with CAP with otherwise unexplained relative bradycardia and loose/watery stools likely have legionnaire's disease because *M pneumoniae* is not associated with relative bradycardia.[8,10,44–46] Similarly, if otherwise unexplained abdominal pain is also present with watery diarrhea, then legionnaire's disease is again likely because *M pneumoniae* does not present with abdominal pain[6,8,45,46,50] (**Table 3**).

CHARACTERISTIC NONSPECIFIC LABORATORY ABNORMALITIES OF LEGIONNAIRE'S DISEASE

Nonspecific laboratory abnormalities characteristic of legionnaire's disease include otherwise unexplained hypophosphatemia (early), a highly increased erythrocyte

Table 3
Legionnaire's disease: community acquired pneumonia radiologic mimics

Noninfectious CAP CXR Mimics		Bacterial CAP LD CXR Mimics	Viral CAP LD CXR Mimics
With Fever	**Without Fever**		
• SLE pneumonitis • CHF (caused by MI) • Pulmonary embolus/ infarction • Pulmonary hemorrhage • Hypersensitivity pneumonitis • Lymphoma (involving the lungs)	• CHF (no MI) • BOOP • Bronchogenic carcinomas • Pulmonary sarcoidosis • PAP • Lung metastases	• *S pneumoniae*[a] • Q fever[a] • *L micdadei*[a] • Pertussis	• Adenovirus • Influenza • Some respiratory viral noninfluenza ILIs ○ HPIV-3[b] ○ hMPV[b] ○ RSV[b]

Abbreviations: BOOP, bronchiolitis obliterans with organizing pneumonia; CXR, chest radiograph; MI, myocardial infarction; PAP, pulmonary alveolar proteinosis.
[a] Adults may have nodular infiltrates.
[b] Adults may have asymmetrical infiltrates.

sedimentation rate (ESR) (>90 mm/h), highly increased serum ferritin levels (>2 × normal), and microscopic hematuria.[53–56] The more such otherwise unexplained characteristic legionnaire's disease findings are present, the more likely is legionnaire's disease.[6,57–59] A less highly increased ESR or ferritin level is consistent with, but not characteristic of, legionnaire's disease and accordingly has no diagnostic specificity.[7,50] Similarly, an otherwise unexplained increased creatine phosphokinase (CPK) level, acute pancreatitis, or acute renal insufficiency (ARI) may occur with legionnaire's disease, but also may be caused by a variety of other disorders.[1–4,7,50,59–61] The diagnostic probability of legionnaire's disease increases with the number of characteristic legionnaire's disease findings present concurrently; that is, the more characteristic findings that are present, the more likely is legionnaire's disease[6,58,60] (**Table 4**).

RELATIVE DIAGNOSTIC WEIGHTS OF CLINICAL CHARACTERISTIC LEGIONNAIRE'S DISEASE FINDINGS

Even characteristic findings have different diagnostic weights or diagnostic importance; for example, otherwise unexplained hypophosphatemia is a highly weighted characteristic finding because no other cause of CAP is associated with decreased serum phosphorus levels.[7,50,57] Characteristic, but less highly weighted, are otherwise unexplained increased serum transaminase levels in patients with CAP.[7,45,58,60] Although no typical cause of CAP is accompanied by mildly/transiently increased serum transaminase levels, increases in transaminase levels are common in Q fever, psittacosis, and legionnaire's disease.[1–4,7,50] Importantly, increased serum transaminase levels are not part of the extrapulmonary organ involvement pattern of *M pneumoniae*; that is, in hepatic involvement manifested by increased serum transaminase levels in patients with CAP, *M pneumoniae* is exceeding unlikely (essentially ruled out).[61] Therefore, the more highly weighted characteristic findings of legionnaire's

Table 4
Legionnaire's disease: pneumonia with nonspecific laboratory abnormalities

	Noninfectious LD Laboratory Mimics	Bacterial LD Laboratory Mimics	Viral LD Laboratory Test Mimics
Leukocytosis	Any pulmonary disorder (with fever)	Any bacterial pneumonia	• Influenza • Respiratory viral ILIs: ○ ILI: RSV, hMPV, HPIV-3 • Adenovirus
Relative lymphopenia	Any pulmonary disorder (on steroids or immunosuppressive drugs)	None	• Influenza • Respiratory viral ILIs: ○ RSV ○ hMPV ○ HPIV-3 • Adenovirus
Highly ↑ ESR (>100 mm/h) and or highly ↑ CRP (>180 mg/L)	Pulmonary emboli/infarction	*S pneumoniae*	None
Highly ↑ serum ferritin levels (>2 × normal)	• Any malignancy involving the lungs • Any cause of renal insufficiency (with pulmonary infiltrates)	• Q fever • PCP	• hMPV • Adenovirus
Hyponatremia	Any pulmonary disorder	Any bacterial pneumonia	Any viral pneumonia
Hypophosphatemia	None	None	• hMPV (rare) • Adenovirus (rare)
Highly increased CPK	SLE	• Leptospirosis • Tularemia	• Influenza • HPIV-3 • Adenovirus
Mildly increased serum transaminases	EBV infectious mononucleosis (with pulmonary involvement)	• Q fever • Psittacosis • Tularemia • Leptospirosis	• Influenza • Respiratory viral ILIs ○ RSV ○ hMPV ○ HPIV-3 • Adenovirus

Abbreviations: CRP, C-reactive protein; ILIs, influenza like illnesses; LD, Legionnaire's disease; PCP, *Pneumocystis* (*carinii*) *jiroveci* pneumonia.

disease are present, the more likely it is that the condition is caused by legionnaire's disease or one of its mimics.[4,58,60]

When should clinicians suspect a mimic of legionnaire's disease? First, as explained, clinicians must be familiar with the relative diagnostic importance (ie, diagnostic weights) of characteristic legionnaire's disease findings; for example, hypophosphatemia versus hyponatremia. If otherwise unexplained hyponatremia is present, mimicking is less likely because hyponatremia may occur with any CAP.[7,50,58] Mimics of legionnaire's disease should be suspected when 1 or more characteristic legionnaire's disease findings are present, when there is often sufficient time for increases in *Legionella* antibody titers and urinary antigen tests are negative[44,45,62,63] (**Table 5**).

Table 5
Pneumonias with increased ferritin levels and other infectious and noninfectious disorders

Infectious Causes	
Pneumonias	**Nonpneumonias**
• LD[a,b] • Adenovirus pneumonia[a,b] • PCP[a,b]	• WNE • EBV • CMV • Toxoplasmosis • *Staphylococcus aureus* ABE • Malaria • Babesiosis • Ehrlichiosis/anaplasmosis
Noninfectious Causes	
May Have Lung Involvement	**No Lung Involvement**
• Chronic renal failure (fluid overload) • Rheumatoid arthritis (rheumatoid lung) • Bronchogenic carcinomas (or any pulmonary malignancy)	• Nonpulmonary malignancies • MPD • Adult Still's disease • SLE • TA • AOCD • Hemochromatosis • Chronic hepatitis (HCV)

Abbreviations: ABE, acute bacterial endocarditis; AOCD, anemia of chronic disease; CMV, cytomegalovirus; EBV, Epstein-Barr virus; HCV, hepatitis C virus; MPD, myeloproliferative disorders; TA, temporal arteritis; WNE, West Nile encephalitis.

[a] Otherwise unexplained and not caused by other disorders associated with increased ferritin levels.

[b] Acute phase ferritin level increases (n $\leq$186 ng/mL) are transient minimal increases, (eg, 187–200 ng/mL). In contrast, diagnostically important non–acute phase ferritin level increases are much higher; for example, greater than 2 $\times$ normal (>375 ng/mL) and persist for days.

Adapted from Cunha CB. Infectious disease differential diagnosis. In: Cunha CB, Cunha BA, editors. Antibiotic essentials. 15th edition. New Delhi: JayPee Medical Publishers: 2017; and Kroll V, Cunha BA. Diagnostic significance of serum ferritin levels in infectious and non-infectious diseases. Infectious Disease Practice 2003;27:199–2.

Among admitted adults with CAP, some have used increased serum procalcitonin (PCT) levels as indicators of legionnaire's disease. However, increased PCT levels are not specific for legionnaire's disease and may be caused by a variety of infectious and noninfectious disorders.[50] The diagnostic uselessness of PCT levels is shown in severe CAP in the intensive care unit. Any cause of ARI may result in increased PCT levels.[50] Legionnaire's disease is often accompanied by ARI, making interpretation of increased PCT levels in this setting unhelpful at best.[64,65]

DIAGNOSTIC IMPORTANCE OF THE TIME COURSE OF CLINICAL FINDINGS

Diagnostically, clinicians should also take into account the time course of findings; that is, clinical as well as most nonspecific test abnormalities develop or resolve as a function of time.[66–68] Early laboratory test abnormalities of legionnaire's disease include otherwise unexplained hypophosphatemia and microscopic hematuria.[53,56] In contrast, otherwise unexplained relative lymphopenia, as with viral ILI mimics, may be present at any time during hospitalization.[26] Other laboratory test abnormalities may occur later or become more increased over time; for example, otherwise unexplained highly increased serum ferritin levels in legionnaire's disease or thrombocytosis in Q fever or *M pneumoniae* CAP.[47,55,66] The diagnostic approach takes into account that, if a particular characteristic laboratory abnormality is not present in a particular case, it may not be present, may have been positive but missed in early testing, or may have yet to become increased or may become more increased over time.[46,66] If a disease is typically associated with characteristic laboratory test abnormalities that are not initially abnormal, it is prudent to repeat these studies during the hospital stay to detect these abnormalities if not present early in hospitalization.[43,44]

LEGIONNAIRE'S DISEASE DIAGNOSTIC TESTING

Specific diagnostic tests for legionnaire's disease are a different matter. An early diagnosis confirmed by sputum culture, increased *Legionella* serum titers, or a positive *Legionella* urinary antigen test is always hoped for. However, positive results with these tests are also time (and species) dependent. In untreated patients, *Legionella* diagnostic titer increases usually occur after 4 to 6 weeks.[57] Titer increases are a function of the host's immune response later in the time course of infection. Furthermore, effective anti-*Legionella* antimicrobial therapy may blunt, delay, or eliminate titer increases. Some individuals never develop a titer increase.[1–4,50]

Legionella urinary antigen tests only for *Legionella pneumophila* (serogroup 1), but do not detect non–*L pneumophila* species.[7] Commonly, the *Legionella* urinary antigen test may be negative initially and may take days to weeks to become positive but then remains positive for weeks to months.[7,62,63]

In patients with several characteristic legionnaire's disease findings present, and persistently negative *Legionella* titers and urinary antigen testing may be clues to a legionnaire's disease mimic. Depending on other clinical findings present, specific diagnostic tests should be ordered to diagnose the causes of the pneumonia masquerading as legionnaire's disease.

THE CLINICAL USEFULNESS OF DIAGNOSTIC ELIMINATORS

The clinical application of the concept of diagnostic eliminators may be helpful in identifying potential legionnaire's disease mimics. Diagnostic eliminators have the important but opposite diagnostic significance of characteristic findings. Diagnostic eliminators are not the same as the absence of characteristic findings in clinical syndromic diagnosis.[42] Diagnostic eliminators are characteristic features that argue strongly against the diagnosis; for example, if legionnaire's disease is being considered in the differential diagnosis of pneumonia, then fever greater than 38.9°C (102°F) without relative bradycardia should be considered as a diagnostic eliminator.[6,14,58]

Consistent, but not characteristic, hematologic findings in legionnaire's disease are leukocytosis with a left shift and a normal platelet count.[1,50] However, either otherwise unexplained leukopenia with thrombocytosis or thrombocytopenia may be used as a diagnostic eliminator for legionnaire's disease.[7,50] In hospitalized adults with CAP in which legionnaire's disease is being considered in the differential diagnosis, these findings should suggest a viral etiology and effectively eliminate legionnaire's disease from further consideration.[14–16,50,67–69] Diagnostic tests should be ordered to identify other causes of CAP in which these finding are characteristic; for example, influenza or viral ILI pneumonias.[31–39] Similarly, as with influenza A, otherwise unexplained relative lymphopenia is a characteristic legionnaire's disease test abnormality. In contrast, the finding of otherwise unexplained lymphocytosis is in effect a diagnostic eliminator for legionnaire's disease. Diagnostic eliminators may provide important clues to legionnaire's disease mimics.[7,50]

COMMON LEGIONNAIRE'S DISEASE MIMICS

The zoonotic atypical CAPs pneumonias most likely to mimic legionnaire's disease are Q fever and psittacosis.[7,9,41,70–76] The zoonotic atypical pneumonias less likely to mimic legionnaire's disease are leptospirosis and tularemia.[7,77–79] Typically, tularemia pneumonia is not accompanied by relative bradycardia but is accompanied by a bloody pleural effusion and hilar adenopathy, which are not features of legionnaire's disease.[7,78,79]

The nonzoonotic atypical pneumonia often confused with legionnaire's disease is caused by *M pneumoniae*.[7,45,47,80] Although *M pneumoniae* has some consistent features in common with legionnaire's disease, there are too many important clinical differences and diagnostic eliminators to be considered as a mimic; for example, hospitalized adults with *M pneumoniae* CAP usually have fever less than 38.9°C (102°F) without relative bradycardia.[7,45–49] Throat or ear pain are common with *M pneumoniae* and are diagnostic eliminators for legionnaire's disease. Otherwise unexplained increased transaminase levels are the rule in legionnaire's disease but are not a feature with *M pneumoniae*.[7,80] *M pneumoniae* diagnostic eliminators include a highly increased ESR (>90 mm/h), highly increased ferritin level (>2 × normal), hypophosphatemia, and microscopic hematuria, which are characteristic findings in legionnaire's disease but are not features of *M pneumoniae* CAP.[7,48,49] However, otherwise unexplained highly increased cold agglutinin titers are a diagnostic eliminator for legionnaire's disease, but should suggest *M pneumoniae* or a less likely viral a pneumonia cause[48,50] (**Table 6**).

Table 6
Legionnaire's disease: clinical predictors and diagnostic eliminators in hospitalized adults with pneumonia

Diagnostic Predictors	Diagnostic Eliminators	
Clinical predictors[a]: • Fever >38.9°C (102°F) (with relative bradycardia) Laboratory predictors[a]: • Highly increased ESR (>90 mm/h) or CRP level (>180 mg/L) • Highly increased ferritin levels (>2 × normal) • Hypophosphatemia (on admission/early) • Highly increased CPK level (>2 × normal) • Microscopic hematuria (on admission)	Chest film eliminators: • CXR (with no infiltrates) • CXR (only if with segmental/lobar infiltrates)	Clinical eliminators[a]: • Fever >38.9°C (102°F) (without relative bradycardia) • Sore throat • Hoarseness • Severe myalgias • Splenomegaly Laboratory eliminators[a]: • Leukopenia • Lymphocytosis • Thrombocytopenia • Thrombocytosis • Highly increased cold agglutinin titers (>1:64)
LD highly likely if >3 (1 clinical plus ≥2 laboratory) clinical predictors present	LD unlikely if <3 clinical predictors present	LD very unlikely if >3 clinical eliminators (ie, 1 clinical eliminator [relative bradycardia] plus >2 laboratory diagnostic eliminators) present

[a] Otherwise unexplained. If finding caused by another disorder, it should not be used as a diagnostic predictor or diagnostic eliminator.

Adapted from Cunha BA, Wu G, Raza M. Clinical diagnosis of legionnaire's disease: six characteristic criteria. Am J Med 2015;128:e21–2.

Among the viral pneumonias, influenza, ILIs (hMPV, RSV, HPIV-3), and adenoviral pneumonia are the most common legionnaire's disease mimics.[17,26,34] In hospitalized adults, ILI viral pneumonias may resemble the radiologic appearance of legionnaire's disease (eg, bilateral multifocal infiltrates), and, if other findings of legionnaire's disease are present, the stage is set for mimicking legionnaire's disease. Some viral ILIs occasionally have nonspecific laboratory abnormalities in common with legionnaire's disease, providing added potential to mimic legionnaire's disease.

The nonviral CAPs most likely to be considered in the differential diagnosis of legionnaire's disease are bacteremic *S pneumoniae* pneumonia, Q fever, and psittacosis.[45,70–76] Bacteremic pneumococcal pneumonia may be accompanied by a highly increased ESR, but may readily be differentiated from legionnaire's disease by the absence of relative bradycardia, abdominal pain, hypophosphatemia, increased ferritin and transaminase levels, ARI, or microscopic hematuria, and is readily diagnosed by blood cultures or pneumococcal urinary antigen.[7,50] For Q fever or psittacosis to be considered in the differential diagnosis of a zoonotic atypical CAP, a history of recent vector contact is required. However, particularly with Q fever, sheep and other animal contact aside, most patients do not have a cat, and often fail to mention being in recent close proximity to a parturient cat.[7,9,74]

If Q fever versus legionnaire's disease is in the differential diagnosis, there is another potential problem with serologic diagnosis. Clinicians should be aware of potential cross reactivity between Q fever and *Legionella* titers, particularly with *L micdadei*.[81–83] Rarely, there may be coinfection with legionnaire's disease and bacteremic *S pneumoniae* pneumonia.[84] Alternately, coinfection with Q fever and legionnaire's disease may also be considered but is reportedly rare. *Legionella* and Q fever cross reactivity is common and is much more likely than bona fide coinfection.[81–85]

REFERENCES

1. Lattimer GL, Rhodes LV 3rd. Legionnaire's disease. Clinical findings and one-year follow-up. JAMA 1978;240:169–71.
2. Woodhead MA, Macfarlane JT. The protean manifestations of Legionnaire's disease. J R Physi 1985;19:224–30.
3. Woodhead MA, Macfarlane JT. Legionnaire's disease: a review of 79 community acquired cases in Nottingham. Thorax 1986;41:635–40.
4. Strampfer MA, Cunha BA. Clinical and laboratory aspects of Legionnaire's disease. Semin Respir Infect 1987;2:228–34.
5. Cunha BA. Clinical features of Legionnaire's disease. Semin Respir Infect 1998; 13:116–27.
6. Cunha BA. The clinical diagnosis of Legionnaire's disease: the diagnostic value of combining non-specific laboratory tests. J Infect 2008;56:395–7.
7. Cunha BA, editor. Pneumonia essentials. 3rd edition. Sudbury (MA): Jones & Bartlett; 2010.
8. Cunha BA. The diagnostic significance of relative bradycardia in infectious disease. Clin Microbiol Infect 2000;6:633–4.
9. Lattimer GL, Rhodes LV 3rd. Psittacosis or Legionnaire's disease? Lancet 1979; 1:724.
10. Gacouin A, Revest M, Letheulle J, et al. Distinctive features between community acquired pneumonia due to *Chlamydophila psittaci* and CAP due to *Legionella pneumophila* admitted to the intensive care unit. Eur J Clin Microbiol Infect Dis 2012;31:2713–8.

11. Cunha BA, Syed U, Mickail N. Systemic lupus erythematosus pneumonitis mimicking swine influenza pneumonia during the swine influenza (H1N1) pandemic. Heart & Lung 2011;40:482–6.
12. Rizzo C, Caporali MG, Rota MC. Pandemic influenza and pneumonia due to *Legionella pneumophila*: a frequently underestimated coinfection. Clin Infect Dis 2010;51:115.
13. Cunha BA, Syed U, Strollo S. Swine influenza (H1N1) pneumonia in hospitalized adults: chest film findings. Heart & Lung 2011;40:253–6.
14. Falsey AR, Walsh EE. Viral pneumonia in older adults. Clin Infect Dis 2006;42: 518–24.
15. Ruuskanen O, Lahti E, Jennings LC, et al. Viral pneumonia. Lancet 2011;377: 1264–75.
16. Cesairo TC. Viruses associated with pneumonia in adults. Clin Infect Dis 2012;55: 107–13.
17. Cunha BA. Severe adenovirus mimicking legionella community acquired pneumonia (CAP). Eur J Clin Microbiol Infect Dis 2009;28:313–5.
18. Coletta FS, Fein AM. Radiological manifestations of *Legionella*/*Legionella*-like organisms. Semin Respir Infect 1998;13:109–15.
19. Zhang z, Liu X, Chen L, et al. Chest radiographic characteristics of community acquired *Legionella* pneumonia in the elderly. Chin Med J 2014;127:2270–4.
20. Kim KW, Goo JM, Lee HJ, et al. Chest computed tomographic findings and clinical features of legionella pneumonia. J Comput Assist Tomogr 2007;31:950–5.
21. Yu H, Higa F, Hibiya K, et al. Computed tomographic features of 23 sporadic cases with *Legionella pneumophila* pneumonia. Eur J Radiol 2010;74:e73–8.
22. Haroon A, Higa F, Hibiya K, et al. Organizing pneumonia pattern in the follow-up CT of *Legionella*-infected patients. J Infect Chemother 2011;17:493–8.
23. Cunha BA, Gran A, Simon J. Round pneumonia in a 50-year old man. Respir Care 2013;58:e80–2.
24. Gobbo PN, Strampfer MA, Schoch P, et al. *Legionella micdadei* pneumonia in normal hosts. Lancet 1986;2:969.
25. Cunha BA, Pherez FM, Strollo S. Swine influenza (H1N1): diagnostic dilemmas early in the pandemic. Scand J Infect Dis 2009;41:900–2.
26. Cunha BA. Swine influenza (H1N1) pneumonia: clinical considerations. Infect Dis Clin North Am 2010;24:203–28.
27. Cunha BA, Mickail N, Thekkel V. Unexplained increased incidence of Legionnaire's disease during the "Herald Wave" of the H1 N1 influenza pandemic. Infect Control Hosp Epidemiol 2010;31:562–3.
28. Cunha BA, Klein NC, Strollo S, et al. Legionnaire's disease mimicking swine influenza (H1N1) pneumonia during the "herald wave" of the pandemic. Heart & Lung 2010;39:242–8.
29. Cunha BA, Pherez FM, Schoch P. Diagnostic importance of relative lymphopenia as a marker of swine influenza (H1N1) in adults. Clin Infect Dis 2009;49:1454–6.
30. Karadag-Oncel E, Ciblak MA, Ozsurekci Y, et al. Viral etiology of influenza-like illnesses during the influenza season between December 2011 and April 2012. J Med Virol 2014;86:865–71.
31. Ong DS, Faber TE, Klein Klouwenberg PM, et al. Respiratory syncytial virus in critically ill adult patients with community acquired respiratory failure: a prospective observational study. Clin Microbiol Infect 2014;20:505–7.
32. Volling C, Hassan K, Mazzulli T, et al. Respiratory syncytial virus infection-associated hospitalization in adults: a retrospective cohort study. BMC Infect Dis 2014;14:655.

33. Widmer K, Griffen MR, Zhu Y, et al. Respiratory syncytial virus and human metapneumovirus-associated emergency department and hospital burden in adults. Influenza Other Respir Viruses 2014;8:347–52.
34. Falsley AR, McElhaney JE, Beran J, et al. Respiratory syncytial virus and other respiratory viral infections in older adults with moderate to severe influenza-like illness. J Infect Dis 2014;209:1873–81.
35. Jain B, Singh AK, Dangi T, et al. High prevalence of human metapneumovirus subtype B in cases presenting as severe acute respiratory illness: an experience at tertiary care hospital. Clin Respir J 2014;8:225–33.
36. Johnstone J, Majumdar SR, Fox JD, et al. Human metapneumovirus pneumonia in adults: results of a prospective study. Clin Infect Dis 2008;46:571–4.
37. Souza JS, Watanabe A, Carraro E, et al. Severe metapneumovirus infections among immunocompetent and immunocompromised patients admitted to hospital with respiratory infection. J Med Virol 2013;85:530–6.
38. Kroll JL, Weinberg A. Human metapneumovirus. Semin Respir Crit Care Med 2011;32:447–53.
39. Cunha BA, Irshad N, Connolly JJ. Adult human metapneumonovirus (hMPV) pneumonia mimicking Legionnaire's disease. Heart & Lung 2016;45:270–2.
40. Cunha BA, Raza M. During influenza season: all influenza like illnesses (ILIs) are not due to influenza: dengue mimicking influenza. J Emerg Med 2015;48: e117–20.
41. Cunha BA, Quintiliani R. The atypical pneumonias: a diagnostic and therapeutic approach. Postgrad Med 1979;66:95–102.
42. Cunha BA, Ortega AM. Atypical pneumonia. Extrapulmonary clues guide the way to diagnosis. Postgrad Med 1996;99:123–8.
43. Cunha BA. Atypical pneumonias: current clinical concepts focusing on Legionnaire's disease. Curr Opin Pulm Med 2008;14:183–94.
44. Cunha BA. Legionnaire's disease: clinical differentiation from typical and other atypical pneumonias. Infect Dis Clin North Am 2010;24:73–105.
45. Woodhead MA, Macfarlane JT. Comparative clinical and laboratory features of legionella with pneumococcal and mycoplasma pneumonias. Br J Dis Chest 1987; 81:133–9.
46. Cotton LM, Strampfer MJ, Cunha BA. Legionella and mycoplasma pneumonia–a community hospital experience with atypical pneumonias. Clin Chest Med 1987; 8:441–53.
47. Cunha BA, Pherez FM. *Mycoplasma pneumoniae* community acquired pneumonia in the elderly: diagnostic significance of acute thrombocytosis. Heart & Lung 2009;38:444–9.
48. Cunha BA. The clinical diagnosis of *Mycoplasma pneumoniae*: the diagnostic importance of highly elevated serum cold agglutinins. Eur J Clin Microbiol Infect Dis 2008;27:1017–9.
49. Clyde WA Jr. Clinical overview of *Mycoplasma pneumoniae* infections. Clin Infect Dis 1993;1:s32–6.
50. Cunha CB. Infectious disease differential diagnosis. In: Cunha CB, Cunha BA, editors. Antibiotic essentials. 15th edition. New Delhi (India): Jay Pee Med Pub; 2016.
51. Cunha BA, Patel A, Grendell J, et al. The gastrointestinal manifestations with swine influenza (H1N1) in hospitalized adults. Scand J Infect Dis 2011;43:79–80.
52. Cunha BA, Pherez FM, Durie N. Swine influenza (H1N1) and acute appendicitis. Heart & Lung 2010;39:544–6.

53. Cunha BA. Hypophosphatemia: a diagnostic significance in Legionnaire's disease. Am J Med 2006;119:e5–6.
54. Cunha BA, Strollo S, Schoch P. Extremely elevated erythrocyte sedimentation rates (ESRs) in Legionnaire's disease. Eur J Clin Microbiol Infect Dis 2010;29:1567–9.
55. Cunha BA. Highly elevated serum ferritin levels as a diagnostic marker for *Legionella* pneumonia. Clin Infect Dis 2008;46:1789–91.
56. Cunha BA, Strollo S, Schoch P. *Legionella pneumophila* community acquired pneumonia (CAP): incidence and intensity of microscopic hematuria. J Infect 2010;61:275–6.
57. Cunha BA. Characteristic predictors that increase the pretest probability of Legionnaire's disease: "Don't order a test just because you can" revisited. South Med J 2015;108:761.
58. Cunha BA, Wu G, Raza M. Clinical diagnosis of Legionnaire's disease: six characteristic criteria. Am J Med 2015;128:e21–2.
59. Cunha BA. Severe legionella pneumonia: rapid diagnosis with Winthrop-University Hospital's Weighted Point Score System (Modified). Heart & Lung 2008;37:312–21.
60. Westblom TU, Hamory BH. Acute pancreatitis caused by *Legionella pneumophila*. South Med J 1988;81:1200–1.
61. Brewster UC. Acute renal failure associated with legionellosis. Ann Intern Med 2004;140:406–7.
62. Phin N, Parry-Ford F, Harrison T, et al. Epidemiology and clinical management of Legionnaire's disease. Lancet Infect Dis 2014;14:1011–21.
63. Cunha BA, Burillo A, Bouza E. Legionnaire's disease. Lancet 2016;387:376–85.
64. Cunha BA. Empiric antimicrobial therapy of community acquired pneumonia: clinical diagnosis versus procalcitonin levels. Scand J Infect Dis 2009;41:782–4.
65. Cunha BA, Syed U, Strollo S. Swine influenza (H1N1) pneumonia: elevated serum procalcitonin levels not due to superimposed bacterial pneumonia. Int J Antimicrob Agents 2010;35:515–6.
66. Cunha BA. Swine influenza (H1N1) pneumonia: bacterial airway colonization common but fatalities due to bacterial pneumonia remain relatively rare. J Clin Virol 2010;47:199–200.
67. Cunha BA, Nausheen S, Busch L. Severe Q fever community-acquired pneumonia mimicking Legionnaire's disease: clinical significance of cold agglutinins, anti-smooth muscle antibodies and thrombocytosis. Heart & Lung 2009;38:354–62.
68. Cunha BA, Corbett M, Mickail N. Human parainfluenza virus type 3 (HPIV-3) viral community-acquired pneumonia (CAP) mimicking swine influenza (H1N1) during the swine flu pandemic. Heart & Lung 2011;40:76–80.
69. Cunha BA, Connolly JJ, Irshad N. The clinical usefulness of lymphocyte:monocyte ratios in differentiating influenza from viral non-influenza like illnesses in hospitalized adults during the 2015 influenza A (H3N2) epidemic: the uniqueness of HPIV-3 mimicking influenza A. Eur J Clin Microbiol Infect Dis 2016;35:155–8.
70. Wspejo E, Gil-Diaz A, Oteo JA, et al. Clinical presentation of acute Q fever in Spain: seasonal and geographical differences. Int J Infect Dis 2014;26:162–4.
71. Nett RJ, Helgerson SD, Anderson AD. Clinician assessment for *Coxiella burnetii* infection in hospitalized patients with potentially compatible illnesses during Q fever outbreaks and following a health alert, Montana, 2011. Vector Borne Zoonotic Dis 2013;13:128–30.

72. Schack M, Sachse S, Rodel J, et al. *Coxiella burnetii* (Q fever) as a cause of community acquired pneumonia during the warm season in Germany. Epidemiol Infect 2014;142:1905–10.
73. Keijemel SP, Krijger E, Delsing CE, et al. Differentiation of acute Q fever from other infections in patients presenting to hospitals, the Netherlands. Emerg Infect Dis 2015;21:1348–56.
74. Nausheen S, Cunha BA. Q fever community acquired pneumonia in a patient with Crohn's disease on immunosuppressive therapy. Heart & Lung 2007;36:300–3.
75. Branley JM, Weston KM, England J, et al. Clinical features of endemic community-acquired psittacosis. New Microbes New Infect 2014;2:7–12.
76. Spoorenberg SM, Bos WJ, van Hannen EJ, et al. *Chlamydia psittaci*: a relevant cause of community-acquired pneumonia in two Dutch hospitals. Neth J Med 2016;74:75–81.
77. Teglia OF, Battagliotti C, Villavicencio RL, et al. Leptospiral pneumonia. Chest 1995;108:874–5.
78. Gill V, Cunha BA. Tularemia pneumonia. Semin Respir Infect 1997;12:61–7.
79. Thomas LD, Schaffner W. Tularemia pneumonia. Infect Dis Clin North Am 2010; 24:43–55.
80. Cunha BA. Elevated serum transaminases in patients with *Mycoplasma pneumoniae* pneumonia. Clin Microbiol Infect 2005;11:1051–2.
81. Dwyer DE, Gibbons VL, Brady M, et al. Serological reaction to *Legionella pneumophila* group 4 in a patient with Q fever. J Infect Dis 1988;158:499–500.
82. Finidori JP, Raoult D, Bornstein N, et al. Study of cross-reaction between *Coxiella burnetii* and *Legionella pneumophila* using indirect immunofluorescence assay and immunoblotting. Acta Virol 1992;36:459–65.
83. Musso D, Raoult D. Serological cross-reactions between *Coxiella burnetii* and *Legionella micdadei*. Clin Diagn Lab Immunol 1997;4:208–12.
84. Tan MJ, Tan JS, File TM Jr. Legionnaire's disease with bacteremic coinfection. Clin Infect Dis 2002;35:533–9.
85. Khatib R, Fakih MG. Optimal criteria for the diagnosis of *Legionella* coinfection. Clin Infect Dis 2003;36:384.

Severe Pneumonia Caused by *Legionella pneumophila*

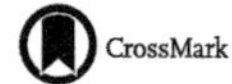

Differential Diagnosis and Therapeutic Considerations

Abdullah Chahin, MD[a,b,*], Steven M. Opal, MD[a,b]

KEYWORDS

- Legionnaire's disease • Severe community-acquired pneumonia
- *Legionella pneumophila* • Pneumonia complications • Hospital-acquired pneumonia
- *Legionella pneumophila* outbreaks

KEY POINTS

- Severe legionella pneumonia poses a diagnostic challenge and requires early intervention.
- Legionnaire's disease can have several presenting signs, symptoms, and laboratory abnormalities that suggest that *Legionella pneumophila* is the pathogen, but none of these are sufficient to distinguish *L pneumophila* pneumonia from other respiratory pathogens.
- *L pneumophila* is primarily an intracellular pathogen and needs treatment with antibiotics that efficiently enter the intracellular space.

Legionnaire's disease is one of the most important nonzoonotic, atypical infections that affect humans. Pneumonia is the predominant clinical manifestation of *Legionella* spp infection in humans. Legionellosis is consistently reported among the top 3 most commonly identified respiratory pathogens in community-acquired pneumonia, in addition to being a reported cause of hospital-acquired pneumonia.[1–4] *Legionella pneumophila* pneumonia is associated with high morbidity, as shown by the high proportion of patients requiring intensive care unit (ICU) admission. However, mortalities for severe *Legionella* spp pneumonia have decreased significantly with the realization that early, targeted therapy that covers this pathogen improves outcome.[4,5] This article focuses on severe legionella pneumonia epidemiology, clinical manifestations, laboratory findings, treatment and outcomes, and the differential diagnostic considerations.

[a] Critical Care Division, Miriam Hospital, Brown University Alpert School of Medicine, Providence, RI, USA; [b] Infectious Disease Division, Rhode Island Hospital, Brown University Alpert School of Medicine, Providence, RI, USA
* Corresponding author. Memorial Hospital of Rhode Island, 111 Brewster Street, Pawtucket, RI 02860.
E-mail address: Abdullah_Chahin@brown.edu

Infect Dis Clin N Am 31 (2017) 111–121
http://dx.doi.org/10.1016/j.idc.2016.10.009

EPIDEMIOLOGY

Legionella pneumonia accounts for about 2% to 15% of all community-acquired pneumonias that require hospitalization in Europe and North America.[6] Patients with legionnaire's disease are more likely to have severe community-acquired pneumonia (SCAP) than those with most other atypical respiratory pathogens. SCAP is defined by more severely abnormal vital signs, more extensive infiltrates on chest radiography, and the need for admission to the ICU.[7–11] For nosocomial legionella pneumonia, the epidemiology has shifted from large outbreaks in tertiary care centers in the 1980s to sporadic cases in community hospitals in more recent years.[12]

The incidence of nosocomial legionella pneumonia is directly related to the lack of availability of in-house testing and lack of due diligence to carefully monitor for the presence of a contaminated water source in the hospital. These nosocomial infections are preventable by careful environmental management in the hospital setting.[13] A single case of nosocomial legionellosis is a priori evidence of a contaminated water supply within the institution. Such an occurrence should immediately prompt an environmental investigation by infection control and environmental services to identify the contaminated water supply and rectify the source of contamination. Person-to-person transmission does not occur and hospital outbreaks indicate a common source of exposure to contaminated water supplies within the hospital.

Factors that have been associated with high severity and mortality in legionella are extremes of age (infants and old patients), nosocomial acquisition, underlying conditions (eg, chronic lung disease, immunodeficiency, solid organ transplants, human immunodeficiency virus, end-stage renal disease, malignancies, and diabetes mellitus), and delayed initiation of proper antimicrobial therapy.[14] Possible predisposing factors and prognostic factors for severe *L pneumophila* pneumonia are listed in **Table 1**.

CLINICAL MANIFESTATIONS AND LABORATORY DIAGNOSIS

Legionella is one of the most commonly misdiagnosed pathogens as a cause severe community-acquired pneumonia. Multiple studies have shown it to be underdiagnosed and undertreated.[15] *Legionella* spp cause an array of respiratory illnesses but this article focuses on SCAP and nosocomial infections. SCAP is operationally defined as community-acquired pneumonia of sufficient severity to warrant ICU care for ventilatory and/or hemodynamic support. Delayed diagnosis of legionellosis is partly

Table 1
Predisposing factors and prognostic factors

Predisposing Factors	Prognostic Indicators
Extremes of age	Extremes of age
Smoking	Chronic lung disease
Chronic lung disease	Immune compromised states
Immunocompromised states	Multilobar involvement and severe hypoxia with need for ventilatory support
Solid organ transplantation	Delay in appropriate antibiotics
Exposure to contaminated water supplies	End-stage kidney disease
Human immunodeficiency virus	Human immunodeficiency virus
Late summer and early autumn months in northern hemisphere	Diabetes
Male gender	Septic shock
	Hyponatremia

Data from Refs.[1–7,11–13,15,16,19]

related to the lack of readily accessible diagnostic tools to help with early identification of legionella infection. The clinical manifestations and radiographic findings are nonspecific and do not accurately distinguish *L pneumophila* from other respiratory pathogens. In addition, typical empiric antibiotic therapy often lacks proper antimicrobial coverage against *Legionella*.[16] Several clinical and laboratory abnormalities have been linked in the past to the diagnosis of legionellosis. These abnormalities include hyponatremia, hypophosphatemia, increased liver enzyme levels, acute mental status changes, headache, diarrhea, early onset of pleuritic pain (sometimes confused with a pulmonary embolus), and acute increase in creatine phosphokinase level. However, follow-up clinical studies have been largely unsuccessful in reliably identifying and verifying clinical and laboratory parameters that are specific for legionella infection. Note that hyponatremia has been a fairly reproducible indictor of severe legionellosis in several studies. Individually, clinical and laboratory abnormalities lack diagnostic specificity. Nonetheless, the specificity of clinical and laboratory findings is increased when those parameters are combined[5] (**Table 2**). Respiratory symptoms tend to be less prominent initially in patients with legionnaire's disease.[17–20]

Legionella pneumonia shares with other intracellular pathogens the propensity to produce relative bradycardia in the presence of fever. This temperature-pulse abnormality with relative bradycardia in response to fever (Faget sign) is uncommon with typical bacterial pneumonia. Pulse rate usually increases by about 15 beats/min for every 1°C increase in body temperature. Faget sign has been frequently described in older adult patients with more severe pneumonia[19] but this finding is not highly specific for legionellosis. Gastrointestinal manifestations such as watery diarrhea and sudden abdominal pain can sometimes be the presenting symptoms in patients with legionella pneumonia. Another clue to the possibility of SCAP from legionellosis is the finding of numerous neutrophils on Gram strain of respiratory specimens with the absence of visible bacteria. Legionella spp are gram-negative pathogens but do not stain well with the standard Gram stain.

Diagnosis is based mainly on the isolation of the pathogen from sputum, bronchoalveolar lavage fluid, pleural fluid, and occasionally from blood cultures. Nonculture, molecular diagnostic methods promise to improve the laboratory diagnosis of

Table 2
Diagnostic clues to the possibility of legionellosis

Factor	Comments	Frequency of Occurrence
Hyponatremia	Fairly reliable in several studies	≥2
Hypophosphatemia	—	≥1
Gastrointestinal symptoms	Diarrhea, abdominal pain, vomiting	≥2
Altered mental status	Confusion, lethargy, head ache	≥1
Increased liver enzyme levels	—	—
Neutrophils on Gram stain with no bacteria identified	Helpful but can be found in viral and mycoplasma pneumonia	≥3
Temperature-pulse dissociation with relative bradycardia	Helpful but not specific	≥3
Acute kidney injury	—	≥1
Nosocomial outbreaks	*Legionella* in hospital water supply	≥2

≥1, uncommon; ≥2, occasionally observed; ≥3, frequently reported.
Data from Refs.[4,5,7,11–13]

legionellosis in the future, but this molecular diagnostic technique has not yet proved sufficiently superior to cultures to supplant the diagnostic accuracy of cultures on standard buffered charcoal yeast extract plates. The urinary antigen is highly specific but primarily detects serotype 1 *L pneumophila* and does not detect other *Legionella* species. Imaging studies, histopathologic findings, and other laboratory methods are of limited use. A 4-fold or greater increase in serum antibody level is useful for epidemiologic purposes but not as a diagnostic test for patients presenting with SCAP. The direct fluorescent antigen test performed on respiratory specimens can be useful in laboratories proficient with the technique and with available reagents.

In a US Centers for Disease Control and Prevention (CDC) report from 2001, only 35 of the first 1000 cases of sporadic legionella pneumonia reported to the CDC were confirmed by culture, and only 19 from specimens obtained before death.[21] Culturing for *Legionella* spp is the single most important laboratory test. This test should be routinely available in all clinical microbiology laboratories given the frequency of *Legionella* as a causative organism. Increased procalcitonin level was found to be a potentially useful biomarker for severity of illness from legionella infection.[22,23]

There is no specific radiological finding that can help identify legionella pneumonia on chest imaging. *Legionella* is typically associated with rapidly worsening infiltrates on chest radiography that may continue to worsen despite antimicrobial treatment.[24,25]

L pneumophila serotype 1 accounts for about 90% of all *Legionella* spp. Infections with serotypes 1, 4, and 6 are the most common isolates from patients with severe community-acquired pneumonia. Other *Legionella* spp, such as *Legionella micdadei, Legionella bozemanae*, *Legionella longbeachae, and Legionella dumoffii*, account for the remaining 10% of human cases of legionella pneumonia.

DIFFERENTIAL DIAGNOSIS CONSIDERATIONS

Mycoplasma pneumoniae

Mycoplasma pneumonia is typically a disease of gradual onset with persistent cough for several days to weeks. Patients characteristically do not appear toxic, despite having significant disease infiltrates on chest radiography, hence the walking pneumonia appellation. Mild pharyngeal injection with minimal or no cervical adenopathy can be seen with mycoplasma pneumonia, but upper respiratory tract symptoms are not common with legionella infections. *Mycoplasma pneumoniae* has long been associated with bullous myringitis, but recent literature has disproved this association.[26] Similar to legionella pneumonia, atypical pneumonia with mycoplasma can be associated with extrapulmonary symptoms such as myalgia, abdominal pain, and diarrhea. Mycoplasma is frequently associated with additional cardiovascular abnormalities such as myocarditis, pericarditis, and heart block.[27] Such cardiac manifestations are not commonly seen in legionella infections. Mycoplasma infection has been associated with several skin manifestations, including erythema multiforme, macular and vesicular exanthems, urticaria, erythema nodosum, and Stevens-Johnson syndrome.[28] Dermatologic findings are uncommon in legionella pneumonia.

Although not exclusive to mycoplasma infection, increased cold agglutinin titers of 1:64 or higher are highly associated with community-acquired pneumonia from *Mycoplasma*. The cold agglutinin titers occur early in presentation (day 1–3). Rarely, meningoencephalitis from *M pneumoniae* can be seen, and is usually associated with very high agglutinin titers (1:1052 or higher).[29] If untreated, mycoplasma pneumonia can lead to the development of asthma in nonasthmatic patients, or an asthma exacerbation in known asthmatics.[30,31] Electrolyte abnormalities are not usually seen in cases of *M pneumoniae* disease.

Streptococcus pneumoniae

Streptococcus pneumoniae is the most common bacterial cause of community-acquired pneumonia. *S pneumoniae* can cause a wide variety of clinical symptoms because of its ability to cause disease by either direct extension from the nasopharynx into surrounding anatomic structures or vascular invasion and hematogenous spread. It can result in meningitis, bacteremia, otitis media, sinusitis, septic arthritis, osteomyelitis, peritonitis, and endocarditis.

Pneumococcal pneumonia typically presents with an acute onset of high fever, rigors, productive cough, and dyspnea. Respiratory symptoms dominate the presentation in cases of *S pneumoniae* infection. Unlike in legionella, extrapulmonary symptoms are uncommon in pneumococcal pneumonia. Patients are typically very sick looking. Patients have rales and dullness to percussion on examination. Concomitant pleural effusion is the most common complication with *S pneumoniae*, but pleural effusions can be seen in many other microorganisms causing pneumonia. The characteristic chest radiography finding in pneumococcal pneumonia is lobar consolidation, whereas sharply marinated peribronchial consolidations within ground-glass opacities are more specific finding with *Legionella*.[32] To differentiate legionella from *S pneumoniae* community-acquired pneumonia, cardiac, hepatic, and renal abnormalities are helpful because they are expected to be normal with *S pneumoniae* but frequently abnormal in legionnaire's disease.

Zoonotic Atypical Pneumonias

Chlamydophila psittaci (psittacosis), *Francisella tularensis* (tularemia), and *Coxiella burnetii* (Q fever), are 3 zoonotic pathogens that can cause atypical pneumonia in humans. Acquisition of these zoonotic infections can only occur with direct contact with animal hosts or laboratory exposure. Therefore, zoonotic pneumonias can be eliminated from diagnostic consideration with a negative contact history. In *C burnetii*, cattle, sheep, and goats are the primary reservoirs. Transmission to humans occurs primarily through inhalation of aerosols from soil contaminated with animal waste. Psittacosis is usually an occupational disease seen in zoo and pet-shop employees, ranchers, and poultry farmers. Human-to-human transmission has been reported but is very rare. Tularemia pneumonia is an uncommon condition that may develop in laboratory workers. It is rarely acquired naturally nowadays and its occurrence should suggest the possibility of a bioterrorist event.

Atypical pneumonia from Q fever and psittacosis are probably underdiagnosed because patients with mild cases may not seek medical attention or may not be reported because pneumonia can sometimes be an incidental finding. It often presents with dry cough, pleuritic chest pain, and dyspnea. The incubation period varies from 2 to 6 weeks.[32] Symptoms are more abrupt in pneumonic tularemia and tend to be more severe. Rash and pharyngitis can be part of the presentation. Association with gastrointestinal symptoms and hepatitis presenting with pain and mild transaminitis can be seen with Q fever and psittacosis. Unlike legionella, no diarrhea is often associated with zoonotic pneumonias. Relative bradycardia in zoonotic community-acquired pneumonia should suggest Q fever or psittacosis but not tularemia.

Leukopenia can sometimes be seen in psittacosis. All zoonotic pneumonias can result in hyponatremia. Transaminitis can be seen with either Q fever or psittacosis. Chest radiology can show bilateral hilar adenopathy and lobar infiltrates or round/oval densities in pneumonic tularemia. Psittacosis and Q fever tend to be associated with patchy consolidation on chest imaging.[33]

Viral Pneumonia

Because of improved diagnostic techniques, the reported incidence of viral pneumonia has increased during the past decade. Recent studies have shown viruses to cause 13% to 50% of pathogen-identified community-acquired pneumonia as sole pathogens and around 8% to 27% of cases as mixed bacterial-viral infections.[34–37] Several viruses have been identified as causes of pneumonia. Among those viruses are influenza virus types A and B (accounting for more than 50% of all viral pneumonias), parainfluenza virus (2%–3%), respiratory syncytial virus (RSV; 1%–4%), coronavirus (1%–14%), adenovirus (1% to 4%), and human metapneumovirus (hMPV; 0%–4%).[34–36,38] Viral pneumonias show seasonal variations and outbreaks can be identified by possible exposure to sick contacts.

Viral pneumonias usually present with nonspecific constitutional symptoms such as fever, chills, rhinitis, dry cough, myalgia, fatigue, and headaches. Later, patients might develop dyspnea and productive cough. Hoarseness of voice and diffuse wheezes are frequent findings on examination in cases of viral pneumonia (especially with RSV and hMPV),[37] findings that are not seen with legionella pneumonia. Chest pain and rigors are not common with viral pneumonias. Extrapulmonary symptoms are not commonly seen in viral pneumonia, with the exception of nausea, vomiting, and diarrhea, which can be seen with adenovirus. Secondary bacterial pneumonia can happen in cases of viral pneumonia, especially with influenza pneumonia. It is characterized by the relapse of high fever, with purulent sputum and cough. This relapse usually occurs after initial improvement.

TREATMENT CONSIDERATIONS

Macrolides, Quinolones, Rifampin, Combinations, Steroids?

Legionella pneumonia should be treated in most patients with a respiratory quinolone and/or a macrolide such as azithromycin (**Table 3**). No randomized controlled trials have directly compared fluoroquinolones versus macrolides in treating legionellosis. A retrospective study has suggested that the use of azithromycin alone or a quinolone alone was associated with a similar mortality and length of stay.[39] However, quicker defervescence and fewer complications were observed with quinolone treatment.[40–44] As a result, levofloxacin is thought to be the empiric drug of choice in severe pneumonia with suspected *Legionella* spp as well as in nosocomial cases.

Some laboratory studies and case reports have suggested possible therapeutic benefits with the combination of antimicrobial therapy with a quinolone plus azithromycin or rifampin. However, clinical observational studies of antimicrobial therapies for legionella have yet to validate the benefits of combination treatment compared with monotherapy. Combination therapy of a quinolone plus azithromycin can be considered in critically ill patients as well as in extrapulmonary legionellosis. One review article suggested considering rifampin therapy for patients with severe disease or significant comorbid conditions and immunocompromised hosts who are refractory to conventional monotherapy regimens.[45]

Despite comparative bioavailability in oral and parenteral treatment, the latter is recommended initially for all patients with severe legionella pneumonia. Vomiting, impaired gastric mobility, nasogastric suctioning, and alkalization of the gastrointestinal tract for stress-ulcer prophylaxis are all factors that can result in compromised absorption of these medications in critical care settings.[46–49]

Table 3
Therapeutic options for adult patients with severe pneumonia from *Legionella pneumophila*

Therapy	Normal Adult Dose	Comments
Macrolides	Azithromycin 500 mg IV every 24 h or clarithromycin 500 mg IV every 12 h	Preferred regimen in most settings, or a fluoroquinolone
Fluoroquinolones	Levofloxacin (500 mg IV/d) or moxifloxacin 400 mg IV once daily	Generally well tolerated and effective
Rifampin	300–600 mg IV every 12 h	Multiple drug interactions, including warfarin, opiates, cyclosporine, antiretroviral protease inhibitors; used with a macrolide or quinolone
Doxycycline	200-mg IV loading dose followed by 100 mg IV every 12 h	Limited clinical experience shows activity
Combinations	Levofloxacin (500 mg IV/d) or another fluoroquinolone + azithromycin (500 mg IV every 24 h); consider adding rifampin to monotherapy despite many drug interactions	No clear evidence of efficacy of combination therapy compared with monotherapy; often used in SCAP with extensive disease in high-risk patients failing monotherapy
Corticosteroids	0.5–1 mg/kg/d	No clinical evidence of benefit at present in patients with SCAP from legionellosis; awaiting clinical trial evidence

Abbreviation: IV, intravenous.
Data from Refs.[11–13,40–55]

In contrast with the 5-day course of atypical coverage in empiric regimens for community-acquired pneumonia, confirmed cases of legionella require longer courses of treatment. Levofloxacin or azithromycin for 7 to 10 days are recommended in cases of moderate to severe legionella pneumonia. For immunocompromised hosts, a 21-day course of levofloxacin is usually recommended.

A recent randomized controlled study found that low-dose corticosteroid therapy was effective in treating community-acquired pneumonia.[50] A series of recent systematic reviews and meta-analyses have appeared in the literature recently that indicate that steroids might be of some benefit in community-acquired pneumonia.[51–54] However, there are no specific data for the effect of corticosteroids in legionella pneumonia. One case study reported that using high-dose corticosteroid is effective for treating severe legionella pneumonia,[55] but sufficient data are not available to validate the use of corticosteroids in the treatment of SCAP caused by *Legionella* spp. Further observational studies, or preferably controlled trials, will be needed to justify the use of glucocorticoids, with their attendant risks, in this clinical setting.

OUTCOMES/MORTALITY

In one study, mortality in cases of legionella pneumonia admitted to the ICU was around 33%. In another study, SAPS (Simplified Acute Physiology Score) II score higher than 46, duration of symptoms before ICU admission longer than 5 days, and intubation were associated with increased mortality.[56] The same study also suggested that early initiation of fluoroquinolone therapy within 8 hours of ICU admission reduces mortality. With early initiation of appropriate antibiotics, mortality decreases to less than 5%.[14] Delay in initiation of appropriate antibiotics is associated with a worse prognosis.[57] Treatment failure tends to occur in patients with severe disease at the time of admission[41] or in immune compromised patients.[58] Legionellosis can leave patients with long-term adverse health effects and morbidity. In one study, survivors of severe legionella pneumonia reported persisting fatigue (75%), neurologic symptoms (66%), and neuromuscular symptoms (63%) at 17 months' follow-up.[59] The same study also reported that health-related quality of life (HRQL) was impaired in 7 of the 8 dimensions assessed by the HRQL questionnaire, and 15% of patients reported symptoms of PTSD.

REFERENCES

1. Viasus D, Di Yacovo S, Garcia-Vidal C, et al. Community-acquired *Legionella pneumophila* pneumonia: a single-center experience with 214 hospitalized sporadic cases over 15 years. Medicine (Baltimore) 2013;92(1):51–60.
2. Roig J, Domingo C, Morera J. Legionnaire's disease. Chest 1994;105:1817–25.
3. Edelstein PH. Legionnaire's disease. Clin Infect Dis 1993;16:741–7.
4. Bartlett JG. Legionnaire's disease: overtreated, underdiagnosed. J Crit Illn 1993; 8:755–68.
5. Cunha BA. Severe *Legionella* pneumonia: rapid presumptive clinical diagnosis with Winthrop-University Hospital's weighted point score system. Heart Lung 2008;37(4):311–20.
6. Muder RR, Yu VL, Fang GD. Community-acquired Legionnaire's disease. Semin Respir Infect 1989;4:32–9.
7. Falcó V, Fernández de Sevilla T, Alegre J, et al. *Legionella pneumophila*: a cause of severe community-acquired pneumonia. Chest 1991;100:1007–11.
8. Community-acquired pneumonia in adults in British hospitals in 1982-1983: survey of aetiology, mortality, prognostic factors, and outcome. The British Thoracic Society and the Public Health Laboratory Service. Q J Med 1987;62:195–220.
9. Rello J, Quintana E, Ausina V, et al. A three-year study of severe community-acquired pneumonia with emphasis on outcome. Chest 1993;103:232–5.
10. Fang GD, Fine M, Orloff J, et al. New and emerging etiologies for community-acquired pneumonia with implications for therapy: a prospective multicenter study of 359 cases. Medicine (Baltimore) 1990;69:307–16.
11. Torres A, Serra-Batlles J, Ferrer A, et al. Severe community-acquired pneumonia: epidemiology and prognostic factors. Am Rev Respir Dis 1991;144:312–8.
12. Stout JE, Yu VL. Legionellosis. N Engl J Med 1997;337:682–7.
13. Vergis EN, Akbas E, Yu VL. Legionella as a cause of severe pneumonia. Semin Respir Crit Care Med 2000;21(4):295–304.
14. Heath CH, Grove DI, Looke DF. Delay in appropriate therapy of *Legionella* pneumonia associated with increased mortality. Eur J Clin Microbiol Infect Dis 1996; 15(4):286–90.
15. Donowitz GR, Mandell GL. Acute pneumonia. In: Mandell GL, Bennet JE, Dolin R, editors. Principles and practice of infectious diseases. 4th edition. New York: Churchill Livingstone; 1995. p. 619–37.
16. England AC, Fraser DW, Plikaytis BD, et al. Sporadic legionellosis in the United States: the first thousand cases. Ann Intern Med 1981;94:164–70.
17. Mulazimoglu L, Yu VL. Can Legionnaires disease be diagnosed by clinical criteria? A critical review. Chest 2001;120:1049–53.

18. Roig J, Aguilar X, Ruiz J, et al. Comparative study of *Legionella pneumophila* and other nosocomial-acquired pneumonias. Chest 1991;99:344–50.
19. Yu VL, Kroboth FJ, Shonnard J, et al. Legionnaire's disease: new clinical perspective from a prospective pneumonia study. Am J Med 1982;73:357–61.
20. Johnstone J, Majumdar SR, Fox JD, et al. Viral infection in adults hospitalized with community-acquired pneumonia: prevalence, pathogens, and presentation. Chest 2008;134(6):1141–8.
21. Karakousis PC, Trucksis M, Dumler JS. Chronic Q fever in the United States. J Clin Microbiol 2006;44(6):2283–7.
22. Haeuptle J, Zaborsky R, Fiumefreddo R, et al. Prognostic value of procalcitonin in *Legionella* pneumonia. Eur J Clin Microbiol Infect Dis 2009;28:55–60.
23. de Jager CP, de Wit NC, Weers-Pothoff G, et al. Procalcitonin kinetics in *Legionella pneumophila* pneumonia. Clin Microbiol Infect 2009;15:1020–5.
24. Coletta FS, Fein AM. Radiological manifestations of *Legionella*/*Legionella*-like organisms. Semin Respir Infect 1998;13:109–15.
25. Boermsa WG, Daneils JM, Lowenberg A, et al. Reliability of radiologic findings and the relation to etiologic agents.
26. Mellick LB, Verma N. The *Mycoplasma pneumoniae* and bullous myringitis myth. Pediatr Emerg Care 2010;26:966–8.
27. Cunha BA. Atypical pneumonias: current clinical concepts focusing on legionnaire's disease. Curr Opin Pulm Med 2008;14:183–94.
28. Yachoui R, Kolasinski SL, Feinstein DE. *Mycoplasma pneumoniae* with atypical Stevens-Johnson syndrome: a diagnostic challenge. Case Rep Infect Dis 2013; 2013:457161.
29. Sotgiu S, Pugliatti M, Rosati G, et al. Neurological disorders associated with *Mycoplasma pneumoniae* infection. Eur J Neurol 2003;10:165–8.
30. Nisar N, Guleria R, Kumar S, et al. *Mycoplasma pneumoniae* and its role in asthma. Postgrad Med J 2007;83:100–4.
31. Sutherland ER, Brandorff JM, Martin RJ. Atypical bacterial pneumonia and asthma risk. J Asthma 2004;41:863–8.
32. Nambu A, Ozawa K, Kobayashi N, et al. Imaging of community-acquired pneumonia: roles of imaging examinations, imaging diagnosis of specific pathogens and discrimination from noninfectious diseases. World J Radiol 2014;6(10): 779–93.
33. Kirby BD, Snyder KM, Meyer RD, et al. Legionnaire's disease: report of sixty-five nosocomially acquired cases of review of the literature. Medicine (Baltimore) 1980;59:188–205.
34. Marcos MA, Camps M, Pumarola T, et al. The role of viruses in the aetiology of community-acquired pneumonia in adults. Antivir Ther 2006;11:351–9.
35. Templeton KE, Scheltinga SA, van den Eeden WC, et al. Improved diagnosis of the etiology of community-acquired pneumonia with real-time polymerase chain reaction. Clin Infect Dis 2005;41(3):345–51.
36. Dowell SF, Anderson LJ, Gary HE Jr, et al. Respiratory syncytial virus is an important cause of community-acquired lower respiratory infection among hospitalized adults. J Infect Dis 1996;174(3):456–62.
37. Falsey AR, Erdman D, Anderson LJ, et al. Human metapneumovirus infections in young and elderly adults. J Infect Dis 2003;187(5):785–90.
38. Jennings LC, Anderson TP, Beynon KA, et al. Incidence and characteristics of viral community-acquired pneumonia in adults. Thorax 2008;63(1):42–8.

39. Gershengorn HB, Keene A, Dzierba AL, et al. The association of antibiotic treatment regimen and hospital mortality in patients hospitalized with *Legionella* pneumonia. Clin Infect Dis 2015;60:e66.
40. Blázquez Garrido RM, Espinosa Parra FJ, Alemany Francés L, et al. Antimicrobial chemotherapy for Legionnaires disease: levofloxacin versus macrolides. Clin Infect Dis 2005;40:800.
41. Mykietiuk A, Carratalà J, Fernández-Sabé N, et al. Clinical outcomes for hospitalized patients with *Legionella* pneumonia in the antigenuria era: the influence of levofloxacin therapy. Clin Infect Dis 2005;40:794–9.
42. Sabrià M, Pedro-Botet ML, Gómez J, et al. Fluoroquinolones vs macrolides in the treatment of Legionnaires disease. Chest 2005;128:1401–5.
43. Haranaga S, Tateyama M, Higa F, et al. Intravenous ciprofloxacin versus erythromycin in the treatment of *Legionella* pneumonia. Intern Med 2007;46:353–7.
44. Garrido R, Espinosa Parra FJ, Francés LA, et al. Antimicrobial chemotherapy for Legionnaires disease: levofloxacin versus macrolides. Clin Infect Dis 2005;40(6):800–6.
45. Varner TR, Bookstaver PB, Rudisill CN, et al. Role of rifampin-based combination therapy for severe community-acquired *Legionella pneumophila* pneumonia. Ann Pharmacother 2011;45(7–8):967–76.
46. Emami S, Hamishehkar H, Mahmoodpoor A, et al. Errors of oral medication administration in a patient with enteral feeding tube. J Res Pharm Pract 2012;1(1):37–40.
47. Heyland DK, Tougas G, King D, et al. Impaired gastric emptying in mechanically ventilated, critically ill patients. Intensive Care Med 1996;22:1339–44.
48. Mimoz O, Binter V, Jacolot A, et al. Pharmacokinetics and absolute bioavailability of ciprofloxacin administered through a nasogastric tube with continuous enteral feeding to critically ill patients. Intensive Care Med 1998;24:1047–51.
49. Dellinger RP, Carlet JM, Masur H, et al. Surviving Sepsis Campaign guidelines for management of severe sepsis and septic shock. Crit Care Med 2004;32:858–73 [Erratum appears in Crit Care Med 2004;32:1448; Erratum appears in Crit Care Med 2004;32:2169–70.].
50. Confalonieri M, Urbino R, Potena A, et al. Hydrocortisone infusion for severe community-acquired pneumonia: a preliminary randomized study. Am J Respir Crit Care Med 2005;171:242–8.
51. Siemieniuk RA, Meade MO, Alonso-Coello P, et al. Corticosteroid therapy for patients hospitalized with community-acquired pneumonia: a systematic review and meta-analysis. Ann Intern Med 2015;163(7):519–28.
52. Chen LP, Chen JH, Chen Y, et al. Efficacy and safety of glucocorticoids in the treatment of community-acquired pneumonia: a meta-analysis of randomized controlled trials. World J Emerg Med 2015;6(3):172–8.
53. Marti C, Grosgurin O, Harbarth S, et al. Adjunctive corticotherapy for community acquired pneumonia: a systematic review and meta-analysis. PLoS One 2015;10(12):e0144032.
54. Wan YD, Sun TW, Liu ZQ, et al. Efficacy and safety of corticosteroids for community-acquired pneumonia: a systematic review and meta-analysis. Chest 2016;149(1):209–19.
55. Yonemaru R, Homma S, Yamasawa F, et al. A case of Legionnaire's disease cured with a combination of erythromycin and steroid therapy. Nihon Kyobu Shikkan Gakkai Zasshi 1991;29:1499–504 [in Japanese].

56. Gacouin A, Le Tulzo Y, Lavoue S, et al. Severe pneumonia due to *Legionella pneumophila*: prognostic factors, impact of delayed appropriate antimicrobial therapy. Intensive Care Med 2002;28(6):686–91.
57. Fernández JA, López P, Orozco D, et al. Clinical study of an outbreak of Legionnaire's disease in Alcoy, southeastern Spain. Eur J Clin Microbiol Infect Dis 2002; 21:729–35.
58. Pedro-Botet ML, Sabria-Leal M, Sopena N, et al. Role of immunosuppression in the evolution of Legionnaire's disease. Clin Infect Dis 1998;26:14–9.
59. Lettinga KD, Verbon A, Nieuwkerk PT, et al. Health-related quality of life and post-traumatic stress disorder among survivors of an outbreak of Legionnaires disease. Clin Infect Dis 2002;35:11–7.

Legionnaire's Disease in Compromised Hosts

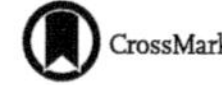

Fanny Lanternier, MD, PhD[a,*], Florence Ader, MD, PhD[b,c], Benoit Pilmis, MD[a], Emilie Catherinot, MD, PhD[d], Sophie Jarraud, MD, PhD[b], Olivier Lortholary, MD, PhD[a,*]

KEYWORDS

• TNF-alpha • Tobacco • TNF blockers • TLR-5 • Legionellosis

KEY POINTS

- Clinicians should be aware that, in immunocompromised patients, (1) legionnaire's disease is a frequent cause of pneumonia, (2) cavitation and empyema may occur, (3) extrapulmonary disease is possible, (4) urine antigen is less sensitive.
- Prompt antibiotic treatment is mandatory.
- Surgery is rarely required in refractory cases or in order to manage pleural or cutaneous involvement.
- Few data are available on these populations and further studies concerning epidemiology, clinical presentation, and diagnosis would be helpful.

OVERVIEW OF ANTI-*LEGIONELLA* IMMUNITY

Legionella spp are intracellular gram-negative bacteria with an environmental origin.[1] The genus *Legionella* comprises more than 60 species. However, *Legionella pneumophila* serogroup 1 alone causes more than 90% of legionnaire's disease (LD). On inhalation through contaminated aerosols, *L pneumophila* can infect and replicate within lung alveolar macrophages. Following phagocytosis, *L pneumophila* generates a unique vacuole that evades fusion with lysosomes and accumulates endoplasmic reticulum protein markers, leading to intracellular replication.[2] The delivery of bacterial proteins into the host cell cytosol, which modulates normal endosomal trafficking and prevents lysosome-mediated killing of the bacteria, is mediated by the immunogenic Dot/Icm secretion apparatus, a type IV secretion system (T4SS) encoded by the *dot* and *icm* genes.[3] In response, multiple pattern recognition systems from host

[a] AP-HP, Hôpital Necker-Enfants malades, Centre d'Infectiologie Necker-Pasteur, IHU Imagine, Université Paris Descartes, 149, rue de Sevres, Paris 75015, France; [b] Legionelles, Inserm 1111 Centre International Recherche en Infectiologie (CIRI), Université Claude Bernard Lyon 1, Lyon, France; [c] Hospices Civils de Lyon, Lyon, France; [d] Hopital Foch, Suresnes, France
* Corresponding author
E-mail addresses: Fanny.lanternier@aphp.fr; olivier.lortholary@aphp.fr

Infect Dis Clin N Am 31 (2017) 123–135
http://dx.doi.org/10.1016/j.idc.2016.10.014
id.theclinics.com

innate immunity are activated. The ectodomains of transmembrane Toll-like receptors (TLR) recognize various agonists produced by *L pneumophila* during engulfment at the cell surface or in an early endosomal compartment. Overall, TLR can generate a rapid and potent response against a pathogen through induction of the transcription factor nuclear factor kappa-B, leading to events that include production of inflammatory cytokines (eg, tumor necrosis factor alpha [TNF-α], interleukin [IL]-6), activation of macrophages, and maturation of dendritic cells. The cytoplasmic adapter protein MyD88 is required by many TLR for signal transduction that generates a functional inflammatory response.[4,5] At the plasma membrane level, TLR5 detects *L pneumophila* flagellin.[6,7] A common stop codon polymorphism in the ligand-binding domain of TLR5 (TLR^{5392STOP}) is associated with human susceptibility to pneumonia caused by *L pneumophila* because of the inability to mediate flagellin signaling.[7] TLR4 detects lipopolysaccharide (LPS) of gram-negative bacteria and TLR2 detects bacterial lipopeptides as well as the unique lipid A fraction of *L pneumophila* LPS.[8–10] At the phagosome membrane level, TLR9 detects unmethylated CpG DNA motifs of bacteria.[11]

Consistent with the determinant role of human TLR in the defense against *L pneumophila*, the authors have reported that the incidence of LD among patients receiving TNF-α antagonists was significantly increased compared with that in controls.[12]

By contrast, the nucleotide-binding domain, leucine-rich repeat (NLR) proteins, constitute a surveillance mechanism capable of responding to microbial products delivered into the host cytosol.[13] A subset of NLR induces the formation of multiprotein complexes known as inflammasomes. Inflammasomes are multiprotein complexes that include members of the NLR family and cysteine protease caspase-1. They mediate pyroptotic cell death and release of IL-1 family cytokines.[14] *L pneumophila* triggers robust T4SS-dependent inflammasome responses in primary human macrophages with caspase-1–dependent release of IL-1β. An alternative noncanonical inflammasome, including human caspase-4, elicits the release of IL-1α and cell death through pyroptosis activation without any requirement for caspase-1.[15,16] Thus, human caspase-1 and caspase-4 are critical mediators of inflammasome activation against *L pneumophila* that allow bacterial growth restriction in human primary macrophages.

Hematological diseases featuring quantitative and qualitative defects of the monocytic-macrophagic system, notably hairy cell leukemia, are a predisposing factor for developing LD. Moreover, specific adaptive immunity is also involved in the control of *L pneumophila* pulmonary infection thanks to various experimental models.[17–23] Human T lymphocytes may be a key requirement for effective anti-*Legionella* control. It has been shown that the acute phase of LD is characterized by absolute lymphocytopenia, which recovers in the subacute phase with an increase in numbers of absolute T cells and reemergence of activated CD4+ and CD8+ T cells.[24] No *L pneumophila*–specific human T-cell epitopes have been identified so far. However, the proof of concept of innate instruction of adaptive immunity in *L pneumophila* infection has been acquired through murine models.[25] On airway infection with *L pneumophila*, engagement of TLR was sufficient for initial T-cell activation and proliferation and MyD88-mediated signals were crucial for Th17 differentiation. In addition, cytosolic NLR recognition was required for effector T-cell differentiation. Another study has determined that murine bone marrow–derived macrophages infected with *Legionella* actively suppressed interferon gamma production by Ag-specific CD4+ and CD8+ T cells, thus repressing effector T-cell function.[26] Overall, precise mechanisms governing human T-cell response in LD remain largely uncovered.

Regarding human adaptive humoral immunity, *L pneumophila* generates a robust antibody response.[27] In murine models, the antibodies elaborated during

L pneumophila infection are protective.[28,29] The immunoglobulins (Ig) IgG2c and IgG1 have been identified as the most protective subclasses of antibody during *Legionella* infection.[30] Nonetheless, the exact contribution of B cell–driven antibodies to host defenses in LD is largely uncovered and there is no increased susceptibility to LD reported among patients with primary or secondary humoral immune deficiencies.[31]

EPIDEMIOLOGY

The surveillance of LD in France relies on data collected by mandatory notification (French acronym). All cases diagnosed by clinicians and biologists must be notified to the regional health agencies that validate the information, conduct an enquiry to identify risk exposures, look for other cases related to these exposures, and when necessary implement measures of control and prevention. France participates in the European LD surveillance network related to travel-associated cases, coordinated by the European Centre for Disease Prevention and Control. In France in 2014 there were 1348 cases of LD reported.[32] The median age was 63 years and male/female sex ratio was 2.7. The incidence increased with age and the highest incidence rate was observed in patients more than 80 years of age. Regarding risk factors, 74% of patients had at least 1 known risk factor and smoking was the only risk factor reported in 45% of cases, 11%% had cancer or hematological malignancies, 9% were on corticosteroids or immunosuppressive treatment, and 17% had diabetes mellitus. The death rate in 2014 was 9.5%.

PRIMARY IMMUNODEFICIENCIES

There is no known primary immunodeficiency during which an increased susceptibility against LD is reported. Anecdotally, a case of lung cavitary pneumonia caused by *L pneumophila* was reported in a 35-year-old patient with hyper-IgE syndrome presenting with hemoptysis.[33] In addition, a case of fatal disseminated *L pneumophila* infection with lung, brain, liver, and spleen abscesses was also reported in a child with severe combined immunodeficiency at the age of 5 years.[34]

SOLID ORGAN TRANSPLANT

LD incidence in the solid organ transplant population is highly variable depending on transplanted organ, and lung and heart transplant recipients harbor the highest risk.[35–37] A Spanish series of LD from 1985 to 2007 reported 14 cases out of 1946 solid organ transplant recipients[38] involving 0.5% of all patients and 0.8% of heart, 0.5% of kidney, and 0.3% of liver recipients. Five cases were nosocomial. LD occurred a median time of 912 days after transplant but 21% occurred within 3 months after transplant. Forty-three percent of patients had allograft rejection and the fatality rate was 14%.

BIOLOGIC THERAPIES

Biologic therapies such as tumor necrosis factor blocker are associated with an increased risk of infections, including legionellosis. Emergence of legionellosis in patients treated with anti–TNF-α therapy was first shown by reporting of a 1-year consecutive series of 10 cases of *L pneumophila* infection in France in patients treated with anti–TNF-α therapy.[39] A prospective French study described legionellosis incidence and risk factors associated with anti–TNF-α therapy between 2004 and 2007. It reported 27 cases and showed that anti–TNF-α therapy was associated with 13-fold increased risk to develop legionellosis, with a higher risk with monoclonal antibodies (15-fold for infliximab or 38-fold for adalimumab) compared with soluble antibody (3-fold for etanercept).[12] All patients had fever and pneumonia, 28% of patients had bilateral pneumonia and 24% had acute respiratory distress, 33% were hospitalized in intensive care unit, and only 1 patient died of legionellosis. Anti–TNF-α was stopped in all patients and restarted in 13 after 6 months and none relapsed. Patients were treated with anti-TNF for a median of 20 months before LD, 67% had received an immunosuppressive treatment during the last year, and 70% were on steroids. A recent literature review from 2004 to 2011 reported 105 cases of LD in patients treated with biologic therapies. Infliximab was the treatment most frequently used (65.3% of cases), followed by adalimumab (23.5%), etanercept (5%), rituximab (3%), and natalizumab (1 patient). However, patients could have received concomitant immunosuppressive drugs. LD occurred a median of 4 months after initiation of biologic therapy. The interval was shorter for patients treated with infliximab than for those treated with etanercept or adalimumab.[40] The fatality rate was 19%, whereas in community-acquired LD in nonimmunosuppressed patients mortality is between 2.5% and 6%.[41,42]

A case of pulmonary LD was also reported in a patient treated with tocilizumab (anti–IL-6 receptor) for rheumatoid arthritis.[43] To our knowledge, no cases of LD were reported with other monoclonal antibodies. Therefore, occurrence of pneumonia in a patient treated with anti–TNF-α therapy, but currently not with other antibodies, requires *Legionella* urinary antigen testing and antibiotic treatment against *L pneumophila*.[44]

HEMATOLOGICAL MALIGNANCIES AND CANCER

LD is an important cause of pneumonia in patients with cancer or hematological malignancies. For example, nosocomial legionellosis was reported to be responsible for 29% of cases of nosocomial pneumonia in patients with head and neck cancer.[45] A 4-year (1977–1980) retrospective study was conducted in a cancer center reporting 36 cases of LD. Forty-two percent of patients had hematological malignancy and 22% had lung cancer. Neutropenia and steroid treatment were risk factors for LD. Fifty-three percent of patients died. Thirty percent of patients had mixed infections and 73% of them died.[46]

Two monocentric retrospective studies were conducted at MD Anderson Cancer Center.[47,48] The first, between 1991 and 2003, reported 50 patients with LD. Eighty-four percent of patients had most of them (80%) relapsing at time of LD diagnosis. Forty percent had and LD occurred 390 days after transplant. Two patients had persistent positive culture despite appropriate antibiotic treatment. At LD diagnosis, 31% of patients had neutropenia and 49% had lymphopenia. A recent study reviewed 33 cases of LD between 2002 and 2014: 27 had HM (13 acute leukemia, 5 chronic lymphocytic leukemia), 23 had neutropenia, 6 had allogeneic hematopoietic stem cell transplant (allo HSCT), and all patients except 1 had lung infection.[48]

Relapse and antimicrobial failures were reported in patients with allo HSCT, as shown by the following case reports. A 19-year-old patient with graft-versus-host disease (GVHD) had cavitating pneumonia 109 days after BMT. Antimicrobial therapy failed and pneumonectomy was required.[49] An adult patient developed lung LD because of *L pneumophila* serogroup 1 at 6 months after allogeneic stem cell transplant complicated with GVHD. Clinicoradiological and bacteriologic failure was documented despite 4 weeks of antibiotics treatment. Surgical resection was necessary for cure.[50] A 9-year-old girl with acute lymphoblastic leukemia developed lung LD and relapsed after allogeneic stem cell transplant.[51]

Two patients with allogeneic stem cell transplant developed pericarditis caused by *L pneumophila* non–serogroup 1.[52,53]

Because of monocytopenia and monocyte functional defect,[54] hairy cell leukemia has been reported as being associated with legionellosis since 1980.[55,56] Since then, several other cases have been reported from different countries.[57]

HUMAN IMMUNODEFICIENCY VIRUS

LD has been infrequently described in patients with human immunodeficiency virus (HIV) and acquired immunodeficiency syndrome, and whether HIV infection is a risk factor for LD is unclear.[58]

CLINICAL PRESENTATION

The incubation period is 2 to 14 days. Symptoms of LD are similar to those of other causes of bacterial pneumonia: fever (67%–100%), cough (41%–92%), chills (15%–77%), and dyspnea (36%–56%) are frequent.[57,59,60] In particular, fever is usually accompanied by relative bradycardia; associated neurologic manifestations consisting of myalgia and arthralgia (20%–43%), headache (17%–43%), and nausea or vomiting (9%–25%)[61–64] are more frequent and suggestive of the diagnosis in patients with pneumonia. Gastrointestinal symptoms can be prominent.

LD can present with various patterns as consolidation, interstitial infiltrates, cavitary lesions, pleural effusion, and multilobar or/and bilateral lung involvement.[47,65] In immunosuppressed patients such as transplant recipients, round nodular opacities can appear, expand, and cavitate.[66] Pleural effusion is present in 15% to 50% of cases.

Cavitation has been associated with *L pneumophila* serotypes 1, 3, 4, 5, 6, and 8 as well as other *Legionella* species: *Legionella micdadei*, *Legionella bozemanae*, *Legionella dumoffii*, and *Legionella longbeachae*.[64,67] In a review of lung abscesses caused by *Legionella* species, glucocorticosteroid therapy was the most frequent risk factor (82.5%). Abscesses frequently arise within 4 weeks after starting high-dose corticosteroid therapy with a median prednisolone dose of 115 mg/d.[68] Most lung abscesses caused by *L pneumophila* resolve without a drainage procedure and spontaneous discharge of cavities may also occur. The need for debridement and drainage is based on individual patient factors. Open or video-assisted thoracoscopic surgery may be indicated for large abscesses, failed medical therapy, empyema, or loculated pleural disease. Overall, surgical or thoracoscopic drainage has been required in approximatively 20% of 57 lung abscesses caused by *L pneumophila* reported in 2011, including cases with empyema.[68] Solid organ transplant recipients more commonly presented pleural effusions, lung abscesses, and/or empyema.[38]

Legionella can cause pulmonary and/or extrapulmonary infection in transplant recipients, although extrapulmonary manifestations are more common in immunocompromised hosts.[69] Neurologic symptoms are classic in LD, including meningoencephalitis, cerebellitis, aseptic meningitis, and transverse myelitis. However, they are no more frequent in immunocompromised patients. Cutaneous legionellosis is an unusual location reported in 13 cases,[70] most of them immunocompromised: 4 received corticosteroids, 2 had solid organ transplants, 2 had allogeneic stem cell transplants, 1 had follicular lymphoma, 1 had chronic lymphocytic leukemia, and 1 had IgA gammapathy. Clinical presentation was erythema, abscess, nodules, induration, ulcer, cellulitis, or masses. Most immunocompromised patients had concomitant lung infection. Five patients had surgery, consisting of drainage, or amputation. Most infections were related to *L pneumophila* (7) serotype 1, 3, 4, 5, 8, or *L micdadei* (3).

L pneumophila aortitis occurred 16 months after heart transplant with *L pneumophila* serogroup 6. Combined surgery and antibiotics were associated for treatment.[71] Twelve cases of pericarditis associated with legionellosis were reported in 1994. All patients but 2 had lung infection. Five patients had immunodepression, including cancer, liver transplant, bone marrow transplant, and hemodialysis.[53] A patient with allogeneic stem cell transplant developing pericarditis caused by *L pneumophila* non–serogroup 1 was reported later.[33]

LEGIONELLOSIS DIAGNOSIS

More than 60 *Legionella* species have been identified, but the species *L pneumophila* is responsible for more than 90% of LD cases diagnosed worldwide. This species can be subdivided into 16 serogroups and most human disease (84% worldwide) is caused by *L pneumophila* serogroup 1 (Lp1).[72–74] The diagnosis of LD is currently based on urinary antigen detection, culture, and polymerase chain reaction (PCR) for respiratory samples. There is currently limited interest in serology.

The LD of immunocompromised (IC) patients has some features that could be considered for the diagnosis of the disease. First, *L pneumophila* non-sg1 and other species of *Legionella* are sparsely involved in LD but these infections do occur, especially in severely IC patients. Among these species, the authors observe mainly *L longbeachae*, *L bozemanae*, *L micdadei*, *L dumoffii*, *Legionella feelei*, *Legionella wadsworthii*, and *Legionella anisa*, but it is speculated that all species could potentially infect humans depending on immune status. *L longbeachae* has increased, despite being known in Australia and New Zealand since the 1980s. The source is associated with composts.[75] Second, the nosocomial LD cases that occurred mainly in IC patients are known to be associated with particular *L pneumophila* sg1 (Lp1) strains that are less well diagnosed by urinary antigen tests. In addition, the extrapulmonary forms of legionellosis are observed mainly in IC patients and concern all species of *Legionella*.

Two methods are of major interest for early diagnosis: the detection of urinary antigen and the use of molecular techniques. Urinary antigen tests account for 70% to 80% of cases that are diagnosed in Europe and United States.[32] This method has many advantages: urine samples are easy to obtain, testing is rapid (15 minutes with immunochromatography test), and antigens appear early (within 2–3 days after the onset of clinical symptoms). Studies showed a specificity of nearly 99% for the better tests. The major drawback is a sensitivity estimated at 80% to 90% for diagnosis of LD caused by Lp1, and from 14% to 69% for other Lp strains.[76–78] These tests do not detect the other species of *Legionella*. Moreover, LD caused by some Lp1 strains, called the Lp1 mAb 3/1-negative strains (non-Pontiac group), are significantly less frequently diagnosed by commercially available assays.[79] The second drawback is that the excretion of antigen may persist for 3 to 4 weeks (up to 1 year) after appropriate antibiotic therapy.[80,81] The persistence of antigenuria does not reflect a failure of treatment but it is significantly associated with immunosuppressive therapy.[81] This late excretion may allow the LD diagnosis of an initially unsuspected case but also may allow a misdiagnosis of the current pneumonia.

The use of PCR on respiratory samples allows a rapid detection of *L pneumophila* by targeting the *mip* gene (macrophage infectivity potentiator) and all *Legionella* species by using specific 16S ribosomal DNA (rDNA) targets. The specificity is near 100% for *L pneumophila*. The specificity of 16S rDNA PCR needs to be better evaluated because some studies did not confirm all PCR positive results by DNA sequencing.[82] The sensitivity of PCR (80%–100%) is higher than that of the culture method when performed on respiratory samples.[83] Regarding Lp1 cases, PCR is less sensitive than UAT[83,84] but the use of PCR can improve LD diagnosis by detecting other serogroups and species. PCR performed on serum showed lower sensitivity (11% to 85%) than for respiratory samples[83,84]; it could be useful for patients who do not expectorate but these samples have to be restricted. The diagnosis of extrapulmonary forms of LD, such as arthritis or endocarditis, can be diagnosed by universal 16S rDNA PCR and sequencing even if the *Legionella* infection had not been suspected.

Isolation of *Legionella* species from a clinical specimen on selective media provides a definitive diagnosis for all species of *Legionella* and is the gold standard. Efforts to obtain a respiratory specimen for culture are still indicated to perform further epidemiologic investigations. The amebic coculture method with *Acanthamoeba* has been described to recover *Legionella* from clinical culture-negative specimens.[85,86]

In addition, regarding IC patients, urinary antigen detection could remain the first-line diagnostic test because it is the fastest and easiest method. Even if there is greater likelihood of Lp non-sg1 and *Legionella* species other than *L pneumophila* in IC patients, Lp1 remains the main agent of LD for these patients. However, if the urinary antigen is negative, PCR of respiratory samples must be performed. The use of culture must be continued for epidemiologic reasons, especially when urinary detection or PCR results are positive.[87]

TREATMENT

The activity and efficacy of different antimicrobials are addressed elsewhere in this issue, so this article focuses on LD treatment in immunocompromised patients because data are scarce.

At the MD Anderson Cancer Center, in a series described earlier, mean treatment duration in 49 patients with HM and cancer was 25 days, whereas clinical response was achieved after a median of 8 days. Two patients had persistent positive cultures and the failure rate was 34% with monotherapy and 27% with combination. Higher failure rates were observed with co-trimoxazole (50%) and erythromycin (60%). None of the 7 patients treated with clarithromycin or azithromycin failed.

An LD outbreak occurred in a cancer reference center in Spain in 2005 over 4 weeks. All patients were in the same wards and all patients in the hospital with respiratory symptoms were tested with *L pneumophila* antigen. In case of antigen positivity, they received levofloxacin treatment, except the index patient, who was treated with clarithromycin. Twelve patients were involved in the outbreak; 5 had solid cancer and the other had HM. All except 2 had lung infiltrate. Three died, and 1 death was legionellosis related (index case). Attributable mortality was 8.3% and the overall case fatality rate was 25%. These results show that early detection and treatment with levofloxacin are associated with low mortality.[88]

Because of scarce data, community-acquired pneumonia guidelines (except for the French guidelines) give imprecise recommendations for legionellosis treatment in immunocompromised patients. Different guidelines are listed in **Table 1** and vary according to the country with a recommendation of longer treatment duration in immunocompromised patients. The addition of rifampicin to macrolide or fluoroquinolone has to be carefully used in severe LD occurring in transplant patients because of interaction with immunosuppressive drugs. Because of these data, azithromycin of fluoroquinolone can be prescribed as a first-line treatment of LD in IC patients. Because of relapse risk, prolonged treatment for up to 21 days is recommended. In cases of lung abscess or empyema, cases were reported to be treated for up to 11 months.[68] In

Table 1
Legionellosis treatment guidelines

	Severity	Antibiotics	Length	Commentary	Reference
French	Mild to moderate	Azithromycin	5 d 10 d in IC patients	—	http://ansm.sante.fr/var/ansm_site/storage/original/application/5e0a0a6ce0725ba42387dc31a14551eb.pdf
	Severe	Fluoroquinolone	8–14 d 21 d in IC patients	Alternative: association fluoroquinolone and macrolide	
ESCMID	—	Levofloxacin or macrolide (azithromycin preferred)	8 d	—	Woodhead et al,[89] 2011
HNEH	—	Azithromycin	—	—	—
USA	—	Fluoroquinolone Azithromycin	8 d	—	Mandell et al,[90] 2007

Abbreviation: ESCMID, European Society for Clinical Microbiology and Infectious Diseases.

principle, 6 to 8 weeks of treatment (3–4 weeks after surgery), adjusted from case to case, could be reasonable.

SUMMARY

Clinicians should be aware that in immunocompromised patients: (1) LD is a frequent cause of pneumonia, (2) cavitation and empyema may occur, (3) extrapulmonary disease is possible, and (4) urine antigen is less sensitive. Prompt antibiotic treatment is mandatory. Surgery is rarely required in refractory cases or in order to manage pleural or cutaneous involvement. Few data are available on these populations and further studies concerning epidemiology, clinical presentation, and diagnosis would be helpful.

REFERENCES

1. Doebbeling BN, Wenzel RP. The epidemiology of *Legionella pneumophila* infections. Semin Respir Infect 1987;2:206–21.
2. Roy CR, Tilney LG. The road less traveled: transport of *Legionella* to the endoplasmic reticulum. J Cell Biol 2002;158:415–9.
3. Shin S, Roy CR. Host cell processes that influence the intracellular survival of *Legionella pneumophila*. Cell Microbiol 2008;10:1209–20.
4. Kawai T, Akira S. The role of pattern-recognition receptors in innate immunity: update on Toll-like receptors. Nat Immunol 2010;11:373–84.
5. Archer KA, Alexopoulou L, Flavell RA, et al. Multiple MyD88-dependent responses contribute to pulmonary clearance of *Legionella pneumophila*. Cell Microbiol 2009;11:21–36.
6. Hawn TR, Verbon A, Lettinga KD, et al. A common dominant TLR5 stop codon polymorphism abolishes flagellin signaling and is associated with susceptibility to legionnaire's disease. J Exp Med 2003;198:1563–72.
7. Hayashi F, Smith KD, Ozinsky A, et al. The innate immune response to bacterial flagellin is mediated by Toll-like receptor 5. Nature 2001;410:1099–103.

8. Akamine M, Higa F, Arakaki N, et al. Differential roles of Toll-like receptors 2 and 4 in in vitro responses of macrophages to *Legionella pneumophila*. Infect Immun 2005;73:352–61.
9. Hawn TR, Smith KD, Aderem A, et al. Myeloid differentiation primary response gene (88)- and toll-like receptor 2-deficient mice are susceptible to infection with aerosolized *Legionella pneumophila*. J Infect Dis 2006;193:1693–702.
10. Girard R, Pedron T, Uematsu S, et al. Lipopolysaccharides from *Legionella* and *Rhizobium* stimulate mouse bone marrow granulocytes via Toll-like receptor 2. J Cell Sci 2003;116:293–302.
11. Bhan U, Trujillo G, Lyn-Kew K, et al. Toll-like receptor 9 regulates the lung macrophage phenotype and host immunity in murine pneumonia caused by *Legionella pneumophila*. Infect Immun 2008;76:2895–904.
12. Lanternier F, Tubach F, Ravaud P, et al. Incidence and risk factors of *Legionella pneumophila* pneumonia during anti-tumor necrosis factor therapy: a prospective French study. Chest 2013;144:990–8.
13. Barbé F, Douglas T, Saleh M. Advances in Nod-like receptors (NLR) biology. Cytokine Growth Factor Rev 2014;25:681–97.
14. Miao EA, Leaf IA, Treuting PM, et al. Caspase-1-induced pyroptosis is an innate immune effector mechanism against intracellular bacteria. Nat Immunol 2010;11:1136–42.
15. Akhter A, Caution K, Abu Khweek A, et al. Caspase-11 promotes the fusion of phagosomes harboring pathogenic bacteria with lysosomes by modulating actin polymerization. Immunity 2012;37:35–47.
16. Casson CN, Yu J, Reyes VM, et al. Human caspase-4 mediates noncanonical inflammasome activation against gram-negative bacterial pathogens. Proc Natl Acad Sci U S A 2015;112:6688–93.
17. Horwitz MA. Cell-mediated immunity in Legionnaire's disease. J Clin Invest 1983;71:1686–97.
18. Blander SJ, Breiman RF, Horwitz MA. A live avirulent mutant *Legionella pneumophila* vaccine induces protective immunity against lethal aerosol challenge. J Clin Invest 1989;83:810–5.
19. Blander SJ, Horwitz MA. Vaccination with *Legionella pneumophila* membranes induces cell-mediated and protective immunity in a guinea pig model of Legionnaire's disease. Protective immunity independent of the major secretory protein of *Legionella pneumophila*. J Clin Invest 1991;87:1054–9.
20. Blander SJ, Horwitz MA. Vaccination with the major secretory protein of *Legionella* induces humoral and cell-mediated immune responses and protective immunity across different serogroups of *Legionella pneumophila* and different species of *Legionella*. J Immunol 1991;147:285–91.
21. Weeratna R, Stamler DA, Edelstein PH, et al. Human and guinea pig immune responses to *Legionella pneumophila* protein antigens OmpS and Hsp60. Infect Immun 1994;62:3454–62.
22. Susa M, Ticac B, Rukavina T, et al. *Legionella pneumophila* infection in intratracheally inoculated T cell-depleted or -nondepleted A/J mice. J Immunol 1998;160:316–21.
23. Neild AL, Roy CR. Legionella reveal dendritic cell functions that facilitate selection of antigens for MHC class II presentation. Immunity 2003;18:813–23.
24. de Jager CPC, Gemen EF, Leuvenink J, et al. Dynamics of peripheral blood lymphocyte subpopulations in the acute and subacute phase of Legionnaire's disease. PLoS One 2013;8:e62265.

25. Trunk G, Oxenius A. Innate instruction of CD4+ T cell immunity in respiratory bacterial infection. J Immunol 2012;189:616–28.
26. Neild AL, Shin S, Roy CR. Activated macrophages infected with *Legionella* inhibit T cells by means of MyD88-dependent production of prostaglandins. J Immunol 2005;175:8181–90.
27. Casadevall A, Pirofski L. A reappraisal of humoral immunity based on mechanisms of antibody-mediated protection against intracellular pathogens. Adv Immunol 2006;91:1–44.
28. Joller N, Spörri R, Hilbi H, et al. Induction and protective role of antibodies in *Legionella pneumophila* infection. Eur J Immunol 2007;37:3414–23.
29. Weber SS, Joller N, Küntzel AB, et al. Identification of protective B cell antigens of *Legionella pneumophila*. J Immunol 2012;189:841–9.
30. Weber SS, Ducry J, Oxenius A. Dissecting the contribution of IgG subclasses in restricting airway infection with *Legionella pneumophila*. J Immunol 2014;193: 4053–9.
31. Schlossberg D, Bonoan J. Legionella and immunosuppression. Semin Respir Infect 1998;13:128–31.
32. European Centre for Disease Control and Prevention. Legionnaire's disease in Europe, 2011. (2011).
33. Di Stefano F, Verna N, Di Gioacchino M. Cavitary legionella pneumonia in a patient with immunodeficiency due to Hyper-IgE syndrome. J Infect 2007;54: e121–3.
34. Cutz E, Thorner PS, Rao CP, et al. Disseminated *Legionella pneumophila* infection in an infant with severe combined immunodeficiency. J Pediatr 1982;100:760–2.
35. Singh N, Gayowski T, Wagener M, et al. Pulmonary infections in liver transplant recipients receiving tacrolimus. Changing pattern of microbial etiologies. Transplantation 1996;61:396–401.
36. Singh N, Stout JE, Yu VL. Prevention of Legionnaire's disease in transplant recipients: recommendations for a standardized approach. Transpl Infect Dis 2004;6: 58–62.
37. Chow JW, Yu VL. Legionella: a major opportunistic pathogen in transplant recipients. Semin Respir Infect 1998;13:132–9.
38. Gudiol C, Garcia-Vidal C, Fernández-Sabé N, et al. Clinical features and outcomes of Legionnaire's disease in solid organ transplant recipients. Transpl Infect Dis 2009;11:78–82.
39. Tubach F, Ravaud P, Salmon-Céron D, et al. Emergence of *Legionella pneumophila* pneumonia in patients receiving tumor necrosis factor-alpha antagonists. Clin Infect Dis 2006;43:e95–100.
40. Bodro M, Carratalà J, Paterson DL. Legionellosis and biologic therapies. Respir Med 2014;108:1223–8.
41. Viasus D, Di Yacovo S, Garcia-Vidal C, et al. Community-acquired *Legionella pneumophila* pneumonia: a single-center experience with 214 hospitalized sporadic cases over 15 years. Medicine (Baltimore) 2013;92:51–60.
42. Mykietiuk A, Carratalà J, Fernández-Sabé N, et al. Clinical outcomes for hospitalized patients with *Legionella* pneumonia in the antigenuria era: the influence of levofloxacin therapy. Clin Infect Dis 2005;40:794–9.
43. Arinuma Y, Nogi S, Ishikawa Y, et al. Fatal complication of *Legionella pneumophila* pneumonia in a tocilizumab-treated rheumatoid arthritis patient. Intern Med 2015;54:1125–30.

44. Goëb V, Ardizzone M, Arnaud L, et al. Recommendations for using TNFα antagonists and French Clinical Practice Guidelines endorsed by the French National Authority for Health. Jt Bone Spine Rev Rhum 2013;80:574–81.
45. Johnson JT, Yu VL, Wagner RL, et al. Nosocomial *Legionella* pneumonia in a population of head and neck cancer patients. Laryngoscope 1985;95:1468–71.
46. Nunnink JC, Gallagher JG, Yates JW. Legionnaire's disease in patients with cancer. Med Pediatr Oncol 1986;14:81–5.
47. Jacobson KL, Miceli MH, Tarrand JJ, et al. *Legionella* pneumonia in cancer patients. Medicine (Baltimore) 2008;87:152–9.
48. Han XY, Ihegword A, Evans SE, et al. Microbiological and clinical studies of legionellosis in 33 patients with cancer. J Clin Microbiol 2015;53:2180–7.
49. Larru B, Gerber JS, Ota KV. Medical treatment failure and complete left pneumonectomy after *Legionella pneumophila* pneumonia in a bone marrow transplant recipient. Pediatr Infect Dis J 2012;31:979–81.
50. Schindel C, Siepmann U, Han S, et al. Persistent *Legionella* infection in a patient after bone marrow transplantation. J Clin Microbiol 2000;38:4294–5.
51. Gonzalez IA, Martin JM. *Legionella pneumophilia* serogroup 1 pneumonia recurrence postbone marrow transplantation. Pediatr Infect Dis J 2007;26:961–3.
52. Schaumann R, Pönisch W, Helbig JH, et al. Pericarditis after allogeneic peripheral blood stem cell transplantation caused by *Legionella pneumophila* (non-serogroup 1). Infection 2001;29:51–3.
53. Scerpella EG, Whimbey EE, Champlin RE, et al. Pericarditis associated with Legionnaire's disease in a bone marrow transplant recipient. Clin Infect Dis 1994;19:1168–70.
54. Nielsen H, Bangsborg J, Rechnitzer C, et al. Defective monocyte function in Legionnaire's disease complicating hairy cell leukaemia. Acta Med Scand 1986;220:381–3.
55. Dournon E, Cordonnier C, DesForges L, et al. Case 52-1982: legionnaire's disease complicating hairy-cell leukemia. N Engl J Med 1983;308:1100.
56. Berlin G, Frydén A, Maller R, et al. Legionnaire's disease in leukaemic reticuloendotheliosis. Scand J Haematol 1980;25:171–4.
57. Cunha BA, Munoz-Gomez S, Gran A, et al. Persistent Legionnaire's disease in an adult with hairy cell leukemia successfully treated with prolonged levofloxacin therapy. Heart Lung J Acute Crit Care 2015;44:360–2.
58. Sandkovsky U, Sandkovsky G, Suh J, et al. Legionella pneumonia and HIV: case reports and review of the literature. AIDS Patient Care STDs 2008;22:473–81.
59. Cunha BA, Burillo A, Bouza E. Legionnaire's disease. Lancet 2016;387:376–85.
60. Mulazimoglu L, Yu VL. Can Legionnaires disease be diagnosed by clinical criteria? A critical review. Chest 2001;120:1049–53.
61. Kirby BD, Snyder KM, Meyer RD, et al. Legionnaire's disease: report of sixty-five nosocomially acquired cases of review of the literature. Medicine (Baltimore) 1980;59:188–205.
62. Roig J, Aguilar X, Ruiz J, et al. Comparative study of *Legionella pneumophila* and other nosocomial-acquired pneumonias. Chest 1991;99:344–50.
63. Yu VL, Kroboth FJ, Shonnard J, et al. Legionnaire's disease: new clinical perspective from a prospective pneumonia study. Am J Med 1982;73:357–61.
64. Fang GD, Fine M, Orloff J, et al. New and emerging etiologies for community-acquired pneumonia with implications for therapy. A prospective multicenter study of 359 cases. Medicine (Baltimore) 1990;69:307–16.
65. Ampel NM, Wing EJ. *Legionella* infection in transplant patients. Semin Respir Infect 1990;5:30–7.

66. Ernst A, Gordon FD, Hayek J, et al. Lung abcess complicating *Legionella micdadei* pneumonia in an adult liver transplant recipient: case report and review. Transplantation 1998;65:130–4.
67. Rudin JE, Wing EJ. A comparative study of *Legionella micdadei* and other nosocomial acquired pneumonia. Chest 1984;86:675–80.
68. Guy SD, Worth LJ, Thursky KA, et al. *Legionella pneumophila* lung abscess associated with immune suppression. Intern Med J 2011;41:715–21.
69. Sivagnanam S, Pergam SA. Legionellosis in transplantation. Curr Infect Dis Rep 2016;18:9.
70. Padrnos LJ, Blair JE, Kusne S, et al. Cutaneous legionellosis: case report and review of the medical literature. Transpl Infect Dis 2014;16:307–14.
71. Guyot S, Goy JJ, Gersbach P, et al. *Legionella pneumophila* aortitis in a heart transplant recipient. Transpl Infect Dis 2007;9:58–9.
72. Beauté J, Zucs P, de Jong B, European Legionnaire's Disease Surveillance Network. Legionnaires disease in Europe, 2009-2010. Euro Surveill 2013;18: 20417.
73. Fields BS, Benson RF, Besser RE. *Legionella* and Legionnaire's disease: 25 years of investigation. Clin Microbiol Rev 2002;15:506–26.
74. Yu VL, Plouffe JF, Pastoris MC, et al. Distribution of *Legionella* species and serogroups isolated by culture in patients with sporadic community-acquired legionellosis: an international collaborative survey. J Infect Dis 2002;186:127–8.
75. Whiley H, Bentham R. *Legionella longbeachae* and legionellosis. Emerg Infect Dis 2011;17:579–83.
76. Helbig JH, Uldum SA, Lück PC, et al. Detection of *Legionella pneumophila* antigen in urine samples by the BinaxNOW immunochromatographic assay and comparison with both Binax Legionella Urinary Enzyme Immunoassay (EIA) and Biotest Legionella Urin Antigen EIA. J Med Microbiol 2001;50:509–16.
77. Helbig JH, Uldum SA, Bernander S, et al. Clinical utility of urinary antigen detection for diagnosis of community-acquired, travel-associated, and nosocomial legionnaire's disease. J Clin Microbiol 2003;41:838–40.
78. Benson RF, Tang PW, Fields BS. Evaluation of the Binax and Biotest urinary antigen kits for detection of Legionnaire's disease due to multiple serogroups and species of *Legionella*. J Clin Microbiol 2000;38:2763–5.
79. Helbig JH, Uldum SA, Luck PC, et al. in Legionella 204–206 (2002).
80. Kohler RB, Winn WC, Wheat LJ. Onset and duration of urinary antigen excretion in Legionnaires disease. J Clin Microbiol 1984;20:605–7.
81. Sopena N, Sabrià M, Pedro-Botet ML, et al. Factors related to persistence of *Legionella* urinary antigen excretion in patients with legionnaire's disease. Eur J Clin Microbiol Infect Dis 2002;21:845–8.
82. von Baum H, Ewig S, Marre R, et al. Community-acquired *Legionella* pneumonia: new insights from the German competence network for community acquired pneumonia. Clin Infect Dis 2008;46:1356–64.
83. Mentasti M, Fry NK, Afshar B, et al. Application of *Legionella pneumophila*-specific quantitative real-time PCR combined with direct amplification and sequence-based typing in the diagnosis and epidemiological investigation of Legionnaire's disease. Eur J Clin Microbiol Infect Dis 2012;31:2017–28.
84. Diederen BMW, de Jong CM, Marmouk F, et al. Evaluation of real-time PCR for the early detection of *Legionella pneumophila* DNA in serum samples. J Med Microbiol 2007;56:94–101.
85. Rowbotham TJ. Isolation of *Legionella pneumophila* serogroup 1 from human feces with use of amebic cocultures. Clin Infect Dis 1998;26:502–3.

86. Descours G, Suet A, Ginevra C, et al. Contribution of amoebic coculture to recovery of *Legionella* isolates from respiratory samples: prospective analysis over a period of 32 months. J Clin Microbiol 2012;50:1725–6.
87. Phin N, Parry-Ford F, Harrison T, et al. Epidemiology and clinical management of Legionnaire's disease. Lancet Infect Dis 2014;14:1011–21.
88. Gudiol C, Verdaguer R, Domínguez MA, et al. Outbreak of Legionnaire's disease in immunosuppressed patients at a cancer centre: usefulness of universal urine antigen testing and early levofloxacin therapy. Clin Microbiol Infect 2007;13: 1125–8.
89. Woodhead M, Blasi F, Ewig S, et al. Guidelines for the management of adult lower respiratory tract infections - Full version. Clin Microbiol Infect 2011;17:E1–59.
90. Mandell LA, Wunderink RG, Anzueto A, et al. Infectious Diseases Society of America/American Thoracic Society Consensus Guidelines on the Management of Community-Acquired Pneumonia in Adults. Clin Infect Dis 2007;44:S27–72.

Legionnaire's Disease and Influenza

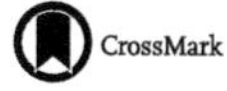

Eleni E. Magira, MD, PhD[a,*], Sryros Zakynthinos, MD, PhD[b]

KEYWORDS

• Legionellosis • Influenza • Coinfection • Secondary infection
• Immunopathogenesis • Host

KEY POINTS

- *Legionella pneumophila* (LP) can be detected in all seasons worldwide.
- In cases of community-acquired pneumonia (CAP), physicians should frequently consider multiple-pathogen infections.
- The impact of dual pulmonary infection usually correlates negatively with the host survival.
- Influenza types A and B viruses pulmonary infection may precede or overlap with legionnaire's disease.

INTRODUCTION

Two significantly important highly pathogenic infection diseases, namely legionellosis and influenza, remain a threat to global health. They can cause severe CAP with respiratory failure but they can also generate hospital-acquired infections.[1] Moreover *Legionella* infection could attribute to influenza infection.[2]

The cause of influenza was definitively resolved back in 1930s with the isolation of swine influenza, a virus which when administered intranasally to susceptible swine induced a mild illness of short duration.[3] The physician Richard Pfeiffer had created the hypothesis that *Bacillus influenzae* (now *Haemophilus influenzae*) was the cause of influenza during the pandemic in 1892.[4] The bacterial origin of influenza was the most prevailing scientific thought. But immunologists failed to consistently isolate *Bacillus influenzae* from patient samples and finally doubted the theory that Pfeiffer's bacillus was the absolute cause of influenza. Bacteria like streptococci and pneumococci were also present among the specimens from cases of clinical influenza.

Disclosures: None.

[a] 1st Department of Critical Care Medicine, Evangelismos General Hospital, National and Kapodistrian University of Athens, 45-47 Ispilandou Street, Athens 10675, Greece; [b] 1st Department of Critical Care and Pulmonary Services, Center of Sleep Disorders, Evangelismos General Hospital, National and Kapodistrian University of Athens, 45-47 Ipsilantou Street, Athens 10676, Greece
* Corresponding author. First Department of Critical Care, National and Kapodistrian University of Athens Medical School, 50 Marathonos, Vrilisia, Athens 15235, Greece.
E-mail address: elmagira@yahoo.com

Infect Dis Clin N Am 31 (2017) 137–153
http://dx.doi.org/10.1016/j.idc.2016.10.010

Nevertheless, the theory that the presence of secondary bacterial invaders in influenza cases contributes negatively in the prognosis of the influenza infection is still relevant today.

The bacterium LD, a fastidious intracellular gram-negative bacillus, was first identified in 1977 as the cause of an outbreak of severe pneumonia in a convention center in Philadelphia in the United States.[5] Although several other species (more than 50) of the genus *Legionella* were subsequently identified, LD is the best-characterized member of the genus *Legionella* and the most frequent cause of human legionellosis.[6]

The exact incidence of legionellosis worldwide is unknown, but in studies involving hospitalized patients with CAP in the United States, Europe, Israel, and Australia, 0.5% to 10% had legionnaire's disease, with an average level of approximately 2%.[7–9] A changing trend in the incidence of legionellosis in the United States was reported to the Centers for Disease Control and Prevention (CDC) over the 2000 to 2009 decade.[10] A recent prospective, population-based study of CAP in hospitalized adults in the United States estimated the annual incidence rates of pathogen detected among 2320 adults with radiographic evidence of pneumonia. The incidence of legionellosis was high among adults 50 to 64 years of age and in those above 80 years old than among younger adults, and the annual incidence of *Legionella* pneumonia–related hospitalization was 0.4 (0.2–0.5) (95% CI).[11]

Statistics from the same study are more comprehensive regarding the influenza incidence. The annual incidence of community-acquired influenza pneumonia requiring hospitalization is 1.5 (1.3–1.8) (95% CI).[11]

VIRULENCE FACTORS OF LEGIONELLA AND INFLUENZA

Influenza viral infection has an extremely highly contagious nature. This remarkable feature results from the capability of the external layer of the influenza virus to be subjected to frequent antigenic changes. The influenza virus structure (**Fig. 1**) is

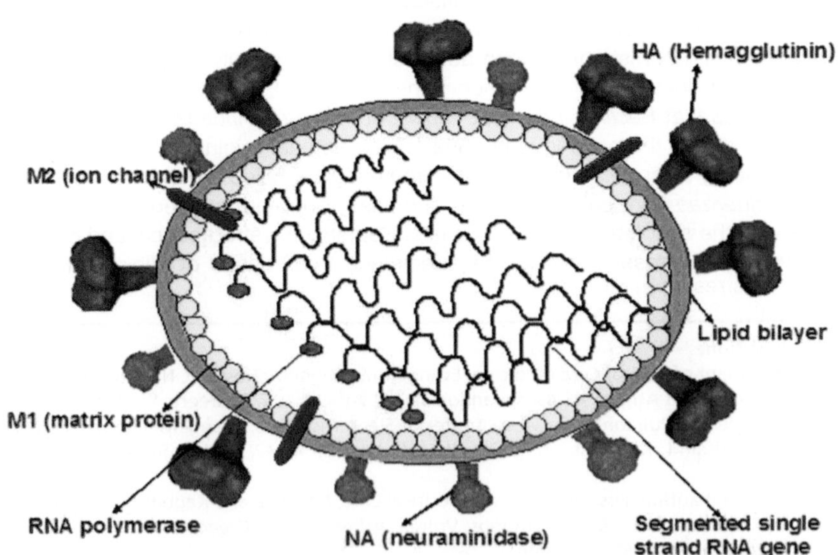

Fig. 1. Structure of influenza: the envelope consists of 3 membrane proteins: (HA glycoprotein, NA neuraminidase, and M2) and a matrix protein (M1) just below the lipid bilayer. The virus contains 8 viral RNA single segments (ribonucleoprotein core).

characterized by its external layer of approximately 500 spikelike projects. The spikes are glycoproteins, neuraminidase (NA) and hemagglutinin (HA), which actually distinguish the influenza virus into 3 main types: influenza A, influenza B, and influenza C. These types have been identified worldwide, with the A and B types causing disease in humans.[12]

Depending on the type of HA and NA glycoproteins, influenza A virus can be subdivided into different serotypes, with subtypes H1N1 and H3N2 the most common to infect humans. The functional role of the HA molecule is that attaches to cell receptors and initiates the process of virus entry into cells. On the other hand, the primary role of the NA glycoproteins is to remove sialic acid from glycoproteins.[13] Sialic acids are cell receptors that are used by many viruses (such as influenza, parainfluenza, mumps, corona, noro, rota, and DNA tumor viruses) as receptors for cell entry.[14] Inhibiting NA with oseltamivir suppresses both viral infection and viral release from cultured human airway epithelial cells.

Although the first human influenza A virus was isolated in 1933, human pandemics also happened in years 1957 and 1968 that possibly resulted from antigenically shifted influenza strains.[15,16] Genes made of RNA, like the influenza viruses, rather than those made of DNA, are more prone to mutations. This is because DNA is a more stable molecule than RNA. Therefore, genome reassortment between different influenza subtypes leads to dramatic alteration in HA and NA glycoproteins, which subsequently give rise to new influenza subtypes. These new subtypes are causing pandemics that occur unpredictably, and frequently these infections are difficult to treat.[16] This phenomenon has been observed only in influenza virus A. In contrast to antigenic shift, antigenic drift occurs as a result of the accumulations of point mutations in the RNA that can alter some antigenic sites of the HA, forming new strain of virus capable of escaping from existing immunity and are usually easy to treat. Influenza viruses A, B, and C have been involved in antigenic drift.[16]

Legionella as an intracellular pathogen has an interesting entering process in the host cells. The *Legionella* bacteria, once phagocytized, reside, without fusion with lysosomes, within a phagosome, which is called *Legionella*-containing vacuole (LCV) (**Fig. 2**), and this is what makes the bacterium resistant to the monocyte microbicidal effects.[11] The same strategy is used by *Salmonella*, *Mycobacterium tuberculosis*, and *Chlamydia*, whereas other intracellular pathogens, such as *Rickettsiae*, *Listeria monocytogenes*, and *Shigella*, contain some clever strategies and escape from the phagosome vacuole.[17]

But how do the *Legionella* bacteria exit and enter other host cells to infect them? During the intracellular growth, LP undergoes structural changes in the envelope that lead to a more highly infectious mature intracellular form that is resistant to environmental stress (see **Fig. 2**). Another mechanism related to the development of infection and the disease progression is contact-dependent cell cytotoxicity induced by LP bacteria and mediated by tiny pores in the host cell membrane.[18]

Genetic analysis has revealed that phagosome biogenesis by LP is controlled by a specialized secretion system that delivers virulence proteins into host cells. *Legionella* has 2 distinct (see **Fig. 2**) protein secretion systems, the Dot/Icm type IV (T4SS) and the Lsp type II (T2SS).[19] The T4SS is required for the intracellular replication, the establishment of the LCV, the inhibition of host cell apoptosis, and the exit of LP from host cells.[20] The secretion system T4SS may transfer nucleic acids and or proteins to cells and, therefore, also plays an important role in horizontal gene transfer.[19] LP also possesses another important secretion system, the Lsp, which is critical for the ability of LP to grow within its natural ameba hosts, including *Acanthamoeba castellanii, Hartmannella vermiformis*, and *Naegleria lovaniensis*.[21] It secretes factors that

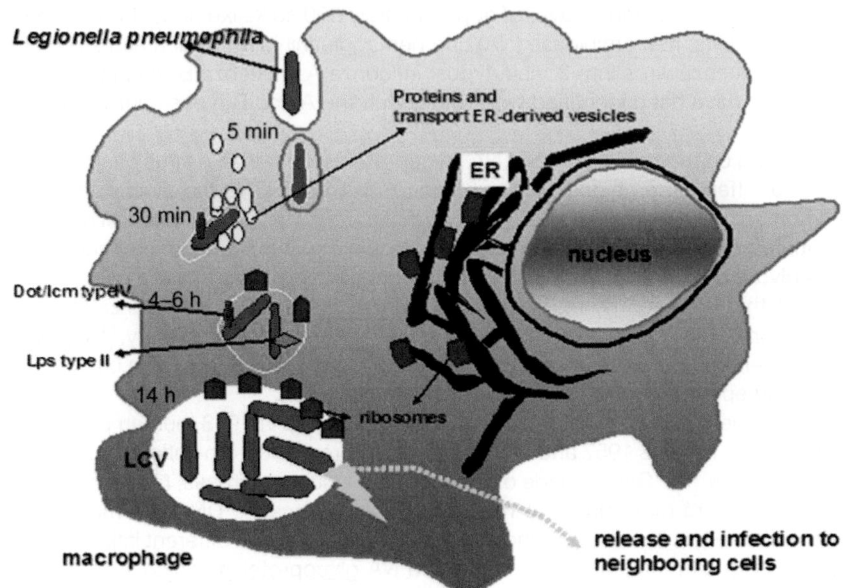

Fig. 2. Intracellular growth of LP (*purple*) in macrophages. On phagocytosis, within 5 minutes, proteins and transport vesicles (*yellow spheres*) are recruited to the LCV. After 15 minutes, the phagosomal membrane becomes thinner and within 4 hours to 6 hours the LCV membrane appears completely comprised of rough endoplasmic reticulum (ER). Eventually, the host cell is lysed, and LP bacteria are released to infect other macrophages.

enables LP to persist in various environmental temperatures and maintain virulence. Besides the T4SS and T2SS, LP harbors other secretion systems that play different roles in contributing to *Legionella* virulence.

INFLUENCE OF ENVIRONMENT IN INFECTION DEVELOPMENT

Legionellosis is a waterborne disease inhabited naturally in freshwater environments. A reservoir that supports the growth of *Legionella* in water is amebas and both (LP and amebas) can survive in a biofilm formation (**Fig. 3**).[22] When biofilm is disrupted, then people potentially became sick after inhalation of bacteria-contaminated water droplets in their air environment. The virulence of LP depends on the size of the particles in which the cells are contained (**Table 1**), the duration of exposure in contaminated water environment, and their site of deposition in the respiratory tract. Interaction of air and water is important in the spreading of the disease. Therefore, airborne transmission of legionellosis with the classical definition does not obviously exist, although a recent report from Portugal implies a probable person-to-person transmission of legionellosis.[23]

Similar to legionellosis infection, several other infectious diseases (*Aspergillosis* spp, *Histoplasmosis capsulatum*, *Coccidioidomycosis, Cryptococcus neoformans*, *Mucorales/Rhizopus* spp, and *Penicillium* spp) are acquired from environmental sources rather than from an infected person.[24]

Transmission of *Legionella* is also possible through municipal water supply. This is facilitated by a high water temperature (*Legionella* multiply at 20°C–40°C) and by modern plumbing systems, where the increased turbulence causes generation of aerosols

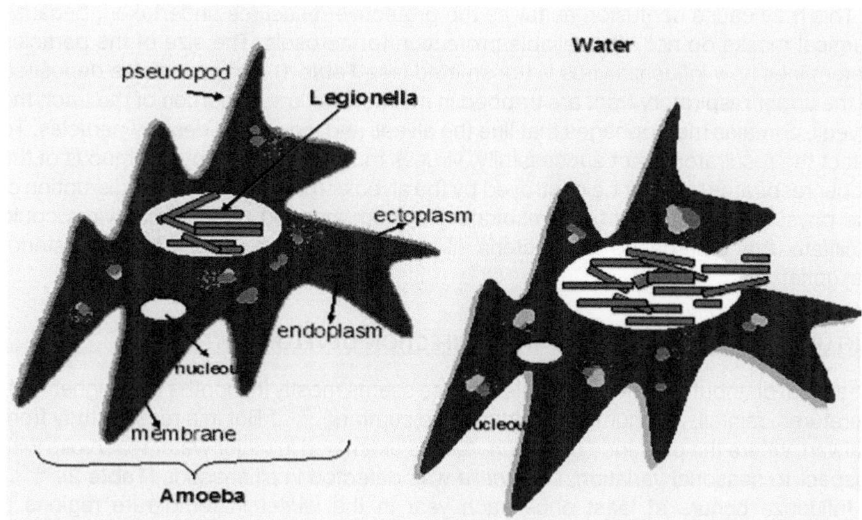

Fig. 3. LP safely carried by ameba (protozoa)-forming biofilm communities. LP are taken up within vacuoles without being digested. When the LP have reached a certain density, the vacuoles release them into the water system.

and droplets. Aerosols and droplets are also common in spa pools, mist machines, and humidifiers. They generate water droplets of appropriate diameter (<5 µm) to transport *Legionella* bacteria deep into the respiratory tract.[25] Oropharyngeal colonization with LP is possible, as previously detected in a total of 186 volunteers including 40 hospital patients, who were proved to have a low prevalence of colonization—4.3% subjects were positive by direct fluorescent antibody test.[26]

On the other hand, there is still a debate whether influenza viruses can be transmitted via only large and even extremely large droplets, approximately 100 µm in diameter (see **Table 1**). The CDC and World Health Organization state that influenza virus transmission occurs primarily by large-particle respiratory droplets (diameter ≥20 µm) that have limited travel distance of approximately 3 m.[27,28] Bischoff and colleagues[29] found that up to 89% of influenza virus–carrying particles were less than 4.7 µm in diameter and that the health care professionals are exposed to mainly small influenza virus particles (<10 µm in mass diameter).

Table 1
Acquisition of legionellosis and influenza linked to particle size inhalation

Approximate Size of Particles	Corresponding Site of Deposition in Respiratory Tract	Particles Containing *Legionella*	Particles Containing Influenzas
Large ≥10°µm	Nose, throat	Yes	Yes
Medium 5–10°µm	Trachea, bronchi	Yes	Yes
Small			
≤5°µm	Deep into the lungs	Yes	Yes
2–4°µm	Ideal for alveolar deposition		
3°µm	Amebic vacuoles		

This may cause confusion as far as the protective measures undertaken, because surgical masks do not offer reliable protection for aerosols. The size of the particles determines how influenza virus is transmitted (see **Table 1**). Large particles deposited in the upper respiratory tract are trapped in mucus. The lowest portion of the tract, the alveoli, contains macrophages that line the alveoli and ingest and destroy particles. To infect the respiratory tract successfully, viruses must not escape by the mucus of the upper respiratory tract or be destroyed by the alveolar macrophages. The disruption of the physiologic barriers of the respiratory system induced by influenza virus could facilitate the emergence of bacteria like *Legionella* that colonize the posterior nasopharynx.

INFLUENCE OF SEASONAL CLIMATE IN INFECTION DEVELOPMENT

Seasonal distribution of legionellosis disease seems mostly in months with higher temperatures, rainfall, and humidity (autumn and summer).[30–34] But in a recent study from Taiwan, where the presence of *Legionella* was examined in major water reservoirs with respect to seasonal variation, *Legionella* was detected in all seasons (**Table 2**).[35]

Influenza occurs at least once each year in the winter in temperate regions,[36] whereas it varies considerably from one location to the other in the tropic regions. For instance, in the southern hemisphere, the winter occurs between June and September. Therefore, the transmission dynamics of influenza virus exist throughout the year and most importantly vary between different countries. People can potentially be exposed to influenza in a constant time fashion worldwide. A definite overlap between legionellosis and influenza could exist at any time.

CLINICAL SIMILARITIES BETWEEN THE TWO PATHOGENS

It is widely accepted that LP serogroup 1 is responsible for a majority of adult *Legionella* infections, with serogroup 6 present in a smaller number of cases; together, both serogroups are responsible for two-thirds of all adult LP infections.[37] Legionellosis by clinical description is associated with 2 clinically and epidemiologically distinct illnesses: legionnaire's disease, which is characterized by fever, myalgia, cough, and

Table 2
Seasonal peak distribution of legionellosis and influenza

Author, Ref	Pathogen	Country	Season	Population
McDonald,[31] 1995	Legionella	Australia	Summer and autumn	14 Cases of 22 (64%)
Colbourne and Dennis,[32] 1989	Legionella	United Kingdom	Summer to early autumn	Sporadic cases
Bhopal and Fallon,[33] 1991	Legionella	Scotland	Autumn	Cooling tower–associated outbreaks
Garbe et al,[34] 1985	Legionella	US	Late summer to autumn	Small cooling towers–associated outbreaks
Kao et al,[35] 2015	Legionella	Taiwan	All seasons	19 Major water reservoirs
Dowel,[36] 2001	Influenza	US	Spring, fall	

clinical or radiographic pneumonia; and Pontiac fever, a milder illness without pneumonia.[38] The most prominent clinical symptoms in patients suffering from legionnaire's disease are[39–43]

Cough in 41% to 92%
Chills in 15% to 77%
Fever greater than 38.8°C in 88% to 90%
Fever greater than 40°C in 21% to 62%
Dyspnea in 25% to 62%
Headache in 40% to 48%
Myalgia/arthralgia in 20% to 40%
Diarrhea in 21% to 50%
Nausea/vomiting in 8% to 49%
Neurologic abnormalities in 4% to 53%
Chest pain in 13% to 35%

As an intracellular pathogen, LP also causes relative bradycardia[44] and, therefore, this symptom, if present, can effectively rule out, for instance, *Mycoplasma pneumoniae* from further diagnostic consideration, which represents extracellular pathogen and does not usually cause bradycardia. Influenza-like illness, which consists of fever greater than 37.7°C, cough, or sore throat, may precede legionnaire's disease and this can create differential diagnostic issues with viral CAPs (adenoviral and swine influenza [H1N1]).[45] **Table 3** shows the clinical and laboratory manifestations of legionnaire's pneumonia and influenza either the same or totally opposed.

Seasonal flu can cause fever, cough, sore throat, runny or stuffy nose, headaches and/or body aches, chills, fatigue. The symptoms of swine influenza are the same but more severe and in addition to the symptoms (discussed previously) several H1N1 flu cases may include vomiting and diarrhea. Therefore, swine flu pneumonia resembles human seasonal influenza but also avian influenza, cytomegalovirus infection, and adenoviral CAP.[50]

DIAGNOSIS OF THE DUAL INFECTION OF INFLUENZA AND LEGIONELLOSIS

Distinguishing viral from bacterial pneumonia can be difficult. This is particularly important because the signs and symptoms of pandemic influenza and legionellosis infection, as discussed previously, are similar. A retrospective analysis of CT scan findings in patients with lower respiratory tract infections demonstrated considerable overlap in findings between those of viral and bacterial origins.[51]

Usually levels of C-reactive protein and procalcitonin (PCT) tend to be higher in patients with bacterial infections compared with those with viral infections. To predict an infection, a prospective, multicenter, observational study in ICU patients with confirmed influenza A infection assessed the role of biomarkers. PCT was the most important variable for coinfection. The investigators concluded that PCT has a high negative predictive value (94%) and lower PCT levels (<0.29 ng/mL) and seems a good tool for excluding coinfection, particularly for patients without shock.[52] No single test, however, can completely distinguish bacterial infections from other infectious causes of pneumonia, because there is considerable overlap in levels between patients with and without bacterial disease.

INFLUENCE OF HOST RISK FACTORS IN DUAL INFECTION DEVELOPMENT

Risk factors for influenza and legionella either as concurrent or as sequential infections are important to identify because this secondary bacterial pneumonia complicating

Table 3
Diagnostic features of legionnaire's pneumonia and influenza pneumonia

Symptoms	Legionellosis	Influenza Pneumonia
Upper respiratory tract	None	Sore throat
Cough	Yes	Yes
Chest radiograph	Single or multiple focal infiltrates rapidly progressive	Central or peripheral ground-glass opacities, consolidations with a patchy or nodular appearance
Lobar consolidation	Yes	No
Wheezing	No	Yes
Rash	Maculopapular, erythematous, or petechial skin lesions[a]	Macular or maculopapular[b]
Hemoptysis	Yes	Possible
Fever >38.8°C	Yes	Yes
Fever + bradycardia	Yes	No
Mental confusion	Yes	Rare
Cardiac involvement	Myocarditis/endocarditis	Myocarditis
Relative bradycardia	Yes	No
Leukocytosis with relative lymphopenia	Yes	Relative lymphopenia
Gastrointestinal symptoms	Loose stools	Vomiting and diarrhea
↑AST/ALT	Yes	↑Mildly
↑CPK	Yes	Yes
Ferritin (>2× normal)	Yes	No
Thrombocytopenia	No	Yes[c]
↑Erythrocyte sedimentation rate	Yes	Yes
↑PCT	Yes	No[49]
Microscopic hematuria	Yes	No
Hypophosphatemia	Yes	No
Pleural effusion	No	No
Hyponatremia	Yes	Yes

Abbreviations: ALT, alanine aminotransferase; AST, aspartate aminotransferase; CPK, creatine kinase.

[a] Ten cases have been reported.[46]
[b] Usually in children in 2%.[47]
[c] Relative thrombocytopenia rarely exists.[48]

influenza infection has been noted to be more severe with higher mortality rates.[53] Individual risk factors for *Legionella* infection include (1) male gender, (2) age over 40 years, (3) smoking, (4) alcohol abuse, (5) certain chronic diseases (eg, diabetes), (6) chronic heart/lung diseases and chronic renal failure, (7) immunosuppressive conditions (eg, corticosteroids, chemotherapy, transplant recipient, and hematological malignancy), (8) iron overload, and (9) a history of recent travel.[30] In a study from Italy of 6 cases of pandemic influenza pneumonia and LP serogroup 1 coinfection, the patients were aged 25 to 70 years, with a median age of 53 years and a male-to-female ratio of 5:1.[54]

Genetic factors may also enhance susceptibility to LP although large studies of genetic host susceptibility and *Legionella* infection are lacking. Polymorphisms of mediators of the immune response to pathogens, like the human Toll-like receptors (TLRs), have recently demonstrated that they are associated with susceptibility to pneumonia caused by LP.[55] Other indirect findings showed that patients with immune deficiencies due to corticosteroid administration, hairy cell leukemia, myelodysplastic syndrome, or AIDS are at an increased risk of severe and persistent legionnaire's disease.[56–58]

Individual risk factors that increase incidence and mortality of influenza are conditions, such as pregnancy and body mass index greater than 35,[59] but genetic risk factors play a significant role in influenza-induced disease. The HLA system, specifically the serotype HLA-A2, confers a protective association against the viral replication after influenza infection compared with those without this HLA serotype.[60]

Another gene, the interferon-inducible transmembrane protein family members, may alter the course of influenza infection in favor of the host.[61] Single nucleotide polymorphism genotyping of the tumor necrosis factor gene was associated with increased incidences of influenza virus infections and increased risk for viral pneumonia during the 2009 pandemic period.[62]

Another important issue regarding the immune ability to fight an infectious pathogen is the immunosenescence phenomenon (**Fig. 4**), which refers to the impact of age-related changes in the immune system.[63] Progressive acquired deterioration of the immune response in people above 65 years has been related to disturbance of both the innate and humoral immune system. Suppression of TLR expression, natural killer cell deficiencies, impaired phagocytic activity of macrophages and neutrophils, and deterioration of the thymic function with subsequent declination of the cell-mediated immunity are some of the most relevant parameters that constitute the puzzle of the aging of the immune system.[64] These impairments, particularly in older people,

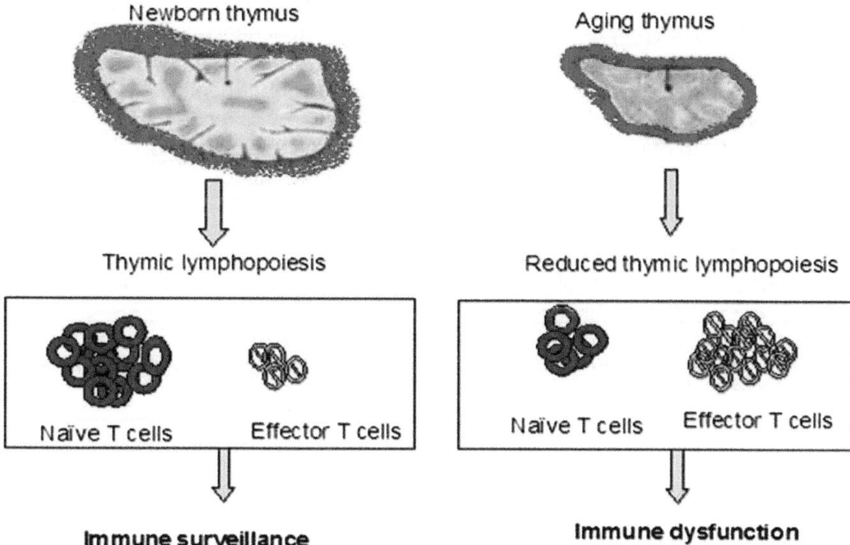

Fig. 4. Immunosenescence. With age, the thymus goes smaller by two thirds and decreases the T cell-lymphocytes content.

potentially are pivotal in the genesis of bacterial complications after an influenza infection insult.

PATHOGENESIS OF THE DUAL INFECTION INFLUENZA AND LEGIONELLOSIS

Two fundamentally different ways in how people can survive infections and in how they affect pathogen prevalence possibly explain the genesis of the secondary infection: resistance and tolerance. Resistance is based on pathogen detection and elimination, whereas tolerance (not to be confused with immunologic tolerance) relies on host adaptation to a certain pathogen burden.[65]

The distinction between these 2 defense mechanisms is crucial because they have different pathologic and epidemiologic effects (**Table 4**). Some patients are capable of tolerating the pathology of the coinfection. An example is individuals with α-thalassemia, who have less severe malaria episodes due to increased tolerance properties because parasite loads are not limited.[66] The coinfection with *Legionella* may be an indication of a patient's low tolerance and weak resistance mechanisms.

These resistance mechanisms are equipped by components of the innate and the adaptive immune system. Initially, the innate immune system recognizes the influenza virus–lung infected cells and the cytokines that are produced activate the antigen-specific adaptive immune responses. This leads to stimulation of TLRs of the macrophages and dendritic cells and subsequent secretion of inflammatory cytokines (eg, interleukin-6 and interferon-γ). Additionally, generation of antibodies by B cells and activation of the $CD4^+$ helper T cells and $CD8^+$ cytotoxic T cells also occur after the host immune response.

But highly pathogenic influenza strains cause severe dysregulation of the host innate immune response, resulting in release of proinflammatory cytokines and chemokines. This cytokine-chemokine storm then leads to collateral damage to the lung tissue.[67] Resistant mechanisms of the host are in jeopardy and, therefore, the burden of influenza increases. This altered cytokine response may also strip sialic acid from the lung, thus exposing receptors for bacterial adherence.[68] This bacterial adherence, in the case of LP, deteriorates the patient. This dual infection (influenza and legionella) negatively affects not only resistance but also tolerance mechanisms (**Fig. 5**). Influenza virus does not exert a protective effect over *Legionella* like the α-thalassemia patients who have less severe malaria. This also means that early treatment with NA inhibitors, which interrupt the cleavage of sialic acids, may increase resistance mechanisms and facilitate clearance of virus.[69] This may also increase the tolerance properties.

BACTERIAL INFECTIONS ASSOCIATED WITH SWINE INFLUENZA

During the 2009 H1N1 influenza pandemic, bacterial pneumonia was present in 4% to 33% of hospitalized or critically ill patients.[70] Bacterial pneumonia peaks anywhere

Table 4
The distinguishing characteristic of resistance and tolerance effects for infectious diseases

Resistance	Tolerance
• Prevents infection • Limits pathogens growth • Clearance infection prevalence • Reduces further transition of infection • Decreases prevalence of pathogen in population • Mediated by the immune response	• Does not inhibit infection • Limits disease severity • Neutral or positive effect on disease prevalence

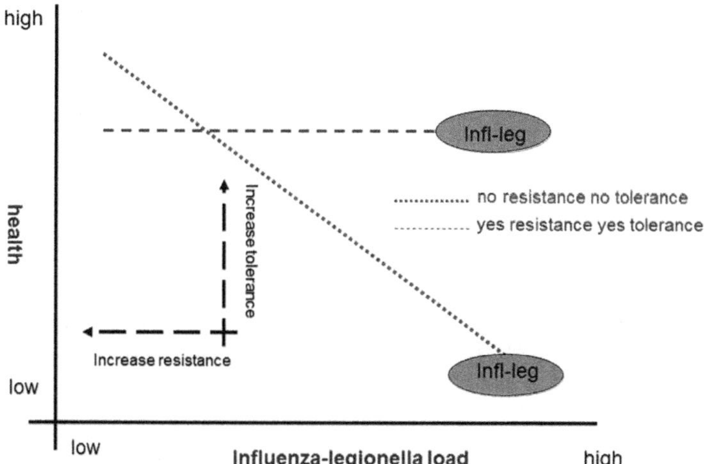

Fig. 5. In this hypothetical scheme, the 2 pathogens, influenza and legionellosis, have similar tolerance and resistance properties (*red dotted line*) but the strain shown in blue has weaker resistance.

from 4 days to 14 days after the primary influenza infection.[71] Bacterial infections may be simultaneous with onset of influenza viral infection or may follow after the influenza virus onset or clearance of the virus. In Australia, bacterial and viral coinfection was identified in approximately 1 in 4 adults and children admitted to ICUs with confirmed influenza A infection in 2009.[72] Bacterial coinfection was identified in 113 of 645 adults in Spanish ICUs with confirmed pandemic influenza A/H1N1.[73] Another study from Argentina identified coexisting bacterial pneumonia in 80 of 325 adults (25%) requiring ventilation with suspected, probable, or confirmed pandemic influenza A/H1N1 infection.[74]

Streptococcus pneumoniae as well as *Staphylococcus aureus* are the most important pathogens causing secondary bacterial pneumonia after influenza.[75,76] Especially when *S pneumoniae* is involved as a secondary bacterial pneumonia, increased morbidity and mortality have been noticed.[74] As far as the methicillin-resistant *Staphylococcus aureus* (MRSA) coinfection, the CDC in 2009 reported only 1 case of MRSA coinfection of the 272 patients hospitalized with pandemic influenza A (H1N1) 2009 influenza virus.[77] But, postmortem lung specimens from 77 cases of fatal influenza A (H1N1) 2009 influenza virus infection demonstrated evidence of concurrent bacterial infection in 22 (29%), 5 of which were MRSA.[78] In contrast, invasive group A *Streptococcus* infection concurrent with either seasonal or 2009 H1N1 influenza has been less frequently reported. Concurrent infection influenza A with *M pneumoniae* has been reported among 1060 patients with respiratory tract infections.[79]

LEGIONELLA PNEUMOPHILA AS SECONDARY OR AS SYNERGISTIC PNEUMONIA ASSOCIATED WITH H1N1 INFLUENZA

Renner and colleagues[79] study had also indicated (**Table 5**) that among the 140 patients (of 1060 patients) with serologic evidence of influenza A virus infection, 21 (15%) patients had confirmed or presumptive evidence of LP infection. Although the diagnosis of viral infection was based on paired sera and, therefore, the sensitivity is increased, cases involving an acute clinical course or early death are missed. This implies that the percentage of LP infection could be more even in this study.

Table 5
Main observational studies evaluating coexistence influenza and legionellosis infections

Ref	Study Design	Population N (Patients) Influenza	N (Patients) Coinfected with *Legionella pneumophila*
Renner et al,[79] 1983	1060 ARTIs, retrospective	140	21 (15%)
Rizzo et al,[54] 2010	2500 Registry of H1N1	1278 hospitalized	6 (18%)
Liu et al,[80] 2015	39,756 ARTIs children, prospective	10,206[a]	87 (0.86%)[b]
Iannuzzi et al,[81] 2011	Case report	2	2
Cunha et al,[83] 2010	Case report	1	1
Citton et al,[82] 2012	Case report	1	1

Abbreviation: ARTIs, acute respiratory tract infections.
[a] Positive for 1 or more respiratory pathogens.
[b] LP plus 1 or more pathogen infections.

In another registry from Italy, in 2500 confirmed cases of pandemic influenza in 2009 to 2010, bacterial coinfection was identified in 33 cases; 6 (18%) cases of bacterial coinfection were caused by LP serogroup 1.[54] The 6 *Legionellosis* cases in a total of 33 bacterial coinfections may indicate that *Legionella* is involved more often than expected. A large study from China with a total of 39,756 children with acute respiratory tract infections showed that 10,206 (25.7%) patients were positive for 1 or more respiratory pathogens. *M pneumoniae* was the most frequent pathogen (19.1%, n = 7585) whereas influenza A virus and B virus were positive in 86 (0.2%) and 1851 (4.7%) patients, respectively. The percentage of influenza coinfections with LP was low, only 21 cases of 1937 patients (1.08%).[80] Two cases of patients in Italy admitted to the ICU with coexisting H1N1 virus and *Legionella* infections have also been reported.[81] Simultaneous development of legionellosis and 2009 H1N1 virus was also reported in another patient with splenic rupture and extensive vascular thrombosis.[82] In contrast, in a nested cohort study conducted in 14 Australian ICUs, among 198 patients admitted to an ICU with polymerase chain reaction–proved influenza A infection, none was complicated with LP coinfection.[72]

Legionnaire's disease may mimic swine influenza pneumonia in many aspects, either laboratory or clinical features (dry cough, headache, high fever, myalgias, increased creatine kinase, myoglobinuria, and so forth) and, therefore, prompt diagnosis of legionnaire's disease, although sometimes difficult, is absolutely necessary. This confusion was noticed during swine influenza (H1N1) pandemic in 2009 when the Winthrop-University Hospital Infectious Disease Division provided the diagnostic legionnaire's disease triad pending *Legionella* test results.[83]

SUMMARY

Legionellosis pneumonia represents a seasonal climate and environment–related respiratory infection. It is disseminated worldwide and can survive in a biofilm formation. Clinicians should be particularly vigilant for possible legionellosis. Simultaneous coinfection and sequential infection with legionellosis has been documented in cases of influenza leading to more severe disease. It may be urgent in CAP to consider multiple-pathogen infections. The immune counteractions between influenza and

Legionella, in particular their interactions with the host, are crucial regarding the prognosis of the dual infection. Manipulation of the immune system, by producing effective pan-influenza strains vaccines or by administrating timely appropriate antiviral and antimicrobial medicines, could possibly increase resistance and tolerance in favor of the host.

REFERENCES

1. Demirjian A, Lucas CE, Garrison LE, et al. The importance of clinical surveillance in detecting legionnaire's disease outbreaks: a large outbreak in a hospital with a Legionella disinfection system-Pennsylvania, 2011-2012. Clin Infect Dis 2015; 60(11):1596–602.
2. Song JY, Cheong HJ, Heo JY, et al. Clinical, laboratory and radiologic characteristics of 2009 pandemic influenza A H1N1 pneumonia: primary influenza pneumonia versus concomitant secondary bacterial pneumonia. Influenza Other Respir Viruses 2011;5(6):e535–43.
3. Shope R. Swine Influenza. III. Filtration Experiments and Etiology. J Exp Med 1931;54:373–85.
4. Roos C. Notes on the bacteriology, and on the selective action of B. influenzae Pfeiffer. J Immunol 1919;4:189–201.
5. Fraser DW, Tsai TR, Orenstein W, et al. Legionnaire's disease: description of an epidemic of pneumonia. N Engl J Med 1977;297:1189–97.
6. Benson RF, Fields BS. Classification of the genus Legionella. Semin Respir Infect 1998;13:90–9.
7. Edelstein PH, Cianciotto NP. Legionella. In: Mandell GL, Bennett JE, Dolin R, editors. Mandell, Douglas, and Bennett's principles and practice of infectious diseases. 6th edition. Philadelphia: Churchill Livingston; 2005. p. 2711–24.
8. Lim WS, Macfarlane JT, Boswell TC, et al. Study of community acquired pneumonia aetiology (SCAPA) in adults admitted to hospital: implications for management guidelines. Thorax 2001;56(4):296–301.
9. Mandell LA, Bartlett JG, Dowell SF, et al. Infectious Diseases Society of America update of practice guidelines for the management of community-acquired pneumonia in immunocompetent adults. Clin Infect Dis 2004;37:1405–33.
10. Centers for Disease Control and Prevention (CDC). Legionellosis - United States, 2000-2009. MMWR Morb Mortal Wkly Rep 2011;60(32):1083–6.
11. Jain S, Self WH, Wunderink RG, et al. Community-Acquired Pneumonia Requiring Hospitalization among U.S. Adults. N Engl J Med 2015;373:415–27.
12. Centers for Disease Control and Prevention. Types of Influenza Viruses. 2014. Available at: http://www.cdc.gov/flu/about/viruses/types.htm. Accessed August, 2014.
13. Stray SJ, Cummings RD, Air GM. Air Influenza virus infection of desialylated cells. Glycobiology 2000;10(7):649–58.
14. Matrosovich M, Herrler G, Klenk HD. Sialic Acid Receptors of Viruses. Top Curr Chem 2015;367:1–28.
15. Smith W, Andrewes CH, Laidlaw PP. A virus obtained from influenza patients. Lancet 1933;222(5732):66–8.
16. Holmes EC, Ghedin E, Miller N, et al. Whole-genome analysis of human influenza A virus reveals multiple persistent lineages and reassortment among recent H3N2 viruses. PLoS Biol 2005;3(9):e300.
17. Gouin E, Welch MD, Cossart P. Actin-based motility of intracellular pathogens. Curr Opin Microbiol 2005;8:35–45.

18. Newton HJ, Ang DK, van Driel IR, et al. Hartland Molecular Pathogenesis of Infections Caused by *Legionella pneumophila*. Clin Microbiol Rev 2010;23(2):274–98.
19. Juhas M, Crook DW, Hood DW. Type IV secretion systems: tools of bacterial horizontal gene transfer and virulence. Cell Microbiol 2008;10(12):2377–86.
20. Losik VP. NF kappaB translocation prevents host cell death after low-dose challenge by Legionella pneumophila. J Exp Med 2006;203:2177–89.
21. Tyson JY, Vargas P, Cianciotto NP. The novel Legionella pneumophila type II secretion substrate NttC contributes to infection of amoebae Hartmannella vermiformis and Willaertia magna. Microbiology 2014;160(Pt 12):2732–44.
22. Declerck P, Behets J, van Hoef V, et al. Replication of Legionella pneumophila in floating biofilms. Curr Microbiol 2007;55(5):435–40.
23. Correia AM, Ferreira JS, Borges V, et al. Probable person-to-person transmission of Legionnaire's Disease. N Engl J Med 2016;374:497–8.
24. Centers for Disease Control and Prevention. Guidelines for environmental infection control in health-care facilities: recommendations of CDC and the Healthcare Infection Control Practices Advisory Committee (HICPAC). MMWR Recomm Rep 2003;52(No. RR-10):1–48.
25. Alhajj M, Nelson NG, McKenzie LB. Hot tub, whirlpool, and spa-related injuries in the U.S., 1990 –2007. Am J Prev Med 2009;37:531–6.
26. Bridge JA, Edelstein PH. Oropharyngeal colonization with Legionella pneumophila. J Clin Microbiol 1983;18(5):1108–12.
27. Centers for Disease Control and Prevention. Prevention strategies for seasonal influenza in healthcare settings. 2010. Available at: www.cdc.gov/flu/professionals/infectioncontrol/healthcaresettings.htm.
28. World Health Organization. Epidemic- and pandemic-prone acute respiratory diseases: infection prevention and control for acute respiratory diseases in health-care facilities. 2008. Available at: http://www.who.int/csr/resour.
29. Bischoff WE, Swett K, Leng I, et al. Exposure to Influenza Virus Aerosols During Routine Patient Care. J Infect Dis 2013;207(7):1037–46.
30. World Health Organization. Legionella and the prevention of legionellosis. Geneva (Switzerland): WHO; 2007. Available at: http://www.who.int/water_sanitation_health/emerging/legionella.pdf.
31. McDonald L. Master of applied epidemiology theses. National centre of epidemiology and population health. Canberra (Australia): Australian National University; 1995. p. 38–9.
32. Colbourne J, Dennis P. The ecology and survival of *Legionella pneumophila*. J Inst Water Environ Manag 1989;3:345–50.
33. Bhopal RS, Fallon RJ. Seasonal variation of Legionnaire's disease in Scotland. J Infect 1991;22:153–60.
34. Garbe PL, Davies BJ, Weisfeld JS, et al. Nosocomial Legionnaire's disease. JAMA 1985;254:521–4.
35. Kao PM, Hsu BM, Chang TY, et al. Seasonal variation of Legionella in Taiwan's reservoir and its relationships with environmental factors. Environ Sci Pollut Res Int 2015;22(8):6104–11.
36. Dowell SF. Seasonal variation in host susceptibility and cycles of certain infectious diseases. Emerg Infect Dis 2001;7:369–74.
37. Yu VL, Plouffe JF, Pastoris MC, et al. Distribution of Legionella Species and Serogroups Isolated by Culture in Patients with Sporadic CommunityAcquired Legionellosis: An International Collaborative Survey. J Infect Dis 2002;186(1):127–8.

38. Legionellosis/Legionnaire's Disease or Pontiac fever (*Legionella pneumophila*). Case Definition Centers for Disease Control and Prevention. 2005. Available at: https://wwwn.cdc.gov/nndss/conditions/legionellosis/case-definition/2005.
39. Yu VL, Kroboth FJ, Shonnard J, et al. Legionnaire's disease: new clinical perspective from a prospective pneumonia study. Am J Med 1982;73:357–61.
40. Fang GD, Fine M, Orloff J, et al. New and emerging etiologies for community-acquired pneumonia with implications for therapy. A prospective multicenter study of 359 cases. Medicine (Baltimore) 1990;69:307–16.
41. Roig J, Aguilar X, Ruiz J, et al. Comparative study of Legionella pneumophila and other nosocomial-acquired pneumonias. Chest 1991;99:344–50.
42. Kirby BD, Snyder KM, Meyer RD, et al. Legionnaire's disease: report of sixty-five nosocomial-acquired cases of review of the literature. Medicine (Baltimore) 1980; 59:188–205.
43. Cunha BA. Clinical features of legionnaire's disease. Semin Respir Infect 1998; 13:116–27.
44. Cunha BA. The diagnostic significance of relative bradycardia in infectious diseases. Clin Microbiol Infect 2000;6:633–4.
45. McCullens J. The co-pathogenesis of influenza viruses with bacteria in the lung. Nat Rev Microbiol 2014;12:252–62.
46. Thalanayar PM, Holguin F. Rash, disseminated intravascular coagulation and legionella: Episode 10 and a rewind into the past. Respir Med Case Rep 2015;15: 95–100.
47. Silva ME, Cherry JD, Wilton RJ, et al. Acute fever and petechial rash associated with influenza A virus infection. Clin Infect Dis 1999;29(2):453–4.
48. Samra T, Pawar M. Reactive thrombocytosis in H1N1 infection. J Lab Physicians 2011;3(2):131–2.
49. Pfister R, Kochanek M, Leygeber T, et al. Procalcitonin for diagnosis of bacterial pneumonia in critically ill patients during 2009 H1N1 influenza pandemic: a prospective cohort study, systematic review and individual patient data meta-analysis. Crit Care 2014;18(2):R44.
50. Cunha B. Antibiotic essentials. 14th edition. Faridabad (India): Jaypee Brothers Medical Publishers; 2015. p. p.63.
51. Miller WT Jr, Mickus TJ, Barbosa E Jr, et al. CT of viral lower respiratory tract infections in adults: comparison among viral organisms and between viral and bacterial infections. AJR Am J Roentgenol 2011;197(5):1088–95.
52. Rodríguez AH, Avilés-Jurado FX, Díaz E, et al. Procalcitonin (PCT) levels for ruling-out bacterial coinfection in ICU patients with influenza: A CHAID decision-tree analysis. J Infect 2016;72(2):143–51.
53. Jamieson AM, Pasman L, Yu S, et al. Role of tissue protection in lethal respiratory viral-bacterial coinfection. Science 2013;340(6137):1230–4.
54. Rizzo C, Caporali MG, Rota MC. Pandemic Influenza and pneumonia due to Legionella pneumophila: a frequent underestimated coinfection. Clin Infect Dis 2010;51:115.
55. Hawn TR, Verbon A, Lettinga KD, et al. A common dominant TLR5 stop codon polymorphism abolishes flagellin signaling and is associated with susceptibility to Legionnaire's disease. J Exp Med 2003;198:1563–72.
56. Higa F, Fujita J, Koide M, et al. Clinical features of two cases of Legionnaire's disease with persistence of Legionella urinary antigen excretion. Intern Med 2008; 47(3):173–8.
57. Schlossberg D, Bonoan J. Legionella and immunosuppression. Semin Respir Infect 1998;13(2):128–31.

58. Cunha BA, Hage JE. *Legionella pneumophila* community-acquired pneumonia (CAP) in a post-splenectomy patient with myelodysplastic syndrome (MDS). Heart Lung 2012;41(5):525–7.
59. Kumar A, Zarychanski R, Pinto R, et al. Critically ill patients with 2009 influenza A(H1N1) infection in Canada. JAMA 2009;302(17):1872–9.
60. Boon AC, de Mutsert G, Graus YM, et al. The magnitude and specificity of influenza A virus-specific cytotoxic T-lymphocyte responses in humans is related to HLA-A and -B phenotype. J Virol 2002;76(2):582–90.
61. Everitt AR, Clare S, Pertel T, et al. IFITM3 restricts the morbidity and mortality associated with influenza. Nature 2012;484:519–23.
62. Antonopoulou A, Baziaka F, Tsaganos T, et al. Role of tumor necrosis factor gene single nucleotide polymorphisms in the natural course of 2009 influenza A H1N1 virus infection. Int J Infect Dis 2012;16(3):e204–8.
63. Danielle AW, Silva AB, Palmer DB. Immunosenescence: emerging challenges for an ageing population. Immunology 2007;120(4):435–46.
64. Joshi SR, Shaw A, Quagliarello VJ. Pandemic influenza H1N1 2009, innate immunity, and the impact of immunosenescence on influenza vaccine. Yale J Biol Med 2009;82:143–51.
65. Schneider DS, Ayres JS. Two ways to survive infection: what resistance and tolerance can teach us about treating infectious diseases. Nat Rev Immunol 2008;8: 889–95.
66. Wambua S, Mwangi TW, Kortok M, et al. The effect of alpha+-thalassaemia on the incidence of malaria and other diseases in children living on the coast of Kenya. PLoS Med 2006;3(5):e158.
67. Oslund KL, Baumgarth N. Influenza-induced innate immunity: regulators of viral replication, respiratory tract pathology & adaptive immunity. Future Virol 2011; 6(8):951–62.
68. Jean C, Louie JK, Glaser CA, et al. Invasive group A streptococcal infection concurrent with 2009 H1N1 influenza. Clin Infect Dis 2010;50(10):e59–62.
69. McCullers JA, Bartmess KC. Role of neuraminidase in lethal synergism between influenza virus and *Streptococcus pneumoniae*. J Infect Dis 2003;187(6):1000–9.
70. Rice TW, Rubinson L, Uyeki TM, et al. Critical illness from 2009 pandemic influenza A virus and bacterial coinfection in the United States. Crit Care Med 2012;40:1487–98.
71. Ballinger MN, Standiford TJ. Postinfluenza bacterial pneumonia: host defenses gone awry. J Interferon Cytokine Res 2010;30(9):643–52.
72. Blyth CC, Webb SAR, Kok J, et al, on behalf of the ANZIC Influenza Investigators, COSI Microbiological Investigators. The impact of bacterial and viral co-infection in severe influenza. Influenza Other Respir Viruses 2013;7(2):168–76.
73. Martin-Loeches I, Sanchez-Corral A, Diaz E, et al. Community-acquired respiratory co-infection (CARC) in critically ill patients infected with pandemic 2009 influenza A (H1N1) virus infection. Chest 2011;139:555–62.
74. Estenssoro E, Rios FG, Apezteguia C, et al. Pandemic 2009 influenza A in Argentina: a study of 337 patients on mechanical ventilation. Am J Respir Crit Care Med 2010;182:41–8.
75. O'Brien KL, Walters MI, Sellman J, et al. Severe pneumococcal pneumonia in previously healthy children: the role of preceding influenza infection. Clin Infect Dis 2000;30:784–9.
76. Grabowska K, Högberg L, Penttinen P, et al. Occurrence of invasive pneumococcal disease and number of excess cases due to influenza. BMC Infect Dis 2006;20(6):58.

77. Jain S, Kamimoto L, Bramley AM, et al. Hospitalized patients with 2009 H1N1 influenza in the United States, April–June 2009. N Engl J Med 2009;361:1935–44.
78. Centers for Disease Control. Bacterial co-infections in lung tissue specimens from fatal cases of 2009 pandemic influenza A (H1N1) – United States, May–August 2009. MMWR Morb Mortal Wkly Rep 2009;58(38):1071–4.
79. Renner ED, Helms CM, Johnson W, et al. Coinfections of Mycoplasma pneumoniae and Legionella pneumophila with Influenza A Virus. J Clin Microbiol 1983; 17(1):146–8.
80. Liu J, Ai H, Xiong Y, et al. Prevalence and correlation of infectious agents in hospitalized children with acute respiratory tract infections in central China. PLoS One 2015;10(3):e0119170.
81. Iannuzzi M, De Robertis E, Piazza O, et al. Respiratory failure presenting in H1N1 influenza with Legionnaire's disease: two case reports. J Med Case Rep 2011; 21(5):520.
82. Citton R, Del Borgo C, Belvisi V, et al. Pandemic influenza H1N1, legionellosis, splenic rupture and vascular thrombosis:a dangerous cocktail. J Postgrad Med 2012;58:228–9.
83. Cunha BA, Mickail N, Syed U, et al. Rapid clinical diagnosis of Legionnaire's disease during the "herald wave" of the swine influenza (H1N1) pandemic: the Legionnaire's disease triad. Heart Lung 2010;39(3):249–59.

Nosocomial (Health Care–Associated) Legionnaire's Disease

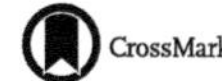

Shanu Agarwal, MD[a,b], Virginia Abell, RN, BA[c],
Thomas M. File Jr, MD, MSc, MACP[a,d,*]

KEYWORDS

• Nosocomial • Health care–associated • *Legionella* • Outbreaks • Prevention

KEY POINTS

- Nosocomial legionellosis is underappreciated as a cause of nosocomial pneumonia especially if there is a lack of awareness of the presence of *Legionella* spp with a hospital water supply.
- Legionnaire's disease should be suspected especially if no other etiology for pneumonia is found.
- Prevention of legionnaire's disease focuses on reducing the reservoir within water systems and includes super heating, ultraviolet light, chlorination, sliver-copper ionization, and distal filtration.

INTRODUCTION

Legionella was first identified in 1976 as a result of a community outbreak of severe pneumonia among participants of the American Legion Convention in Philadelphia, Pennsylvania.[1,2] Since then there have been numerous outbreaks of legionnaire's disease (LD) in health care settings. Outbreaks are commonly associated with facilities that have large water systems, such as hotels and resorts, long-term care facilities, and hospitals. Thus, hospitals are increasingly facing the potential for nosocomial transmission. This article reviews the epidemiology of health care–associated (HCA)

Funding: None.

Conflict of Interest: No conflict (S. Agarwal and V. Abell). Recent research funding, Cempra and Pfizer; Scientific Advisory Board Member, Allergan, Cempra, Merck, MotifBio, Nabriva, Pfizer, and Tetraphase (T.M. File).

[a] Infectious Disease Division, Summa Health, 1077 Forge Boulevard, Akron, OH 44310, USA; [b] Department of Medicine, Northeast Ohio Medical University, 4029 Street Rt 44, Rootstown, OH 44272, USA; [c] Infection Prevention and Clinical Safety, Summa Akron City and St. Thomas Hospitals, 525 East Market Street, Akron, OH 44309-2090, USA; [d] Internal Medicine, Infectious Disease Section, Northeast Ohio Medical University, 4029 Street Rt 44, Rootstown, OH 44272, USA

* Corresponding author. 75 Arch Street, Suite 506 (Suite 105 for Research), Akron, OH 44304.
E-mail address: filet@summahealth.org

Infect Dis Clin N Am 31 (2017) 155–165
http://dx.doi.org/10.1016/j.idc.2016.10.011 id.theclinics.com
0891-5520/17/

LD, reviews characteristics of several HCA outbreaks, and discusses strategies to prevent HCA infection.

EPIDEMIOLOGY

Although *Legionella* spp are uncommon causes of nosocomial infection, the Centers for Disease Control and Prevention (CDC) recommends a high degree of suspicion[3]; this is especially when there are cases of nosocomial pneumonia caused by undefined etiology. Nosocomial LD should be considered whenever there has been a laboratory documented case within a health care facility in the past or *Legionella* has been documented from surveillance cultures of health care water sources. The CDC guidance document on the prevention of HCA pneumonia defines laboratory-confirmed cases to be "definite" HCA LD if a patient has spent equal to or greater than 10 days continuously in a health care facility before the onset of LD, or "possible" HCA LD if a patient has spent 2 to 9 days in a health care facility before the onset of LD.[3] When a single case of laboratory-confirmed definite health care–associated LD is identified, or when two or more cases of laboratory-confirmed, possibly HCA LD occur within 6 months, an outbreak investigation is recommended.[3] In contrast, other policies support a risk assessment of health care transmission of *Legionella* based on quantification of the organism from a facility's water sources.[4] Many facilities apply a "30% action threshold" whereby decontamination of the water system is performed when *Legionella* is recovered from 30% or more of the tested sites.[5] However, the utility of this policy has been questioned; and nosocomial transmission has occurred with less than 30% of sites tested positive. A survey of peer-reviewed publications suggests the 30% cutoff value has a sensitivity of 59% and specificity of 74%, which implies a 41% false-negative rate and 26% false-positive rate.[5]

Within the hospital setting, recognition of nosocomial pneumonia (NP) is crucial to identifying an outbreak. Key to this recognition is the input from microbiology, infectious disease services, and infection control personnel.[6] The documentation of an outbreak within a health care setting to a certain extent depends on identifying identical strains or clones of the organism. Because *Legionella pneumophila* serogroup 1 expresses a conserved genome, the use of standard molecular techniques may be insufficient to accurately monitor an outbreak. Recently Bartley and colleagues[7] have demonstrated the use of whole gene sequencing offers the potential to accurately identify outbreak strains. They used genomic epidemiology and whole gene sequencing to link *L pneumophila* serogroup 1 isolates from 2 patients from an outbreak with a clone that had been present in a hospital water supply.[7]

Nosocomial Sources and Transmission

Because *Legionella* amplifies in man-made water sources in the presence of warm water temperatures (20°C–45°C),[8] nosocomial LD can occur as patients are exposed to such sources. Health care facilities are included in the types of buildings that have been associated with the transmission of *Legionella* to patients. Cases of HCA LD often arise from exposure to *Legionella* bacteria in hospital potable water distribution systems. Surveys have shown that *Legionella* colonizes the hot water distribution system in 12% to 70% of hospitals in specific geographic areas.[9,10] In one study from Hungary, 90% of survey hospitals found *Legionella* in the water supply; most of the hospitals were greater than 30 years old.[11]

Legionella spp are particularly likely to be found in pipes and water tanks of health care facilities when there is stasis, the presence of sediment, or biofilm. In addition, the presence of amebae or algae within water systems is associated with *Legionella* spp because these are natural hosts for *Legionella* and provide essential nutrients.[12] The wide-ranging network of pipes of water distribution systems within hospitals make for ideal conditions for *Legionella* replication. Biofilms often form within the luminal surfaces of water pipes and are made up of a complex matrix of algae and various debris.

The incidence of LD depends on the degree of water reservoir contamination, the intensity of patient exposure to that water, and the susceptibility of the host. Transmission of nosocomial LD has been linked to inhalation or aspiration of water contaminated with *Legionella*; and has been associated with numerous health care water sources including respiratory therapy equipment, decorative fountains, high-pressure water cleaning, whirlpool baths, drinking fountains, and cooling towers.[8,13] Aspiration of contaminated water used to flush nasogastric tubes or inhalation devices has been implicated in nosocomial disease.[9,14] Oropharyngeal colonization by *Legionella* is also possible. *Legionella* spp were detected by direct fluorescent antibody in several sputum samples from patients undergoing solid organ transplantation during a 3-year period.[15]

Patient Host Factors

Because hospitalized patients are often older or have immunocompromising or chronic illnesses, they are at high risk for LD. However, LD can also occur in healthy, immunocompetent individuals. The rate of legionellosis increases with increasing age, although this may be caused by a higher rate of comorbidities in older individuals rather than being a direct association. Smoking has a strong association with the predisposition of acquiring LD.[16] Transplant recipients and patients receiving cancer chemotherapy carry a high risk for *Legionella* spp infection.[17–19] Glucocorticoid administration and other illnesses associated with immunosuppression are also independent risk factors.

LD has only been infrequently reported in patients with human immunodeficiency virus infection.[20] Receipt of biologic therapies increases the risk of *Legionella* infection. A recent review of the literature revealed 105 cases of LD in patients receiving tumor necrosis factor-α inhibitors (infliximab, adalimumab, etanercept) or the anti-B-cell monoclonal antibody, rituximab.[21] Most received the biologic for rheumatologic diseases and most also received other immunosuppressive therapy, such as steroids. The overall mortality was 19%.

Legionnaire's Disease in Long-Term Care Facilities

In long-term care facilities and nursing homes, *Legionella* spp are important but under-recognized causes of pneumonia.[22,23] Two outbreaks of *Legionella sainthelensi* pneumonia were described in nursing homes in Canada; 29 cases occurred during a 2-month period.[22] Four (14%) case-residents had documented pneumonia and four case-residents died. Univariate analysis revealed that a history of stroke (odds ratio [OR], 2.3; 95% confidence interval [CI], 1.0–5.3), eating pureed food (OR, 4.6; 95% CI, 1.6–12.7), and having fluids administered with medication (OR, 2.5; 95% CI, 1.0–5.9) were significant risk factors. Cases were less likely to wear dentures (OR, 0.4; 95% CI, 0.2–0.9) or to eat solid food (OR, 0.3; 95% CI, 0.1–0.6). Only eating pureed food remained significant in a multivariable analysis (OR, 4.6; 95% CI, 1.6–13.0; $P = .01$).

Other Outbreaks (Automobile Plant)

Industrial plants are a source for the propagation and transmission of *Legionella*. LD outbreaks have been reported in industrial settings, including an automotive plant whose workers were exposed to contaminated fluids where an aerosol-producing device was implicated.[24]

HEALTH CARE–ASSOCIATED OUTBREAKS (SELECTED US EXPERIENCE)

1977 Columbus, Ohio

In August 1977, three patients at a community hospital located in Columbus, Ohio, were found to have severe pneumonia with LD. All three patients had been hospitalized or visited the hospital (index hospital) within 2 weeks before the onset of their illness. Marks and colleagues[25] described the outbreak investigation, which involved serologic *Legionella* screening of patients who were hospitalized at the index hospital with pneumonia after July 1, 1977. Serum samples were collected and tested from employees and construction workers of the index hospital. Individuals and health care workers at the index hospital, who were in close contact with the confirmed cases, were also tested to evaluate the risk of secondary spread. Nine confirmed and presumptive *Legionella* cases were identified at the index hospital. Six of these patients were diagnosed with pneumonia and were exposed to the index hospital on 2 or more of the 14 days before the onset of illness. Three nearby hospitals were selected to serve as controls. Five patients at the control hospitals had positive *Legionella* serum titers. Three of the five patients were from the renal transplant service and had been hospitalized for at least 1 month before the onset of pneumonia. The outbreak investigation was able to associate the cluster of cases with recent hospitalization rather than community exposure. In October 1978, water specimens were tested for *Legionella* bacterium and a Philadelphia-type strain was isolated from the cooling towers of the index hospital; however, the air conditioning system and construction sites were also hypothesized as possible sources.

2008 New Brunswick, New Jersey

In 2008, a hospital-associated *Legionella* outbreak was identified at Saint Peter's University Hospital in New Brunswick, New Jersey. Six patients were identified as having LD.[26] The patients were all located in the same area of the hospital and all had immunocompromising conditions. Hospital investigation revealed the isolation of *Legionella* bacteria in the water source that supplied this patient area. Low chlorine levels in the water supply were detected and linked to the cause of the *Legionella* colonization. Subsequently, plans to increase chlorine levels in the water supply were instituted and filters were installed on the showerheads of inpatient rooms.

2011 Pittsburgh, Pennsylvania

An outbreak investigation in 2011 further emphasized the importance of including LD in the differential of HCA pneumonia. Demirjian and colleagues[27] describe a large outbreak at the Veterans Administration Hospital Healthcare System where a *Legionella* disinfection system was in place. In 1994, the hospital installed a copper-silver ionization system to control the persistent presence of *Legionella* in its water distribution system. Laboratory-confirmed *Legionella* cases were identified from January 2011 to December 2012. Cases were further classified into definite HCA (clinical pneumonia with laboratory confirmation of LD and hospitalization for 14 days before onset of symptoms) versus probable HCA LD (clinical pneumonia with exposure to the hospital only during a portion of the 2- to 14-day period before onset). Five definite and 17 probable HCA *Legionella* cases were identified and six patients died of the disease. Multiple water sources at the hospital system were collected for *Legionella* culture.

Water pH, temperature, total chlorine residuals, and copper and silver ion concentrations were also measured. Microbiologic cultures showed growth of *Legionella* in 23 of 25 locations where environmental samples were obtained. Some of the clinical *Legionella* isolates matched the environmental isolates. Despite adequate copper and silver ion concentrations, *Legionella* was isolated from the water samples. Results of the investigation linked the cases to the potable water system and emphasized the importance of including LD in the differential of HCA pneumonia, even in the setting of a long-term disinfection program.

2013 Franklin, Ohio

Susceptible patient populations are not only at risk for HCA *Legionella* in the acute care setting but also at long-term care facilities. In 2013, a total of 39 cases of LD were identified at a retirement community in Columbus, Ohio.[28] Of the 39 confirmed cases, six patients died from LD. A cooling tower that used an automated biocide (biocide injected only during active use) delivery system was identified as the outbreak source. Cooling towers that work on timed biocide delivery systems can become a reservoir for the amplification and dissemination of *Legionella*. The investigation highlighted the importance of cooling tower designs and the need to have ongoing environmental *Legionella* surveillance.

The HCA *Legionella* outbreaks described previously are some of many (**Table 1**) that have been recognized in the last few decades. Information gathered from outbreaks such as these help health care facilities implement strategies to prevent LD through active surveillance. Infection control programs and local and state health departments are vital resources in identifying outbreaks and guiding health care institutions in taking a proactive approach to the prevention of HCA LD.

Nosocomial Legionnaire's Disease: Approach to Diagnosis

LD should be suspected as a cause of nosocomial pneumonia especially if no other etiology is defined. Nosocomial LD is easily overlooked because of a lack of awareness of the presence of LD within a hospital water supply. Guidelines for routine environmental sampling for *Legionella* in hospitals have been adopted in several

Table 1
Some representative United States health care–associated *Legionella* outbreaks

Reference/ Year	City	Location	Source	Cases	Deaths
Marks,[25] 1977	Columbus, OH	Riverside Hospital	Suspected cooling tower and water supply near construction areas	9 at index hospital 5 at control hospital	0
2008[26]	New Brunswick, NJ	Saint Peter's University Hospital	Drinking water	6	2
Demirjian,[27] 2012	Pittsburgh, PA	Veteran's Administration Hospital	Water supply	22	6
Quinn,[28] 2013	Franklin, OH	Long-term care facility	Cooling tower	39	6
Hu,[42] 2015	South Bronx, NY	Hotel	Cooling tower	113	12

states in the United States, by the United States Veterans Affairs Healthcare System, and by many European countries.[2,29–31] The CDC has accepted the concept of routine environmental culturing for institutions with bone marrow transplant programs.

Successful diagnosis requires specialized laboratory tests. In the past, the diagnosis of endemic LD in the hospital setting was often missed because of the lack of availability of specialized laboratory tests. However, the *Legionella* urinary antigen assay has become more readily available, and the diagnosis of *Legionella* pneumonia has therefore increased. The laboratory diagnosis of *Legionella* including specialized culture methods (using CYE agar), serologic, and molecular methods is discussed elsewhere in this issue.

HOSPITAL MANAGEMENT AND PREVENTION

Role of the Water Environment in Legionella Transmission

In cases of HCA *Legionella* pneumonia, the potable water supply is the chief environmental risk factor. Maintaining hospital water systems free of *Legionella* colonization minimizes the risk of infection (**Table 2**).[4]

Monitoring is key to clinical recognition of *Legionella* pneumonia. Patients suspected of community-acquired or HCA pneumonia should have a *Legionella* urinary antigen test. If detected, a lower respiratory specimen, on selective media, should be cultured for *Legionella*.

Some characteristics of the *Legionella* organism and hospital water systems adversely affect the efficacy of water control measures. *Legionella* are present in a large percentage of municipal domestic water systems serving hospital systems. Within the water system infrastructure are many risk factors. Existence of hot water holding tanks, "dead-leg" plumbing that has been altered to prevent water flow, and areas of stagnant water accommodate biofilms in piping providing nutrition and protection for *Legionella* reservoirs.

Table 2
Representative methods to reduce *Legionella* within hospital water systems

Method	Advantages	Disadvantages
Super heat and flush: heat water to 70°C; flush all water outlets for 30 min to suppress *Legionella*	Can be done on recognition of adverse conditions	Time-consuming; labor intensive; temporary fix; risk of burns
Hyperchlorination: raise continuous chlorine levels three-fold providing residual disinfection at distal sites[a]	Provides some residual disinfection at distal sites	Corrosive to pipes; increased leaks causing water shut-offs Potential carcinogen[12]
Silver/copper ionization: ions disrupt the cell wall killing *Legionella*[1,7,41]	Long-term solution Effective killing of organisms Not affected by high water temperatures	Ongoing ion monitoring and electrode replacement Costly installation
Point-of-use filters: provides a barrier at each distal outlet	Prevents the flow of bacteria to the point of use	Need to be provided on every at-risk outlet; need replacement every 30 d

[a] In addition to this free chlorine method, monochloramine and chlorine dioxide formulations are also available for long-term use.

These water systems, often old and complex, are prone to disruption. Routine maintenance, construction work, and emergency situations require shut down and re-establishment of the water. Turbulent flow disturbs the reservoirs and redistributes the *Legionella* toward distal outlets.

Routine Management of the Water System

Because *Legionella* survives at temperatures up to 60°C, keeping hot water storage at a temperature of at least 60°C seems prudent[32]. However, at 60°C water can cause third-degree burns in children in 1 second and in adults in 5 seconds.[33] So hospital regulations require a distal outlet delivery temperature of 49°C. This is a dilemma for facility engineers to manage as follows:

1. Inhibit *Legionella* growth by maintaining proper water temperatures.
   a. Maintain hot water holding tank at temperature = greater than 60°C (140°F).
   b. Where possible, use instantaneous heating devices having a discharge temperature of 60°C (140°F). Instantaneous heating installations are more effective in new systems lacking established biofilms of *Legionella*.
   c. Distal water distribution temperature 49°C (120°F).
2. Chlorine-treated water is widely used and effective against many waterborne pathogens. However, its control of enteric pathogens is more reliable than its ability to control *Legionella*.[34]
3. Ultraviolet light irradiation of recirculating water kills bacterial cells by damaging their DNA. Ultraviolet can supplement chlorine as a protection against *Legionella*.
4. Prevent or eliminate dead-legs at every opportunity during new construction or renovation projects.
5. Routine preventative maintenance programs may not eliminate *Legionella* colonization in old water systems or in those previously colonized.[35]

Environmental Monitoring of the Water System

Routine sampling of water for *Legionella* remains a discordant topic with differing rationale and approaches proposed.

Ascertaining the state of *Legionella* colonization requires environmental surveillance of the water systems. Water sample cultures are the prevalent method for ascertaining colonization. More recently a sensitive, specific polymerase chain reaction assay has been available. It cannot differentiate between live and dead organisms. Therefore, culture remains the best practice test.[36]

The CDC recommends clinical disease monitoring for *Legionella* in HCA pneumonia. If *Legionella* pneumonia is suspected, environmental sampling is begun to identify the source of *Legionella* and the effectiveness of corrective action. CDC reserves baseline environmental sampling for high-risk centers, such as transplant units.

The reasons behind avoiding routine water testing[37] include the following:

1. Environmental sampling results are hard to interpret because some amount of *Legionella* occurs naturally in so many water systems.
2. The *Legionella* colony count likely to produce illness is unknown.
3. *Legionella* is isolated during routine sampling in the absence of disease. This leads to the dilemma of what, if any action to take. A reservoir is only one element in the chain of infection. What is the virulence of the organism? Is there high-risk susceptibility in the resident population? Can the water be aerosolized? Is there opportunity for the host to inhale or aspirate?
4. Negative testing can lead to false security and lax operation and maintenance practices.

Proponents of routine environmental culturing include *Legionella* experts Drs Janet Stout and Victor Yu.[38] This strategy finds routine environmental cultures for *Legionella* are necessary to assess risk even in the absence of disease. Rationale for this proactive approach is as follows:

1. *Legionella* colonization varies over time. Continued environmental surveillance documents this variation
2. Hospital-acquired LD cases have always been associated with *Legionella* in the water system.
3. Positive environmental sampling creates a high degree of suspicion and allows for intensified active surveillance for cases.
4. Routine sampling allows evaluation of effective prevention and control measures.

The CDC has provided guidance for sampling methods, sites, and frequency.[39] These water samples must be tested by a laboratory skilled in environmental testing with ELITE certification from the CDC.[32] Interpretation of *Legionella* testing results varies. Some facilities take an escalating course of action if any testing site has *Legionella* higher than the level of detection (1 colony/test or <1 CFU/mL).[40] Many facilities apply a "30% action threshold" whereby decontamination of the water system is performed when *Legionella* is recovered from 30% or more of the tested sites.[41]

Emergency Management of Legionella Contamination in the Water System

Unacceptable levels of *Legionella* in the water system or clinical cases of HCA *Legionella* pneumonia require corrective action.[29,31,35] In outbreak situations corrective action is needed rapidly. Short-term remediation must be followed by long-term solutions.

Limitations to the Success of Interventions

Many nooks and crannies of a complex water system provide protection for *Legionella* colonies. Combine this with the biofilms common on water contact surfaces and *Legionella* are provided with nutrients. Most water distribution systems eventually develop biofilms that may harbor *Legionella* and promote metal pipe corrosion, scaling, and sediment buildup. The more age to the system, the greater the risk.

1. Reservoirs of *Legionella* are not necessarily eliminated by any of these methods. Continuous processes with silver-copper and chlorine may control regrowth of *Legionella*. However, a recent Pennsylvania hospital *Legionella* outbreak occurred despite the use of copper/silver ionization. The authors emphasized the need for continued vigilant clinical screening for *Legionella*.[7]
2. Super heating and flushing only temporarily eliminates or decreases *Legionella*.
3. Ultraviolet light does not affect distal sites nor does it eradicate hot water tanks or instantaneous heating systems; these affect primarily the initial contamination of a water system.
4. Water shutoff, weather, and water supply intermittently interrupted because of construction or emergencies are likely to disturb *Legionella* reservoirs and limit effectiveness of control measures. There must be a water maintenance risk management plan in place for all of these contingencies.

Successful Interventions

When infection prevention/epidemiology professionals lead a multidisciplinary team of health care and engineering personnel in selecting and evaluating routine, emergency, and long-term *Legionella* control measures, the effort is more likely to be successful.[4,27]

Multiple lines of defense against *Legionella* are needed for continuous clearing of colonization. In hospitals with persistent endemic growth of *Legionella* in the water system, multiple approaches provide a cushion against failure of a system: ultraviolet light and copper/silver ions. Both clinical and epidemiologic identification methods aid a program of water treatment.[13]

Western Pennsylvania Healthcare Initiative[29] and the Veterans Administration Directives[31] provide comprehensive guidelines on all aspects of *Legionella* prevention, treatment, and risk management. These guidelines also emphasize the importance of a multidisciplinary team approach to managing this program of prevention and intervention. The guidelines also emphasize the importance of continuous attention to clinical pneumonias and maintenance of the water system. It is a cliché but true: *Legionella* control is a marathon and a sprint.

REFERENCES

1. Available at: http://www.cdc.gov/legionella/about/history.html. Accessed July 8, 2016.
2. Cunha BA, Burillo A, Bouza E. Legionnaire's disease. Lancet 2016;387:376–85.
3. CDC. Guidelines for preventing health-care-associated pneumonia, 2003: recommendations of CDC and the Healthcare Infection Control Practices Advisory Committee (HICPAC). MMWR Morb Mortal Wkly Rep 2004;53(RR03):1–36.
4. Lin YE, Stout JE, Yu VL. Prevention of hospital-acquired legionellosis. Curr Opin Infect Dis 2011;24:350–6.
5. Cunha BA, Thekkel V, Schoch PE. Community-acquired versus nosocomial *Legionella* pneumonia: lessons learned from an epidemiologic investigation. Am J Infect Control 2011;39:901–3.
6. Allen JG, Myatt TA, Macintosh DL, et al. Assessing risk of health care-acquired Legionnaire's disease from environmental sampling: the limits of using a strict percent positivity approach. Am J Infect Control 2012;40:917–21.
7. Bartley PB, Ben Zakour NL, Stanton-Cook M, et al. Hospital-wide Eradication of a Nosocomial *Legionella* pneumophila serogroup 1 Outbreak. Clin Infect Dis 2016; 62:273–9.
8. Plouffe J, File TM Jr. Update of *Legionella* infections. Curr Opin Infect Dis 1999; 12:127–32.
9. Sabria M, Yu VL. Hospital-acquired legionellosis: solutions for a preventable infection. Lancet Infect Dis 2002;2:368–73.
10. Alessandro DD, Fabiani M, Cerquetani F, et al. Trend of *Legionella* colonization in hospital water supply. Ann Ig 2015;27:460–6.
11. Barna Z, Kádá M, Kálmán E, et al. *Legionella* prevalence and risk of legionellosis in Hungarian hospitals. Acta Microbiol Immunol Hung 2015;62:477–99.
12. Lagana P, Caruso G, Piccione D, et al. *Legionella* spp., amoebae and non-fermenting gram-negative bacteria in an Italian university hospital water system. Ann Agric Environ Med 2014;21:489–93.
13. Palmore TN, Stock F, White M, et al. A cluster of nosocomial Legionnaire's disease linked to contaminated hospital decorative water fountain. Infect Cont Hosp Epidemiol 2009;30:764–8.
14. Venezia RA, Agresta MD, Hanley EM, et al. Nosocomial legionellosis associated with aspiration of nasogastric feedings diluted in tap water. Infect Control Hosp Epidemiol 1994;15:529–33.

15. Jaresova M, Hlozanek I, Striz I, et al. *Legionella* detection in oropharyngeal aspirates of transplant patients prior to surgery. Eur J Clin Microbiol Infect Dis 2006; 25:63–4.
16. Strauss WL, Plouffe JF, File TM Jr, et al. Risk factors for domestic acquisition of Legionnaires disease. Ohio Legionnaires Disease Group. Arch Intern Med 1996;156:1685–92.
17. Singh N, Stout JE, Yu VL. Prevention of Legionnaire's disease in transplant recipients: recommendations for a standardized approach. Transpl Infect Dis 2004;6: 58–62.
18. Guidol C, Garcia-Vidal C, Fernandez-Sabel N, et al. Clinical features and outcomes of Legionnaire's disease in solid organ transplant recipients. Transpl Infect Dis 2009;11:78–82.
19. Han XY, Ihegwood A, Evans SE, et al. Microbiological and clinical studies of legionellosis in 33 patients with cancer. J Clin Microbiol 2015;53:2180–7.
20. Sandkovsky U, Sandkovsky G, Suh J, et al. *Legionella* pneumonia and HIV: case reports and review of the literature. AIDS Patient Care STDS 2008;22:473–81.
21. Bodro M, Carratala J, Paterson DL. Legionellosis and biologic therapies. Respir Med 2014;108:1223–8.
22. Loeb M, Simor AE, Manell L, et al. Two nursing home outbreaks of respiratory infection with *Legionella sainthelensi*. J Am Geriatr Soc 1999;47:547–52.
23. Quinn C, Demirjian A, Watkins LF, et al. Legionnaire's disease outbreak at a long-term care facility caused by a cooling tower using an automated disinfection system—Ohio, 2013. J Environ Health 2015;78:8–13.
24. Allan T, Horgan T, Scaife H, et al. Outbreak of Legionnaire's disease among automotive plant workers. MMWR Morb Mortal Wkly Rep 2001;50:357–9.
25. Marks JS, Tsai TF, Martone WJ. Nosocomial Legionnaire's disease in Columbus, Ohio. Ann Intern Med 1979;90:565–9.
26. Available at: www.nj.com/news/index.ssf/.../legionnaires_disease_strikes_s.htm. Accessed July 8, 2016.
27. Demirjian A, Lucas C, Garrison L, et al. The importance of clinical surveillance in detecting legionnaire's disease outbreaks: a large outbreak in a hospital with a *Legionella* disinfection system-Pennsylvania, 2011-2012. Clin Infect Dis 2015; 60:1596–602.
28. Quinn C, Demirijian A, Lucas C, et al. Legionnaire's disease outbreak at a long-term care facility caused by a cooling tower using an automated disinfection system—Ohio, 2013. J Environ Health 2015;78(5):8–13.
29. Allegheny County Health Department, Pittsburgh Regional Health Initiative. Updated guidelines for the control of *Legionella* in Western Pennsylvania. Santa Monica (CA): RAND Corporation; 2014. Available at: www.legionella.com/files/96532662.pdf. Accessed July 8, 2016.
30. World Health Organization. *Legionella* and the prevention of legionellosis 2007. Available at: www.who.int/water_sanitation_health/.../legionella.pdf. Accessed July 7, 16.
31. Clancy CM. Prevention of healthcare-associated *Legionella* disease and scald injury from potable water distribution systems. Washington, DC: VHA Directive; 2014. 1061. Available at: www.va.gov/vhapublications/ViewPUblication.asp?pub_ID=3033. Accessed July 8, 2016.
32. ANSI/ASHRAE Standards 188–2015. Legionellosis: risk management for building water systems. Approved June 26, 2015. Available at: https://www.ashrae.org/resources–publications/bookstore/ansi-ashrae-standard-188-2015-legionellosis-risk-management-for-building-water-systems. Accessed July 8, 2016.

33. American Burn Association. Prevention scald injury educator's guide. Available at: http://www.ameriburn.org/Preven/ScaldInjuryEducator'sGuide.pdf. Accessed June 30, 2016.
34. Kuchta JM, States SJ, McNamara AM, et al. Susceptibility of *Legionella pneumophila* to chlorine in tap water. Appl Environ Microbiol 1983;46(5):1134–9.
35. Lin YS, Stout JE, Yu VL, et al. Disinfection of water distribution systems for Legionella. Semin Respir Infect 1998;13(2):147–59.
36. Joly P, Falconnet P-A, André J, et al. Quantitative real-time *Legionella* PCR for environmental water samples: data interpretation. Appl Environ Microbiol 2006; 72(4):2801–8.
37. Kozak NA, Lucas CE, Winchell JM. Identification of *Legionella* in the environment. Methods Mol Biol 2013;954:3–25.
38. Stout J, Goetz A, Yu V. Legionella. In: Mayhall C, editor. Hospital epidemiology and infection control. Philadelphia: Lippincott Williams & Wilkins; 2012. p. 535–50.
39. Centers for Disease Control Sampling Procedure and Potential Sampling Sites. Available at: www.cdc.gov/legionella/outbreak-toolkit/. Accessed June 30, 2016.
40. Yang CS. Sampling and controlling *Legionella* bacteria in domestic water systems. Elmhurst (IL): Aerotech P&K; 2004. Available at: https://www.emlab.com/media/resources/Sampling-Controlling-Legionella-Domestic-Water-System.pdf. Accessed June 26, 2016.
41. Kussman MJ. Prevention of *Legionella* disease. VHA directive 2008–10. Washington, DC: Department of Veterans Affairs, Veterans Health Administration; 2008.
42. Hu W, Remnick N. Hotel that enlivened the Bronx is now a hot spot for Legionnaires. New York Times August 11, 2015. p. A1 New York edition.

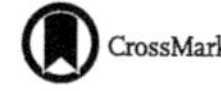

Laboratory Tests for Legionnaire's Disease

W. Michael Dunne Jr, PhD[a], Nathalie Picot, MSc[b], Alex van Belkum, PhD[c,*]

KEYWORDS

- *Legionella pneumophila* • Detection • Characterization • Diagnostics

KEY POINTS

- Despite the fact that *Legionella* is a recently discovered pathogenic genus, many clinically useful culture-based, immunologic, and molecular tests have been developed, although there still is a need for further optimization of the diagnostic process.
- Despite disadvantages including low sensitivity and long incubation times, the excellent specificity of culture of *Legionella* species makes it a valuable addition to any diagnostic algorithm and facilitates downstream antibiotic susceptibility testing.
- Both urine antigen testing and molecular assays for the detection of *Legionella pneumophila* are important but still in need of improvement in terms of sensitivity.
- Combining urine antigen testing with culture or molecular assays currently provides the best algorithm for diagnosis of *Legionella* disease.
- Whole genome sequencing facilitates the epidemiologic association of isolates of *Legionella* species potentially involved in outbreaks of infection.

INTRODUCTION

In 1977, McDade and colleagues[1] first reported on the isolation of a gram-negative, non–acid-fast bacillus from the lung tissue of 4 patients who died of a severe respiratory illness acquired while attending an American Legion convention in Philadelphia in 1976. The tissue from those patients was inoculated intraperitoneally into Guinea pigs, several of which became moribund 3 to 6 days after the onset of fever. Tissue (liver, lung, spleen) taken at necropsy of the animals was then inoculated into embryonated

Disclosure Statement: All authors are employees of bioMérieux and have a business implication in the work presented here. bioMérieux develops and sells a wide variety of diagnostic tests in the field of clinical microbiology and infectious diseases. However, the study was designed and executed independently by the authors and the company had no influence on the overall outcome of the literature studies presented here.

[a] Scientific Office, BioMérieux, 100 Rodolphe Street, Durham, NC 27712, USA; [b] Innovation Group, Info Doc, BioMérieux, Chemin de l'Orme, Marcy-l'Étoile 69280, France; [c] Scientific Office, BioMérieux, 3, Route de Port Michaud, La Balme Les Grottes 38390, France
* Corresponding author.
E-mail address: alex.vanbelkum@biomerieux.com

Infect Dis Clin N Am 31 (2017) 167–178
http://dx.doi.org/10.1016/j.idc.2016.10.012
0891-5520/17/

hen's eggs which, in turn, caused death of the embryos 4 to 7 days after inoculation. Smears of the yolk sacs from those embryos found pleomorphic gram-negative rods that did not grow on routine microbiologic culture media, but viable colonies could be cultivated using Mueller-Hinton agar supplemented with 1% hemoglobin and Isovitalex. Using the cultured organisms as a source of antigen, the group found increasing antibody titers or a single elevated titer from patients with this newly described entity called Legionnaire's disease using an indirect immunofluorescent assay. The same was observed for Guinea pigs who survived inoculation with the cultured organisms. Therefore, the first diagnostic assay for Legionnaire's disease was defined as a 4-fold increase in indirect immunofluorescent assay titer to a level ≥64 or a single antibody titer of 128. Using this assay, 2 previously unidentified but similar outbreaks of febrile illness that occurred in a psychiatric hospital in Washington, DC in 1965 and in a county public health office in Pontiac, Michigan in 1968 were found to have been instigated by the same or similar bacterial species. Within 1.5 years of the initial outbreak, a diagnostic tool and a means of recovering the etiologic agent of Legionnaire's disease was developed, although the true width and breadth of illness caused by the rapidly expanding *Legionella* species was yet to be appreciated. Testing for and characterization of *Legionella pneumophila* is not straightforward, as the bacteria have an intracellular lifestyle within alveolar macrophages and monocytes. One can only wonder how quickly the diagnostic process would have developed had metagenomic sequencing and whole genome analysis been available at the time.

Seven years after this publication, Edelstein,[2] in the *Proceedings of the 2nd International Symposium on Legionella*, reported on the state-of-the-art laboratory diagnosis of Legionnaire's disease. He indicated that one of the major advances was made courtesy of improvements in media formulation, which allowed for improved recovery of *Legionella* from clinical samples and the recognition of new species and recognition of serogroups within the species *L pneumophila*. Among culture media advancements, the successive development of charcoal-yeast extract agar, buffered charcoal-yeast extract (BCYE) agar, and BCYE with α-keto-glutarate with antibiotic inhibitors made recovery of *L pneumophila* and other *Legionella* species possible—even from highly contaminated specimen types. Classical bacteriology played an important role in the first phases of having to identify a novel pathogen and develop methods for its rapid detection. The diversity of *Legionella* spp infection was also beginning to be appreciated at this time, especially extrapulmonary sites including systemic disease with concomitant positive blood cultures. However, in 1984, diagnosis still relied heavily on culture and, more importantly, serologic means or detection in respiratory secretions using direct or indirect immunofluorescent staining. Dr. Edelstein's astute recognition of the potential for urine as a source of soluble bacterial antigen testing generated speculation that "once commercially available, it may replace other immunologic means of diagnosis."[2]

Initially, both radio immunoassays and enzyme immunoassays were developed to detect soluble *L pneumophila* antigens in urine.[3] These were then converted to latex agglutination[4] and lateral flow immune-chromatographic assays[5] for ease of use, the latter of which are currently used today.

FIRST-GENERATION MOLECULAR TESTING SYSTEMS

The fledgling laboratory tool of polymerase chain reaction (PCR) amplification entered *Legionella* diagnostics in the early 1990s for detection of the genus in environmental sources[6] and directly from clinical (broncho-alveolar lavage [BAL]) samples.[7,8] Using the *mip* gene as a target, Jaulhac and colleagues[7] could detect *L pneumophila* serogroups 1 to 14, *Legionella micdadei,* and *Legionella bozmanii* serogroup 1 in a spiked BAL sample at 25 colony-forming units (CFU)/mL. Retrospective analysis of 68 BAL samples from patients with suspected *Legionella* pneumonia identified all 8 culture-positive specimens and an additional 7 culture-negative samples. Four of these came from patients with serologic evidence of disease. Kessler and colleagues,[8] evaluated a commercial kit (EnviroAmp Legionella PCR Amplification Kit, Perkin Elmer Cetus, Norwalk, VA) that used a rapid DNA extraction process, biotinylated primers for genus only, and *pneumophila* species detection and a nonradiolabeled probe system for detection of genus, species, and internal positive control amplicons. In spiked studies, the system had a limit of detection of around 3×10^4 CFU but could detect all *L pneumophila* serogroups and 6 other *Legionella* species. They also tested 52 BAL samples retrospectively, and all 3 positive PCR samples were culture positive as well. There were no false-positive or false-negative results.

TESTS FOR TODAY AND THE FUTURE

With this brief review of a few things past, fast forward to the current decade. How much have the tools changed and what are the current recommendations on the best approach toward the diagnosis of *Legionella* disease (LD). The current diagnostic entities that can be used to identify/confirm possible cases of LD include culture, antigen detection, serology, and nucleic amplification testing (NAAT).

Culture and Specific Detection of Bacterial Cells

From the standpoint of culture, the technology had fairly matured by the early 1980s, yet it is still considered the reference standard for diagnostic purposes because of versatility.[9–11] It can be used to isolate all *Legionella* species, serotypes, and serogroups from any specimen type—patient or environment. It would seem reasonable then to include culture in combination with other methods such as urinary antigen testing (UAg) for difficult-to-obtain samples such as lung biopsy, pleural fluid, and BAL for patients with undiagnosed causes of pneumonia. Although the sensitivity of culture varies widely depending on specimen type and species(<10%–80%), the specificity for all practical purposes is nearly 100%. BCYE supplemented with α-ketoglutarate (BCYEα) and L-cysteine remains the medium of choice. Selection from contaminating upper respiratory tract flora can be enhanced by brief acid pretreatment or the addition of a cocktail of antimicrobial agents to the medium (ie, BMPA or modified Wadowski-Yee agar[9]). Although not widely used, coculture with *Acanthamoeba* spp can allow for the growth of fastidious *Legionella* spp that will not grow on BCYEα. This is a labor-intensive process that is not likely to be performed in routine clinical microbiology laboratories. Growth of *L pneumophila* usually takes 3 to 5 days to generate visible colonies on BCYEα and perhaps a bit longer for other *Legionella* species. Colonial growth can be grossly inspected for a characteristic opalescent sheen using indirect lighting or autofluorescence when illuminated with long-wave ultraviolet light. Confirmatory identification of growth can be accomplished using serologic reagents, NAAT, or, most recently, matrix-assisted laser desorption time of flight (MALDI-TOF) mass spectrometry (MS).[9] Although culture remains a necessary adjunct for the diagnosis of non–*L pneumophila* serogroup 1 (LP1) disease, the routine use of UAg assays or NAAT has decreased over the years as a primary means of diagnosis.

In addition, the detection of bacterial cells, sometimes with high sensitivity, can also be performed with other technologies. Using magnetic nanoparticles for labeling of bacterial cells in combination with amperometric magneto-immunoassays allows for the sensitive detection of bacterial cells (up to 10 CFU/mL).[12] For epidemiologic purposes, culture remains essential for strain typing, whole genome sequence analysis, or antimicrobial susceptibility testing.[9–11]

Urine Antigen Assay

Because resistance to macrolides and fluoroquinolones is rare among clinically significant *Legionella* species,[11] prompt identification of LD regardless of species is key to administration of recommended primary antimicrobial therapy including parenteral azithromycin, levofloxacin, or moxifloxacin.[13] Because LP1 is responsible for nearly 90% of all LD cases globally (not as dominant in the European Union or southeast Asia), the UAg assay, which detects soluble exopolysaccharide from LP1, has nearly displaced all other methods of diagnosis as a first-pass screen for LD.[10] Several factors have increased the use of UAg, including ease of use and sample collection, low cost, rapid results, and US Food and Drug Administration clearance and Conformité Européenne marking. However, a negative UAg test result does not rule out LD caused by other species.[10,11] For these cases, adjunct methods such as culture or PCR amplification and sequencing must be used in combination. As mentioned earlier, the evolution of UAg detection led to several platforms including a 96-well enzyme immunoassay (EIA) format and immune-chromatographic (ICT; lateral flow) assays developed by a variety of manufacturers.[10] Although the sensitivity of ICTs can vary significantly (usually in the range of 70%–90% depending on specimen processing), the specificity is generally greater than 95%.[10] In 2010, Bruin and colleagues[14] compared the performance of the Legionella V-TesT (Coris BioConcept, Gembloux, Belgium) with that of the BinaxNow Legionella urinary antigen test (Alere, Scarborough, ME). For this study, a panel of nonconcentrated, frozen urine samples collected from 1999 to 2007 containing 118 samples from 118 patients with proven LD and 71 samples from 71 patients with respiratory tract infections (RTIs) from other causes were evaluated. The sensitivity and specificity of V-TesT versus the BinaxNOW assays were 82.2% and 98.6% and 83.9% and 100%, respectively, if read after the prescribed 15 minutes of incubation. The sensitivity for both assays could be increased to 91.5% if the tests were read after 60 minutes, but the change was not statistically significant. Two years later, Svarrer and colleagues[15] compared the Oxoid Xpect Legionella UAg assay (Basingstoke, UK) for *L pneumophila* serogroups 1 and 6 and the BinaxNOW assay with the Binax Legionella EIA assay. The authors used a complex collection of samples including 115 urine samples from 91 cases of LD, 93 of which were from 69 patients with culture-confirmed disease. In this mix, 27 urine samples were from 23 patients with non-Lp1 disease. Ninety-four urine samples from patients with RTI not caused by *Legionella* spp were included as well. At the patient level, the sensitivity of the Binax EIA was 79%, but the BinaxNOW and Oxoid Xpect assays generated a dismal 47% and 32% sensitivity, respectively. The specificity was greater than 97% for all 3 assays. The authors concluded that, in their hands, neither of the ICTs should be used alone for the diagnosis of LD. After this publication, Held[16] noted in a short communication that the sensitivity of the BinaxNOW assay could be increased by making additional readings of the strip for up to 4 hours. He observed no false-positive results by delaying the readings using 60 urine samples from patients having RTIs not caused by *Legionella* spp but cautioned that prolonged incubation should be accompanied by other confirmatory methods of diagnosis. He also noted that mixed results regarding the increased sensitivity generated by extended reading times along with subsequent decreased specificity have been recognized for this and other *Legionella* UAg assays. In a somewhat more complicated trial, Beraud and colleagues[17] compared the Sofia *Legionella* Fluorescent Immunoassay (FIA; Quidel, San Diego, CA) with the BinaxNOW urinary antigen card at 2 reference centers using a panel of 179 prospective samples and 90 frozen repository urine specimens from patients with proven LD. The Sofia assay is an immune-chromatographic test that uses fluorescent tags to increase sensitivity and an automated reader. Although not recommended by the manufacturer, some samples were analyzed after concentration via filter centrifugation or heating at 100°C for 5 minutes followed by brief centrifugation. In the first part of the evaluation using nonconcentrated samples, the sensitivity and specificity of the Sofia assay was determined to be 100% and 97.2% but only after heating discrepant samples, which eliminated 5 false-positive results generated by the FIA assay. The BinaxNOW assay, however, missed 4 true-positive results for a sensitivity of 95.6% with 100% specificity. In the second half of the study, 199 urine samples were used to evaluate the 2 systems: the Sofia FIA using neat specimens, whereas concentrated samples were used for the BinaxNOW system. Under these conditions, the sensitivity of both assays was 100%, whereas the specificities were 97.3% and 100% for the Sofia and BinaxNOW, respectively. The manipulation of urine samples using filter concentration or heating provides additional variability in the performance of *Legionella* UAg and must be taken into account during verification studies. Jørgensen and colleagues[18] examined the performance of the ImmuView ICT assay (bioTrading, Mijdrecht The Netherlands)—the first test to offer detection of LP1 antigen and all 92 *Streptococcus pneumonia* capsular types in urine. For the purpose of this review, only the LP1 UAg detection function of the assay was evaluated and compared with the performance of the Binax *Legionella* urinary antigen EIA assay. For this evaluation, urine samples from 55 culture-confirmed cases of LP1 disease, 44 samples from probable LP1 disease (Binax EIA-positive), and 50 samples from patients with culture-confirmed non-LP1 LD were used. For the 99 samples from proven or probable cases of LP1 LD, the sensitivity of the Binax EIA, BinaxNOW ICT, and ImmuView was 75%, 71%, and 89%, respectively. With the BinaxNOW ICT, 18 of the positive results were recorded as "faintly positive." The sensitivity of the ImmuView ICT was statistically significantly better than the other 2 assays. All 3 assays demonstrated 100% specificity relative to the detection of LP1 antigen in urine. However, the authors noted that LP1 causes only about 60% of LD in Europe; therefore, a negative result does not indicate absence of LD and should be paired with other means of diagnosis echoing the recommendation of others.[10,11]

Nucleic Acid Amplification Tests

Unlike UAg ICT and EIA assays, the development and addition of NAAT offers the potential to detect LP1, LP nonserogroup 1, and *Legionella* spp as agents of LD from any specimen type or from environmental sources. This is especially important in areas of the world in which a higher percentage of cases of LD are caused by non-LP1 strains.[11] Several of such tests use oligonucleotide arrays for species and sometimes even bacterial type identification.[19] Further, PCR amplification paired with sequencing technology can be additionally useful for epidemiologic investigations.[10] The introduction of real-time PCR technology made it possible to quantitate the burden of organisms present in a sample but was unable to differentiate between live and dead organisms. Although several commercial enterprises have developed NAAT for *Legionella,* only one is cleared by the US Food and Drug Administration (BD ProbeTec ET *L pneumophila*, Becton-Dickenson, Sparks, MD) but, as the name suggests, only detects LP serogroups 1 to 14. This assay is a strand displacement amplification assay but is currently not being commercially marketed. In addition, assays other than PCR-based amplification are in various stages of development as well, including isothermal amplification assays such as nucleic acid sequence-based amplification and loop-mediated isothermal amplification.[10] In 2013, Benitez and Winchell[20] designed a multiplex PCR assay capable of distinguishing *Legionella* spp, *L pneumophila,* and LP1 from patient specimens in a single reaction. They used multiple TaqMan primer and probe sets with distinct fluoroprobes to detect individual reactions. The primer targets included the *ssrA* gene for *Legionella* spp, *mip* for *L pneumophila,* and *wzm* for LP1. The RNase P assay was included as an internal control to detect human DNA. Using a panel of 215 clinical and environmental strains including 52 *Legionella* species and 41 non-*Legionella* species, they determined the specificity of the assay to be 100%. The limit of detection of the assay in terms of LP1 genomic DNA was 25 fg. They then tested a panel of clinical samples including 15 culture-positive, direct fluorescent antibody-positive specimens and 6 that were negative for both. The assay showed 100% clinical sensitivity with this panel. The assay took about 4 hours to perform including extraction and provided direct quantification using a reverse transcription PCR format. The assay was designed as an adjunct to other diagnostic modalities to promote a more effective public health response and rapid institution of appropriate antimicrobial therapy. Two years later at the Cleveland Clinic, Chen and colleagues[21] compared the efficacy of UAg (BinaxNOW), culture (BCYEα with acid pretreatment of nonsterile samples), and a laboratory-developed PCR assay targeting the *mip* gene for the diagnosis of LD over a 46-month study period. Verification of isolate identification was accomplished using MALDI-TOF MS after confirming no growth by subculture on blood agar plates but positive growth on BCYEα. Of the 12,569 UAg assays, 3747 cultures, and 3596 PCR assays performed, they obtained 378 positive results. The UAg produced the greatest number of positive results (2.8%) followed by 0.4% positive cultures and 0.8% positive PCR results. Thirty-seven patients had $\geq$2 assays performed with $\geq$1 positive result, and, of these, 32 patients had medical charts available for review, and 84% of those could be classified as either proven or probable LD. Using this patient set, the overall sensitivity and specificity of the 3 methods of diagnosis were as follows: 50% and 100% for culture; 92% and 99.9% for PCR, and 96% and 99.99% for UAg. There was good correlation between UAg and PCR results, but it was clear that most cases evaluated were caused by LP1 based on the sensitivity and specificity of the UAg. The correlation might not have been as positive in areas of the world in which other serogroups of LP and non-LP disease comprise a significant portion of the total. Gadsby and colleagues[22] examined the utility of a first-line PCR assay for *L pneumophila* or *Legionella* species for the diagnosis of LD in Scotland over a 44-month study period. Lower respiratory tract samples were analyzed using a previously described duplex PCR assay for LP and *Legionella* spp (N = 1736), LP only (N = 181), or *Legionella* spp only (N = 27). For the investigation, physicians were instructed to submit urine for LP1 UAg testing (BinaxNOW *Legionella* Urinary Antigen ICT, Alere, Stockport, UK); respiratory samples for culture and syndromic molecular testing for respiratory viruses, *Mycoplasma pneumoniae,* and *Legionella*; and paired acute and convalescent sera for *Legionella* antibody titers. PCR for *Legionella* spp targeted specific 16S rRNA sequences whereas the *L pneumophila* PCR assay was directed against the *mip* gene.[23] BCYE agar was used for culture of *Legionella* spp. Of the 1944 total samples tested by PCR, 49 (2.6%) from 36 patients were positive for *L pneumophila.* Twenty-eight cases (77.8%) were laboratory confirmed, whereas 8 were called *probable cases* based on European Union definitions, and many of these were associated with a major outbreak of LD that occurred during the spring and summer of 2012. *Legionella* spp were identified in 16 (0.9%) specimens from 10 patients (5 confirmed, 5 classified as probable). Interestingly, no viral infections were detected by PCR in patients positive for *L pneumophila/Legionella* spp by PCR. Although PCR had a lower sensitivity and specificity compared with the UAg assay, results from the former were available sooner in several cases and, when combined with the UAg assay, provided a 92.6% and 98.3% sensitivity and specificity, respectively. The authors concluded that PCR should be included as a primary test in patients with possible LD.

Most recently, Benitez and Winchell[24] developed a multiplex assay that can type 9 non-*pneumophila Legionella* spp as an adjunct to their initial PCR assay.[20] This upgrade can detect and discriminate *L micdadei, Legionella bozemanii, Legionella dumoffii, Legionella longbeachae, Legionella feelei, Legionella anisa, Legionella parisensis, Legionella tucsonensis* serogroups 1 and 3, and *Legionella sainthelensis* serogroups 1 and 2. Identification of *L anisa, L parisensis,* and *L tucsonensis* 1 and 3 is accomplished using a high-resolution melt curve analysis of the 112 base-pair amplicon from the *ssrA* gene target. Identification of *L bozemanii, L longbeachae,* and *Legionella feeleii* uses melt curve analysis of different *mip* gene–amplified products from each species. Additional multiplex tests have been described more recently and their usefulness underscored.[25,26] The current reference standard for identification of these species is PCR amplification and sequencing of the *mip* gene, which can be time consuming and expensive, whereas this approach is relatively inexpensive and can be performed quickly. The investigators note that of the non-LP cases of LD observed worldwide, most are caused by *L micdadei, L bozemanii, L dumoffii,* and *L longbeachae* with *L micdadei* being responsible for approximated 60% of these. Using a panel of 300 *Legionella* spp type strains, and clinical and environmental isolates, the authors determined that the assay was 100% specific for differentiation of these species and serogroups. However, the analytical sensitivity differed in terms of limit of detection (LOD) of genomic DNA. For example, the LOD for *L micdadei, L dumoffii, L feeleii,L longbeachae, and L bozemanii* (the most frequent causes of non-*pneumophila* LD) was 50 fg of DNA. For *L anisa, L parisensis,* and *L tucsonensis* 1 and 3, the LOD was 500 fg, whereas for *L sainthelensis* 1 and 2, the LOD was 500 pg and 5 pg respectively. This assay is more likely to be used routinely in public health or reference laboratories in which a higher volume of non-*pneumophila* spp might be encountered or in parts of the world in which these species represent a higher proportion of isolates causing LD.

PCR has a positive impact to the detection of LD (eg, Murdoch and colleagues[27] and Mentasti and colleagues[28]). Recently, Avni and colleagues[29] systematically reviewed the diagnostic accuracy of all the studies describing PCR as a single diagnostic tool and compared its performance to urinary antigen testing. Both prospective and retrospective studies (n = 38) were included. In the end and based on more than 650 LD patients included, the authors concluded that PCR of respiratory samples clearly outperformed that of urinary antigen testing in which PCR detected between 18% and 30% more clinical cases. The authors concluded that at the current state of affairs, PCR of respiratory samples should be regarded as a valid tool for the diagnosis of LD.

Serology and Direct Fluorescent Antibody Staining Methods

Although serologic evaluation of patients with possible LD and direct identification of organisms in tissue or respiratory specimens using direct immune-fluorescent microscopy was once a staple of *Legionella* diagnosis, the advent of more rapid methods such as PCR and UAg assays has, for the most part, displaced these approaches. Because seroconversion necessitates the collection of acute and convalescent sera 4 to 8 weeks apart to show a 4-fold increase in titer to $\geq$1:128, it is definitely not a timely method of diagnosis.[10] A single high titer cannot rule out previous (at an undetermined earlier time point) disease. In-house developed enzyme-linked immunosorbent assay systems have been evaluated using thousands of samples, and still the sensitivity did not go much beyond 60%.[30] Further, antibody responses can be delayed in certain patient populations or not occur at all—even in the presence of positive cultures.[10,11] Serologic evaluation can be of some help in retrospective analysis of possible outbreaks of LD or when other primary diagnostic methods are negative in the face of strong suspicion of LD but is usually only performed in a limited number of public health laboratories.[31] And although direct immune-fluorescent or antibody-tagged latex beads can still be used to identify culture isolates, the advent of MALDI-TOF MS and reverse transcription PCR assays have all but eliminated this approach to colony identification. Application of lateral flow tests and other rapid tests has gained attention but did not really lead to broad acceptation of these tests. Several formats have been proposed, and some of these have been identified as good supplements for fast diagnosis of LD.[18,32,33]

ANTIMICROBIAL SUSCEPTIBILITY TESTING

L pneumophila primarily replicates in alveolar macrophages and monocytes. This implies that antibiotics should be able to first penetrate such host cells and then effectively kill the bacteria. This action also has an impact on antimicrobial susceptibility testing (AST), and many have tried to perform AST using bacteria-internalized cells belonging to different human cell lines (eg, Ref.[34]). Because *L pneumophila* will also grow in axenic cultures, a combination of classical and intracellular testing has been advocated. In the early years after the first detection of *L pneumophila*, therapy mostly included erythromycin, but this was soon followed up with macrolide or quinolone treatment. Hence, most AST research was focused on these latter categories of antibiotics. For instance, there was excellent concordance between broth dilution and intracellular testing using HL60 cells for levofloxacin and telithromycin.[34] These studies led to calibration of methods that were easier to use than the cell culture–based assays. Disk diffusion testing was validated for most antibiotics with the exception of moxifloxacin and rifampin,[35] whereas the use of Etest was found to be reliable as well.[36] These developments improved the ease with which AST could be performed for *L pneumophila*. A recent report also showed that tests could be automated (including the ones that use host cell culture) and that automated synergy testing supports the use of combination therapy[37]—especially for antibiotic-resistant strains of *L pneumophila*.[38]

EPIDEMIOLOGIC TYPING OF *LEGIONELLA* ISOLATES

When an epidemiologic link was suspected, *Legionella* isolates cultured from patients have been analyzed with an assortment of methods permitting detailed comparison of bacterial phenotypes or genotypes. Contemporary approaches mostly use genotyping. Initially, molecular methods were introduced to replace classical serotyping. PCR protocols for differentiating serogroup 1 from the other serogroups became popular and were validated by the European Society for Clinical Microbiology and Infectious Diseases Study Group for Legionella Infections.[39] This group established the accuracy of the test for a variety of PCR platforms, which was also confirmed in independent studies.[40] Serogrouping soon became a diagnostic test more than an epidemiologically relevant subtyping assay.

Pulsed field gel electrophoresis was applied successfully in the epidemiologic analysis of *Legionella* isolates, as were a variety of other classical genomic methods (eg, restriction fragment length polymorphism, amplified ribosomal DNA restriction analysis, and amplified fragment length polymorphism). However, over the last 5 years, more comprehensive, essentially genomewide methods were developed and put into practice. Whole genome maps can be generated by specific electrophoresis of stretched small DNA restriction fragments and sensitive optical imaging. Alignment of the fragments allows for a physical reconstruction of the genomic map of a bacterial strain. This technique has also been applied to the epidemiology of *Legionella* species.[41] In the first validation study, it was shown that genome mapping compared favorably with the more classical methods. However, despite good performance of optical mapping, it is currently suggested that sequence-based typing will likely replace all of the other typing methods.

One example of a sequence-based system exploits repeat diversity in the clustered regularly interspaced short palindromic repeats (CRISPR) locus. Sequencing such repeats confirmed relatedness within outbreak-associated strains or diversity among nonrelated isolates.[42] In addition to sequencing of the CRISPR loci, the size of the PCR product spanning this region can be used as an epidemiologic marker. In a probe hybridization format, CRISPR analysis is better known as *spoligotyping*. A semiautomated spoligotyping assay was developed using the microbead-based Luminex system, and that format was shown to work well.[43] Not all *Legionella* strains contain CRISPR elements, so alternative approaches were developed. One of these uses the Luminex platform for the detection of polymorphic DNA segments.[19] The genomic version of Multi-Locus Sequence Typing schemes as developed by Moran-Gilad and colleagues[44] in 2015 has been more broadly accepted. The authors suggested a core genome typing scheme exploiting 1521 gene targets. This system allows for detailed comparative analyses of strains once their genome sequence was known. This system is very portable and can easily be shared among researchers working in different institutes on different continents. A recent report[45] disclosed the source of an outbreak of LD in New York state showing the public health relevance of the genomic approach.

SUMMARY

The comprehensive reviews of Mercante and Winchell[10] and Cunha and colleagues[11] provide an excellent summary of the utility of the various contemporary means of *Legionella* diagnostics available to clinicians and clinical microbiologists today. These methods are not only useful for the purposes of identifying LD in patients, but also for establishing the source of infection and tracking the spread of LD through epidemiologic approaches. In areas in which LP1 is the predominant cause of LD, the UAg approach to diagnosis seems most attractive based on cost, speed, ease of use, and analytical performance. However, even in a part of the world where LP1 holds a leading role, it would seem prudent to include a nonbiased approach toward the diagnosis of LD such as culture or a multiplex PCR assay that recognizes LP1, LP-non1, and *Legionella* nonpneumophila variants, because treatment modalities would be similar for each even if a specific species was not initially recognized. Clearly, with the rapid development of sequence-based metagenomic analysis and whole genome sequencing, a single approach could be used for the identification of multiple potential causes of community and health care–associated pneumonia.[45] Finally, little is known on the value of human biological response modifiers. The diagnostic value of C-reactive protein, ferritin, or procalcitonin levels has not yet been extensively explored,[46] and more research should be performed to clarify the potential diagnostic value of host markers.

REFERENCES

1. McDade JE, Shepard CC, Fraser DW, et al. Legionnaire's disease: isolation of a bacterium and demonstration of its role in other respiratory disease. N Engl J Med 1977;297:1197–203.

2. Edelstein PH. Laboratory diagnosis of Legionnaires disease. In: Thornsberry C, Balows A, Feely JC, et al, editors. Legionella: proceedings of the 2nd international symposium. Washington, DC: American Society for Microbiology; 1984. p. 3–5.
3. Sathapatayavongs B, Kohler RB, Wheat LJ, et al. Rapid diagnosis of Legionnaire's disease by urinary antigen detection. Comparison of ELISA and radioimmunoassay. Am J Med 1982;72:576–82.
4. Sathapatayavongs B, Kohler RB, Wheat LJ, et al. Rapid diagnosis of Legionnaire's disease by latex agglutination. Am Rev Respir Dis 1983;127:559–62.
5. Domíguez J, Galí N, Matas L, et al. Evaluation of a rapid immunechromatographic assay for the detection of *Legionella* antigen in urine samples. Eur J Clin Microbiol Infect Dis 1999;18:896–8.
6. Mahbubani MH, Bej AK, Miller R, et al. Detection of *Legionella* with polymerase chain reaction and gene probe methods. Mol Cell Probes 1999;4:175–87.
7. Jaulhac B, Nowicki M, Bornstein N, et al. Detection of *Legionella* spp. in bronchoalveolar lavage fluids by DNA amplification. J Clin Microbiol 1992;30:920–4.
8. Kessler HH, Reinthaller FF, Pschaid A, et al. Rapid detection of *Legionella* species in bronchoalveolar lavage fluids with the EnviroAmp *Legionella* PCR amplification and detection kit. J Clin Microbiol 1993;31:3325–8.
9. Jarraud S, Descours G, Ginevra C, et al. Identification of *Legionella* in clinical samples. Methods Mol Biol 2013;954:27–57.
10. Mercante JW, Winchell JM. Current and emerging *Legionella* diagnostics for laboratory outbreak investigations. Clin Microbiol Rev 2015;28:95–126.
11. Cunha BA, Burillo L, Bouza E. Legionnaire's disease. Lancet 2016;387:376–85.
12. Martin M, Salazar P, Jimenez C, et al. Rapid *Legionella pneumophila* determination based on a disposable core-shell Fe(3)O(4)@poly(dopamine) magnetic nanoparticles immunoplatform. Anal Chim Acta 2015;887:51–8.
13. Gilbert DN, Chambers HF, Eliopoulos GM, et al. The Sanford guide to antimicrobial therapy. 45th Edition. Sperryville (VA): Antimicrobial Therapy Inc; 2015.
14. Bruin JP, Peeters MF, Ijzerman EPF, et al. Evaluation of *Legionella* V-TesT for the detection of *Legionella pneumophila* antigen in urine samples. Eur J Clin Microbiol Infect Dis 2010;29:899–900.
15. Svarrer CW, Lück C, Elverdal PL, et al. Immunochromatic kits Xpect *Legionella* and BinaxNOW Legionella for detection of *Legionella pneumophila* urinary antigen have low sensitivities for the diagnosis of Legionnaire's disease. J Med Microbiol 2012;61:213–7.
16. Held J. Increasing the sensitivity of the BinaxNOW Legionella urinary antigen immunochromatographic test by additional readings at later time points. J Med Microbiol 2012;61:884–5.
17. Beraud L, Gervasoni K, Freydiere AM, et al. Comparison of Sofia *Legionella* FIA and BinaxNOW® *Legionella* urinary antigen card in two national reference centers. Eur J Clin Microbiol Infect Dis 2015;34:1803–7.
18. Jørgensen CS, Uldum SA, Sorensen JF, et al. Evaluation of a new lateral flow test for detection of *Streptococcus pneumoniae* and *Legionella pneumophila* urinary antigen. J Microbiol Methods 2015;116:33–6.
19. Cao B, Liu X, Yu X, et al. New oligonucleotide microarray for detection of pathogenic and non-pathogenic *Legionella* spp. PLoS One 2014;9:e113863.
20. Benitez AJ, Winchell JM. Clinical application of a muiltiplex real-time PCR assay for simultaneous detection of *Legionella* species, *Legionella pneumophila*, and *Legionella pneumophila* serogroup 1. J Clin Microbiol 2013;51:348–51.
21. Chen DJ, Procop GW, Vogel S, et al. Utility of PCR, culture, and antigen detection methods for diagnosis of Legionellosis. J Clin Microbiol 2015;53:3474–7.

22. Gadsby NJ, Helgason KO, Dickson EM, et al. Molecular diagnosis of *Legionella* infections – clinical utility of front-line screening as part of a pneumonia diagnostic algorithm. J Infect 2016;72:161–70.
23. Templeton KE, Scheltinga SA, Sillekens P, et al. Development and clinical evaluation of an internally controlled, single-tube multiplex real-time PCR assay for detection of *Legionella pneumophila* and other Legionella species. J Clin Microbiol 2003;41:4016–21.
24. Benitez H, Winchell D. Rapid detection and typing of pathogenic non-pneumophila *Legionella* spp. isolates using a multiplex real-time PCR assay. Diagn Microbiol Infect Dis 2016;84:298–303.
25. Kim SM, Jeong Y, Sohn JW, et al. Multiplex real-time PCR assay for *Legionella* species. Mol Cell Probes 2015;29:414–9.
26. Yang G, Benson R, Pelish T, et al. Dual detection of *Legionella pneumophila* and *Legionella* species by real-time PCR targeting the 23S-5S rRNA gene spacer region. Clin Microbiol Infect 2010;16:255–61.
27. Murdoch DR, Podmore RG, Anderson TP, et al. Impact of routine systematic polymerase chain reaction testing on case finding for Legionnaire's disease: a pre-post comparison study. Clin Infect Dis 2013;57:1275–81.
28. Mentasti M, Fry NK, Afshar B, et al. Application of *Legionella pneumophila*-specific quantitative real-time PCR combined with direct amplification and sequence-based typing in the diagnosis and epidemiological investigation of Legionnaire's disease. Eur J Clin Microbiol Infect Dis 2012;31:2017–28.
29. Avni T, Bieber A, Green H, et al. Diagnostic Accuracy of PCR alone and compared to urinary antigen testing for detection of *Legionella* spp.: a systematic review. J Clin Microbiol 2016;54:401–11.
30. Elverdal PL, Jorgensen CS, Krogfelt KA, et al. Two years' performance of an in-house ELISA for diagnosis of Legionnaire's disease: detection of specific IgM and IgG antibodies against *Legionella pneumophila* serogroup 1, 3 and 6 in human serum. J Microbiol Methods 2013;94:94–7.
31. Simonsen O, Wedege E, Kanestrom A, et al. Characterization of the extent of a large outbreak of Legionnaire's disease by serological assays. BMC Infect Dis 2015;15:163–70.
32. Jorgensen CS, Uldum SA, Elverdal PL. Application of a lateral flow test as an additional serological tool for diagnosis of *Legionella* infections. J Microbiol Methods 2014;96:12–5.
33. Bruin JP, Diederen BM. Evaluation of Meridian TRU *Legionella*(R), a new rapid test for detection of *Legionella pneumophila* serogroup 1 antigen in urine samples. Eur J Clin Microbiol Infect Dis 2013;32:333–4.
34. Stout JE, Sens K, Mietzner S, et al. Comparative activity of quinolones, macrolides and ketolides against *Legionella* species using in vitro broth dilution and intracellular susceptibility testing. Int J Antimicrob Agents 2005;25:302–7.
35. Bruin JP, Diederen BM, Ijzerman EP, et al. Correlation of MIC value and disk inhibition zone diameters in clinical *Legionella pneumophila* serogroup 1 isolates. Diagn Microbiol Infect Dis 2013;76:339–42.
36. De Giglio O, Napoli C, Lovero G, et al. Antibiotic susceptibility of *Legionella pneumophila* strains isolated from hospital water systems in Southern Italy. Environ Res 2015;142:586–90.
37. Chiaraviglio L, Kirby JE. High-throughput Intracellular antimicrobial susceptibility testing of *Legionella pneumophila*. Antimicrob Agents Chemother 2015;59: 7517–29.

38. Bruin JP, Koshkolda T, IJzerman EP, et al. Isolation of ciprofloxacin-resistant *Legionella pneumophila* in a patient with severe pneumonia. J Antimicrob Chemother 2014;69:2869–71.
39. Mentasti M, Kese D, Echahidi F, et al. Design and validation of a qPCR assay for accurate detection and initial serogrouping of *Legionella pneumophila* in clinical specimens by the ESCMID Study Group for *Legionella* Infections (ESGLI). Eur J Clin Microbiol Infect Dis 2015;34:1387–93.
40. Cao B, Tian Z, Wang S, et al. Structural comparison of O-antigen gene clusters of *Legionella pneumophila* and its application of a serogroup-specific multiplex PCR assay. Antonie van Leeuwenhoek 2015;108:1405–23.
41. Bosch T, Euser SM, Landman F, et al. Whole-Genome mapping as a novel high-resolution typing tool for *Legionella pneumophila.* J Clin Microbiol 2015;53: 3234–8.
42. Luck C, Brzuszkiewicz E, Rydzewski K, et al. Subtyping of the *Legionella pneumophila* "Ulm" outbreak strain using the CRISPR-Cas system. Int J Med Microbiol 2015;305:828–37.
43. Gomgnimbou MK, Ginevra C, Peron-Cane C, et al. Validation of a microbead-based format for spoligotyping of *Legionella pneumophila.* J Clin Microbiol 2014;52:2410–5.
44. Moran-Gilad J, Prior K, Yakunin E, et al. Design and application of a core genome multilocus sequence typing scheme for investigation of Legionnaire's disease incidents. Euro Surveill 2015;20:100–12.
45. Raphael BH, Baker DJ, Nazarian E, et al. Genomic resolution of outbreak-associated *Legionella pneumophila* Serogroup 1 isolates from New York State. Appl Environ Microbiol 2016;82:3582–90.
46. Bellmann-Weiler R, Ausserwinkler M, Kurz K, et al. Clinical potential of C-reactive protein and procalcitonin serum concentrations to guide differential diagnosis and clinical management of pneumococcal and *Legionella* pneumonia. J Clin Microbiol 2010;48:1915–7.

Antimicrobial Therapy for Legionnaire's Disease

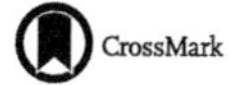

Antibiotic Stewardship Implications

Cheston B. Cunha, MD[a,*], Burke A. Cunha, MD, MACP[b,c]

KEYWORDS

- Legionnaire's disease • Antimicrobial therapy • Community-acquired pneumonia
- Antimicrobial stewardship • Doxycycline

KEY POINTS

- Effective antibiotic therapy for legionnaire's disease is based on anti-*Legionella* activity and high antibiotic concentrations in alveolar macrophages.
- Antibiotics used for legionnaire's disease include doxycycline, quinolones, and azithromycin. Alternately, tigecycline, trimethoprim-sulfamethoxazole, and rifamycin are also effective in legionnaire's disease.
- Legionnaire's disease outcomes depend not only on effective anti-*Legionella* therapy but also, importantly, on host factors (ie, cardiopulmonary function, degree or duration of impaired cell-mediated immunity, and immunomodulatory or immunosuppressive drugs).
- When the pathogen is unknown, empiric therapy for community-acquired pneumonia has been with a ß-lactam plus an anti-*Legionella* antibiotic.
- If legionnaire's disease is likely, based on characteristic extrapulmonary findings, monotherapy with an anti-*Legionella* antibiotic provides effective therapy.

BACKGROUND

Effective antibiotic therapy against legionnaire's disease depends on the antibiotic's degree of anti-*Legionella* activity and ability to concentrate in alveolar macrophages (AMs), the primary site of infection in the lung in legionnaire's disease.[1–10] Antibiotics with anti-*Legionella* activity that do not penetrate into AMs are clinically ineffective.[7,11,12] The anti-*Legionella* antibiotic concentrations in AMs range from 10 to 30 times greater than serum concentrations.[3,4,6] Differences in serum concentration or relative minimum inhibitory concentrations are clinically irrelevant considering the supratherapeutic serum concentrations in AMs.[2,10] (**Table 1**). Effectiveness of

[a] Division of Infectious Disease, Rhode Island Hospital, The Miriam Hospital, Brown University Alpert School of Medicine, Providence, RI 02903, USA; [b] Division of Infectious Disease, Winthrop-University Hospital, Mineola, NY 11501, USA; [c] School of Medicine, State University of New York, Stony Brook, NY 11794, USA
* Corresponding author.
E-mail address: ccunha@lifespan.org

Infect Dis Clin N Am 31 (2017) 179–191
http://dx.doi.org/10.1016/j.idc.2016.10.013

Table 1
Pharmacokinetic determinants of antibiotic penetration into alveolar macrophages in legionnaire's disease

Antibiotic-Penetration Pharmacokinetic Factors into AMs		Clinically Useful Anti-*Legionella* Antibiotics with High AM Levels
Optimal AM Penetration (eg, Doxycycline, Quinolones) Major Factors • Lipid solubility = high V_d (>0.4 L/kg) • Low protein binding • Active intracellular antibiotic transport • Concentrated to AM levels (10–30 × simultaneous serum levels) Minor Factors • Molecular size • pKa • Degree of inflammation	Poor AM Penetration (eg, ß-lactams) • Low lipid solubility = low V_d (~0.2 L/kg) • Relatively high protein binding • Low intracellular AM levels (<10% of simultaneous serum levels)	Preferred Therapy • Doxycycline • Macrolides • Quinolones Alternate Therapy • Tigecycline • TMP-SMX • Rifampin

Abbreviations: pKa, ionization potential; V_d, volume of distribution.

[a] Imipenem has anti-*Legionella* activity in vitro but does not concentrate in AM and is not effective in Legionnaire's disease. Some other antibiotics (eg, clindamycin and chloramphenicol) concentrate in AM but have no anti-*Legionella* activity.

antibiotic therapy for legionnaire's disease also depends on host factors (ie, preexisting cardiopulmonary status, intactness of cell-mediated immunity [CMI], and early initiation of therapy).[13–15] The commonly used antibiotics with demonstrated clinical effectiveness in legionnaire's disease are doxycycline, trimethoprim-sulfamethoxazole (TMP-SMX), rifampin, quinolones, macrolides, and tigecycline.[14–20] These antibiotics have been used in treating legionnaire's disease alone or in combination.[21–25] With effective early therapy, there is slow clinical improvement over 5 to 7 days. Duration of therapy is important to assure cure as well as preventing relapse, not uncommon with less than 2 weeks of therapy.[26,27] Legionnaire's disease severity relates to inoculum size and host factors (ie, degree of decreased T-lymphocyte function or CMI).[27] Decreased CMI may be due to age and concurrent immunomodulating infections; for example, cytomegalovirus or disorders associated with impaired CMI (eg, human immunodeficiency virus, cancer chemotherapy, steroids, and immunomodulatory or immunosuppressive agents such as anti-TNF-α).[28–32] Clearly, early therapy is associated with better outcomes than late therapy and suboptimal therapy results in worse outcomes than optimal antibiotic therapy.[33] Careful analysis is needed in interpreting effectiveness of antibiotic therapy in legionnaire's disease because many nonsevere cases of community-acquired pneumonia (CAP) due to legionnaire's disease will improve or resolve with no therapy or suboptimal therapy (eg, imipenem).[11,12,32]

PHARMACOKINETIC CONSIDERATIONS

Historically, optimal monotherapy for legionnaire's disease has been with doxycycline, a quinolone, or azithromycin.[16,19,20,22,32] Therapeutic failures have been related to host factors.[34,35] Particularly in severe cases, rifampin or TMP-SMX have been used in combination with another anti-*Legionella* antibiotic.[36] However, taking into account the multiple factors previously mentioned, combination therapy in legionnaire's disease has no proven advantage over well-chosen monotherapy (eg, doxycycline, a quinolone, or azithromycin).[11,21,24,32] Clinicians have the tendency to add antibiotics when the diagnosis is uncertain or the disease is severe. Well-selected monotherapy remains the standard treatment of legionnaire's disease.[14–16]

Traditionally, initial antibiotic therapy for legionnaire's disease in hospitalized adults has been given via the intravenous (IV) route. Most anti-*Legionella* antibiotics are also available as oral formulations and have high bioavailability (>90%) and are well-suited for IV-to-oral switch regimens.[34–50] After clinical improvement or defervescence, usually after 5 to 7 days, oral therapy is usually started but may be begun as early as after 3 days in some cases. Oral therapy may be used anytime in the course of legionnaire's disease to complete 2 weeks of therapy (**Table 2**).

ANTIBIOTIC STEWARDSHIP CONSIDERATIONS

In CAPs, if the diagnosis of legionnaire's disease is highly likely or proven, early monotherapy with doxycycline, azithromycin, or a quinolone provides optimal legionnaire's disease therapy.[11,12,50] Reasons to not add another antibiotic to the regimen in legionnaire's disease patients include worsening infiltrates on chest radiograph (CXR), volume depletion, abdominal pain, acute renal failure, or persistent fevers (during the first week of therapy). Because there is no acquired resistance to the commonly used anti-*Legionella* antibiotics, continued fever, leukocytosis, or slow clinical improvement are expected features of legionnaire's disease.[51] Although anti-*Legionella* monotherapy has been shown to be as effective as combination therapy, some clinicians add another anti-*Legionella* antibiotic in hosts with severe pneumonia, iron overload, or markedly impaired CMI. Common combinations include doxycycline

Table 2
Empiric therapy for legionnaire's disease in normal and compromised hosts

Mild Legionnaire's Disease Ambulatory Setting	Moderately Severe Legionnaire's Disease	Severe Legionnaire's Disease in MICU
Preferred Therapy • Doxycycline 100 mg (po) q 12 h × 14 d • Levofloxacin 500 mg (po) q 24 h × 14 d • Moxifloxacin 400 mg (po) q 24 h × 14 d • Azithromycin 500 mg (po) × 1 dose, then 250 mg (po) q 24 h × 10 d[a]	Preferred Therapy • Doxycycline 200 mg (IV) q 12 h × 72 h, then 100 mg (IV) q 12 h × 11 d[b] • Moxifloxacin 400 mg (IV) q 24 h × 14 d • Tigecycline 200 mg (IV) × 1 d then 100 mg (IV) q 24 h × 2 wk[a]	Preferred Therapy • Doxycycline 200 mg (IV) q 12 h × 14 d • Levofloxacin 500 mg (IV) q 24 h × 14 d • Moxifloxacin 400 mg (IV) q 24 h × 14 d Double-drug therapy • TMP-SMX 5 mg/kg (IV) q 6 h × 14 d or rifampin 300 mg (po) q 12 h × 14 d may be used as a 2nd drug

Abbreviation: MICU, medical intensive care unit.

[a] Loading dose required.

[b] Loading regimen recommended with doxycycline. Because it takes 4 to 5 serum half-lives ($t_{1/2}$) to achieve steady state, and the $t_{1/2}$ of doxycycline is 18 to 22 hours, it takes 4 to 5 days to achieve steady state if given as recommended (ie, 100 mg IV or po q 12 h). Therefore, for doxycycline a loading regimen is preferred to treat serious systemic infections.

Adapted from Cunha CB, Cunha BA, editors. Antibiotic essentials. 15th edition. New Delhi (India): Jay Pee Medical Publishers; 2016.

or azithromycin plus a quinolone. Alternately, TMP-SMX or rifampin has been added to a quinolone or azithromycin therapy.[11,14–16]

In hospitalized adults with CAP due to legionnaire's disease or other CAP pathogens, IV-to-oral switching has important antimicrobial stewardship program (ASP) implications.[52–57] At any given dose, it has been shown that 3 days of IV therapy followed by 11 days of oral therapy has the same outcomes as 14 days of oral therapy.[57] Oral therapy is as effective as equivalent IV therapy and much less expensive. From a drug cost standpoint, oral therapy is not only less expensive but the cost of administering IV antibiotic therapy is eliminated with oral therapy. Furthermore, the complications of IV therapy (eg, phlebitis and line-related bacteremias) are eliminated with oral therapy.[50,57] From an ASP perspective, an additional pharmacoeconomic benefit of completing therapy with an oral formulation is decreased hospital length of stay.[52,53,58–62]

COMMUNITY-ACQUIRED PNEUMONIA COMBINATION THERAPY VERSUS MONOTHERAPY

In practice, therapeutic decisions regarding anti-*Legionella* coverage relate to 2 clinical considerations. First, if the diagnosis of legionnaire's disease is most likely clinically based on characteristic clinical findings in legionnaire's disease, then monotherapy with doxycycline, azithromycin, or a quinolone are optimal regardless of legionnaire's disease severity.[50,63] Second, the more common clinical scenario is that of CAP of unknown cause and the decision is whether to add an anti-*Legionella* antibiotic to a beta-lactam (eg, ceftriaxone).[54,64]

Based on habit or guidelines, most practitioners will use empiric double-drug therapy because the physician is not familiar with the clinical features of a legionnaire's disease or diagnostic test results are pending.[63–65] Excluding sputum culture for *Legionella*, *Legionella* titers may not be elevated early and, even if elevated, titer results are commonly reported days into hospitalization. Early therapy may blunt or delay titer elevations and some patients with legionnaire's disease never demonstrate a titer elevation.[14,15,66–69] With *L pneumophila* (serotype 1), *Legionella* urinary antigen testing may be negative initially but usually becomes positive after 1 to 2 weeks. If positive, *L antigenuria* continues for weeks with legionnaire's disease. *Legionella* urinary antigen test is not useful to diagnose non-*L pneumophila* (serotype 1) strains. The best way to diagnose non-*L pneumophila* strains are titers or sputum culture. Although most cases of legionnaire's disease are due to *L pneumophila* (serotype 1), in some areas, non-*L pneumophila* species are common causes of legionnaire's disease (eg, *L micdadei* or *L longbeachae*). For this reason, if the diagnosis of legionnaire's disease is suspected, both *Legionella* sp titers and urinary antibody tests should be ordered. If initially negative, both tests should be repeated weekly until after 4 to 6 weeks after hospital discharge before considering the tests truly negative.[66–70] As polymerase chain reaction tests for *Legionella* sp become widely available, the diagnosis of *L pneumophila* and non-*L pneumophila* strains causing legionnaire's disease will become more accurate and results reported more rapidly. However, as with current diagnostic methods for legionnaire's disease, all patients with CAP should not be shotgun tested for all potential CAP pathogens.[51,71] Legionnaire's disease, in particular, with well-recognized characteristic clinical findings should continue to guide selective testing in CAP cases highly likely to be legionnaire's disease (**Table 3**).[72–75]

If clinical predictors of legionnaire's disease are present (ie, legionnaire's disease is highly likely), then antibiotic monotherapy for legionnaire's disease is effective and

Table 3
Legionnaire's disease: clinical predictors and diagnostic eliminators in hospitalized adults with pneumonia

Diagnostic Predictors	Diagnostic Eliminators	
Clinical predictors[a] Fever >102°F (with relative bradycardia) Laboratory predictors[a] • Highly elevated ESR (>90 mm/h) or CRP (>180 mg/L) • Highly elevated ferritin levels (>2 × n) • Hypophosphatemia (on admission or early) • Highly elevated CPK (>2 × n) • Microscopic hematuria (on admission)	Chest film eliminators • CXR (with no infiltrates) • CXR (only if with segmental/lobar infiltrates)	Clinical eliminators[a] • Fever >102°F (without relative bradycardia) • Sore throat • Hoarseness • Severe myalgias • Splenomegaly Laboratory eliminators[a] • Leukopenia • Lymphocytosis • Thrombocytopenia • Thrombocytosis • Highly elevated cold agglutinin titers (>1:64)
Legionnaire's disease highly likely if >3 clinical predictors present (1 clinical plus ≥2 laboratory)	Legionnaire's disease unlikely if <3 clinical predictors present	Legionnaire's disease very unlikely if >3 clinical eliminators (ie, 1 clinical eliminator [relative bradycardia] plus >2 laboratory diagnostic eliminators present)

Abbreviations: CPK, creatinine phosphokinase; CRP, C-reactive protein; ESR, erythrocyte sedimentation rate.

[a] Otherwise unexplained. If finding due to another disorder, it should not be used as a diagnostic predictor or diagnostic eliminator.

Adapted from Cunha BA, Wu G, Raza M. Clinical diagnosis of legionnaire's disease: six characteristic criteria. Am J Med 2015;128:e21–22.

a ß-lactam is not essential.[71] This determination has important ASP, clinical, and pharmacoeconomic implications.[38–41,46,47,50] If anti-*Legionella* monotherapy is chosen wisely (ie, doxycycline or respiratory quinolone), both *Legionella* and typical bacterial CAP pathogens are effectively treated. These antibiotics are highly effective against all typical and atypical CAP pathogens, as well as legionnaire's disease.[50,51]

Among the types of CAP, pneumococcal and Q fever CAP are most likely to mimic legionnaire's disease.[51,76] Clinically, *Mycoplasma pneumoniae* is less likely to be confused with legionnaire's disease, with fevers of less than 102°F, lack of relative bradycardia, unelevated serum transaminases, lack of hypophosphatemia or hyponatremia, and it is usually less severe.[51] Although doxycycline and respiratory quinolones are effective against *M pneumoniae*, azithromycin should be avoided due to potential macrolide-resistant *M pneumoniae*.[77,78] Doxycycline, not tetracycline, is effective against *Streptococcus pneumoniae*, including penicillin-resistant strains.[48,49] Doxycycline is highly active against *Coxiella burnetii* (Q fever) and is also effective against macrolide-resistant strains of *M pneumoniae*.[50,51] For atypical bacterial CAP due to *S pneumoniae*, *Haemophilus influenzae*, or non-*Legionella* atypical pathogens, azithromycin monotherapy should be avoided because about 30% of *S pneumoniae* strains are macrolide-resistant[79–90] (**Table 4**). For the zoonotic atypical CAPs (eg, psittacosis, tularemia, and Q fever CAP), macrolides are suboptimal therapy.[50,51]

Table 4
Empiric therapy for typical and atypical community-acquired pneumonia: antibiotic stewardship considerations

CAP	CAP Pathogens	Initial Empiric IV Therapy	IV-to-po Switch Options
Pulmonary pathogen unknown (typical vs atypical)	*S pneumoniae* *H influenzae* *Moraxella catarrhalis* *M pneumoniae* *Chlamydophila pneumoniae* Legionnaire's disease	Combination therapy Ceftriaxone plus either doxycycline or respiratory quinolone or azithromycin[a]	Combination therapy Oral 2nd generation cephalosporin plus either doxycycline or respiratory quinolone or azithromycin
Pulmonary Pathogen (known or likely)			
CAP (typical) clinical findings confined to the lungs	Typical *S pneumoniae* *H influenzae* *M catarrhalis*	Monotherapy Ceftriaxone or doxycycline or respiratory quinolone	Monotherapy Oral 2nd GC or doxycycline or respiratory quinolone or azithromycin[a]
CAP (atypical) pneumonia with extrapulmonary organ involvement	Atypical *M pneumoniae* *C pneumoniae* Legionnaire's disease	Monotherapy Doxycycline or respiratory quinolone or azithromycin[a]	Monotherapy Doxycycline or respiratory quinolone or azithromycin[a]
Legionnaire's disease (highly likely by clinical predictors)	*Legionella* sp	Monotherapy Doxycycline or respiratory quinolone or azithromycin or tigecycline	Monotherapy Doxycycline or respiratory quinolone or azithromycin
Legionnaire's disease (severe)	*Legionella* sp	Monotherapy Doxycycline or respiratory quinolone or azithromycin Combination therapy Any of the above plus either rifampin or TMP-SMX	Monotherapy Doxycycline or respiratory quinolone or azithromycin

[a] If *Mycoplasma pneumoniae* unlikely.
[b] If penicillin-resistant, *S pneumoniae* (penicillin-resistant strains) or MDR *S pneumoniae* unlikely.
[c] Duration of therapy (IV + PO): 2 weeks (normal host) or 3 weeks (severe or compromised hosts).
Adapted from Cunha CB, Cunha BA, editors. Antibiotic essentials. 15th edition. New Delhi (India): Jay Pee Medical Publishers; 2016; and Cunha BA, editor. Pneumonia essentials. 3rd edition. Sudbury (MA): Jones & Bartlett Publishers; 2010.

SUMMARY

Therefore, if several clinical predictors are present and suspicion of legionnaire's disease is high, doxycycline, azithromycin, or a respiratory quinolone provides optimal empiric monotherapy. Early IV-to-oral switch completes 2 weeks of therapy for normal hosts and 3 weeks of therapy for those with impaired CMI with legionnaire's disease.

Not all CAP cases should be tested for legionnaire's disease. Only patients with characteristic findings of legionnaire's disease (ie, clinical predictors) should be tested for legionnaire's disease. If present, legionnaire's disease clinical predictors have the effect of increasing pretest probability of legionnaire's disease (ie, selective high-yield *Legionella* testing is preferable to shotgun testing for all possible CAP pathogens).

If there are insufficient characteristic findings that make legionnaire's disease unlikely (ie, low pretest probability), then the practitioner has 2 options. First, a ß-lactam plus doxycycline, a respiratory quinolone, or azithromycin remain the most common approach. ASP recommendations (ie, optimal monotherapy, IV or oral) is cost-effective, clinically effective, and well-received by patients who do not need further IV therapy and can be discharged earlier (ie, decreased length of stay). Using an anti-*Legionella* antibiotic also active against typical bacterial CAP pathogens (eg, doxycycline or a respiratory quinolone), as previously outlined, decreases unnecessary ß-lactam use. Another ASP consideration is to not include a ß-lactam as part of initial double-drug therapy in regard to early IV-to-oral switch therapy. Ceftriaxone, the most often used ß-lactam in CAP protocols, has no oral equivalent and most practitioners complete therapy with an oral second-generation cephalosporin plus oral doxycycline or a respiratory quinolone (see **Table 4**). In hospitalized adults with CAP, if a ß-lactam is not used initially, beginning therapy with IV doxycycline or a respiratory quinolone provides seamless transition from IV-to-oral using the same oral antibiotic, at the same dose IV and po, to complete therapy. From an ASP perspective, this approach minimizes the pill burden and the potential for medication side effects and drug interactions.

The duration of antibiotic therapy has important clinical and ASP implications.[91] There is a trend toward decreasing unnecessary antibiotic use (ie, unnecessary double-drug therapy) if monotherapy is as effective. There is also, from an ASP perspective, a decrease in duration of therapy. For CAP due to typical bacterial pathogens, the traditional 14 days of therapy may be shortened to 5 to 7 days based on clinical response. Levofloxacin has successfully been used to treat typical CAP in 5 days. With CAP, clinical improvement is manifested by decrease in fever, pulmonary symptoms, decrease in leukocytosis, and improvement on the CXR. These parameters have been used to assess clinical improvement and are the basis of early (after clinical defervescence) IV-to-oral switch therapy. Clinicians should rely on their clinical judgment and should not rely on serial inflammatory markers.[51]

With legionnaire's disease, optimal duration of therapy is a more nuanced assessment. First, *Legionella* sp are intracellular AM pathogens. In general, infections due to intracellular pathogens respond more slowly than infections due to extracellular pathogen (eg, *S pneumoniae*). With optimal anti-*Legionella* therapy, fevers decrease slowly, not in the first 72 hours but over 5 to 7 days. Most hospitalized adults with legionnaire's disease are moderately to severely ill with pneumonia during the first 3 days. Even with optimal, anti-*Legionella* therapy, infiltrates on CXR often progress.[92–94] Because of slowly decreasing fevers and infiltrates on CXR not improving quickly, some have used procalcitonin (PCT) levels to guide duration of therapy.[95] Unfortunately, PCT levels are not elevated in all cases of legionnaire's disease. Many intensive care unit patients have reasons, other than legionnaire's disease, to have elevated PCT levels, which may be elevated in a variety of noninfectious disorders (eg, dialysis, drug fever, febrile neutropenia, immunosuppressive therapy or steroids, trauma, hypotension, shock, pancreatitis, and renal insufficiency).[96] From clinical and ASP perspectives in assessing improvement or duration of therapy in legionnaire's disease, PCT determinations may be more misleading than helpful.[96–98] The laboratory test most closely predictive of clinical improvement in legionnaire's disease is the degree of relative lymphopenia. With effective therapy, the degree of relative lymphopenia lessens over time (eg, 4% to 8% to 20%).[45] Relative lymphopenia also has prognostic significance in legionnaire's disease.

Things being equal, immunocompetent hosts with legionnaire's disease are usually treated for 2 weeks, and compromised hosts are treated with decreased CMI for 3 weeks. Because legionnaire's disease is an intracellular pathogen, shorter courses of therapy may result in relapse.[92,94]

REFERENCES

1. Vilde JL, Dournon E, Rajagopalan P. Inhibition of *Legionella* pneumophilia multiplication within human macrophages by antimicrobial agents. Antimicrobial Agents Chemother 1986;30:743–8.
2. Baldwin DR, Wise R, Andrews JM, et al. Azithromycin concentrations at the sites of pulmonary infection. Eur Respir J 1990;3:886–90.
3. Wise R, Baldwin DR, Andrews JM, et al. Comparative pharmacokinetic disposition of fluoroquinolones in the lung. J Antimicrob Chemother 1991;228:65–71.
4. Murdoch MB, Peterson LR. Antimicrobial penetration into polymorphonuclear leukocytes and alveolar macrophages. Semin Respir Infect 1991;6:112–21.
5. Olsen KM, San Pedro G, Gann LP, et al. Intrapulmonary pharmacokinetics of azithromycin in healthy volunteers given five oral doses. Antimicrobial Agents Chemother 1996;40:2582–5.
6. Bergogne-Berezin E. Predicting the efficacy of antimicrobial agents in respiratory infections – is tissue concentration a valid measure? J Antimicrob Chemother 1995;35:363–71.
7. Honeybourne D. Antibiotic penetration in the respiratory tract and implications for the selection of antimicrobial therapy. Curr Opin Pulm Med 1997;3:170–4.
8. Stout JE, Arnold B, Yu VL. Comparative activity of ciprofloxacin, ofloxacin, levofloxacin, and erythromycin against *Legionella* species by broth microdilution and intracellular susceptibility testing in HL-60 cells. Diagn Microbiol Infect Dis 1998;30:37–43.
9. Jonas D, Engels I, Friedhoff C, et al. Efficacy of moxifloxacin, trovafloxacin, clinafloxacin and levofloxacin against intracellular *Legionella pneumophila*. J Antimicrob Chemother 2001;47:147–52.
10. Stout JE, Sens K, Mietzner S, et al. Comparative activity of quinolones, macrolides and ketolides against *Legionella* species using in vitro broth dilution and intracellular susceptibility testing. Int J Antimicrob Agents 2005;25:302–7.
11. Edelstein PH. Antimicrobial chemotherapy for legionnaires disease; a review. Clin Infect Dis 1995;21:S265–76.
12. Edelstein PH. Imipenem therapy for Legionnaires disease. J Infect Chemother 2015;21:76.
13. Pinzone MR, Cacopardo B, Abbo L, et al. Duration of antimicrobial therapy in community acquired pneumonia: less is more. ScientificWorldJournal 2014;2014:759138.
14. Phin N, Parry-Ford F, Harrison T, et al. Epidemiology and clinical management of Legionnaires disease. Lancet Infect Dis 2014;14:1011–21.
15. Cunha BA, Burillo A, Bouza E. Legionnaire's disease. Lancet 2016;387:376–85.
16. Klein NC, Cunha BA. Treatment of Legionnaires disease. Semin Respir Infect 1998;13:140–6.
17. Garcia-Vidal C, Carratala J. Current clinical management of Legionnaires disease. Expert Rev Anti Infect Ther 2006;4:995–1004.

18. Carratala J, Carcia-Vidal C. An update on *Legionella*. Curr Opin Infect Dis 2010;23:152–7.
19. Valve K, Vaalasti A, Anttila VJ, et al. Disseminated *Legionella pneumophila* infection in an immunocompromised patient treated with tigecycline. Scand J Infect Dis 2010;42:152–5.
20. Townsend ML, Pound MW, Drew RH. Potential role of tigecycline in the treatment of community-acquired bacterial pneumonia. Infect Drug Resist 2011;4:77–86.
21. Viasus D, DiYacovo S, Garcia-Vidal C, et al. Community-Acquired *Legionella pneumophila* pneumonia. A single center experience with 214 hospitalized sporadic cases over 15 years. Medicine 2013;92:51–60.
22. Cunha BA. Empiric therapy of community-acquired pneumonia: guidelines for the perplexed? Chest 2004;125:1913–9.
23. Batard E, Lecadet N, Goffinet N, et al. High variability among Emergency Departments in 3rd-generation cephalosporins and fluoroquinolones use for community-acquired pneumonia. Infection 2015;43:681–9.
24. Cunha BA. Current concepts in the antimicrobial therapy of community-acquired pneumonia. Drugs Today (Barc) 1998;34:107–23.
25. Mandell LA, Waterer GW. Empirical therapy of community-acquired pneumonia: advancing evidence or just more doubt? JAMA 2015;314:396–7.
26. The B, Grayson ML, Johnson PD, et al. Doxycycline vs. macrolides in combination therapy for treatment of community-acquired pneumonia. Clin Microbiol Infect 2012;18:E71–3.
27. Scalera NM, File TM. Determining the duration of therapy for patients with community-acquired pneumonia. Curr Infect Dis Rep 2013;15:191–5.
28. Gacouin A, LeTulzo Y, Lavoue S, et al. Severe pneumonia due to *L. pneumophila*: prognostic factors, impact of delayed appropriate antimicrobial therapy. Intensive Care Med 2002;28:686–91.
29. Mercatello A, Frappaz D, Robert D, et al. Failure of erythromycin/rifampicin treatment of *Legionella* pneumonia. J Infect 1985;10:282–3.
30. Kurz RW, Graninger W, Egger TP, et al. Failure of treatment of *Legionella* pneumonia with ciprofloxacin. J Antimicrob Chemother 1988;22:389–91.
31. Bruin JP, Koshkolda T, IJzerman EP, et al. Isolation of ciprofloxacin-resistant *Legionella pneumophila* in a patient with severe pneumonia. J Antimicrob Chemother 2014;69:2869–71.
32. Diederen BMW. *Legionella* spp. and Legionnaires disease. J Infect 2008;56:1–12.
33. Prina E, Ranzani OT, Torres A. Community-acquired pneumonia. Lancet 2015;386:1097–108.
34. Rudin JE, Evans TL, Wing EJ. Failure of erythromycin in treatment of *Legionella micdadei* pneumonia. Am J Med 1984;76:318–20.
35. Tan JS, File TM Jr, DiPersio JR, et al. Persistently positive culture results in a patient with community-acquired pneumonia due to *Legionella pneumophila*. Clin Infect Dis 2001;32:1562–6.
36. Vamer TR, Bookstaver PB, Rudisill CN, et al. Role of rifampin-based combination therapy for severe community-acquired *Legionella pneumophila* pneumonia. Ann Pharmacother 2011;45:967–76.
37. Quintiliani R, Nightingale CH. Transitional antibiotic therapy. Infect Dis Clin Prac 1994;3:161067.
38. Cunha BA. Oral antibiotic therapy of serious systemic infections. Med Clin North Am 2006;90:1197–222.

39. Cunha BA. Intravenous to oral switch therapy in community-acquired pneumonia. Am J Med 2001;111:412–3.
40. Katz E, Larsen LS, Fogarty CM, et al. Safety and efficacy of sequential i.v. to p.o. moxifloxacin versus conventional combination therapies in the treatment of community-acquired pneumonia in patients requiring initial i.v. therapy. J Emerg Med 2004;27:554–9.
41. Kotwant A, Kumar S, Swain PK, et al. Antimicrobial drug prescribing patterns for community-acquired pneumonia in hospitalized patients: a retrospective pilot study from New Delhi, India. Indian J Pharmacol 2015;47:375–82.
42. Torres A, Muir JF, Corris P, et al. Effectiveness of oral moxifloxacin in standard first-line therapy in community-acquired pneumonia. Eur Respir J 2003;21: 135–43.
43. Furlanut M, Brollo L, Lugatti E, et al. Pharmacokinetic aspects of levofloxacin 500 mg once daily during sequential intravenous/oral therapy in patients with lower respiratory tract infections. J Antimicrob Chemother 2003;51:101–6.
44. Dunbar LM, Wunderink RG, Habib MP, et al. High-dose, short course levofloxacin for community-acquired pneumonia: a new treatment paradigm. Clin Infect Dis 2003;37:752–60.
45. File TM, Milkovich G, Tennenberg AM, et al. Clinical implications of 750 mg 5 day levofloxacin for the treatment of community-acquired pneumonia. Curr Med Res Opin 2004;20:1473–81.
46. Rijinders BJ. Moxifloxacin for community-acquired pneumonia. Antimicrobial Agents Chemother 2003;47:444–5.
47. Lode H, Grossman C, Choudhri S, et al. Sequential IV/PO moxifloxacin treatment of patients with severe community-acquired pneumonia. Respir Med 2003;97: 1134–42.
48. Johnson JR. Doxycycline for treatment of community-acquired pneumonia. Clin Infect Dis 2002;35:632–3.
49. Cunha BA. Doxycycline for community-acquired pneumonia. Clin Infect Dis 2003; 37:870.
50. Cunha CB, Cunha BA, editors. Antibiotic essentials. 15th edition. New Delhi (India): Jay Pee Med Publishers; 2016.
51. Cunha BA, editor. Pneumonia essentials. 3rd edition. Sudbury (MA): Jones & Bartlett; 2010.
52. Cunha CB, Varughese CA, Mylonakis E. Antimicrobial stewardship programs (ASPs): the devil is in the details. Virulence 2013;4:147–9.
53. Cunha CB. Principles of Stewardship. In: LaPlante K, Cunha C, Morrill H, et al, editors. Antimicrobial stewardship: principles & practice. London (United Kingdom): CABI Publishers; 2016. p. 1–7.
54. Nussenblatt V, Avdic E, Cosgrove S. What is the role of antimicrobial stewardship in improving outcomes of patients with CAP? Infect Dis Clin North Am 2013;27: 211–28.
55. Hurst JM, Bosso JA. Antimicrobial stewardship in the management of community-acquired pneumonia. Curr Opin Infect Dis 2013;26:184–6.
56. Jenkins TC, Stella SA, Cervantes L, et al. Targets for antibiotic and healthcare resource stewardship in inpatient community-acquired pneumonia: a comparison of management practices with National Guideline Recommendations. Infection 2013;41:135–44.
57. Siegel RE, Halpern NA, Almenoff PL, et al. A prospective randomized study of inpatient iv. antibiotics for community-acquired pneumonia: the optimum duration of therapy. Chest 1996;110:965–71.

58. Davis SL, Delgado G Jr, McKinnon PS. Pharmacoeconomic considerations associated with the use of intravenous-to-oral moxifloxacin for community-acquired pneumonia. Clin Infect Dis 2005;2:S136–43.
59. Jewesson P. Cost-effectiveness and vale of an IV switch. Pharmacoeconomics 1994;5:20–6.
60. Cunha CB. Pharmacoeconomic considerations in antimicrobial stewardship programs. In: LaPlante K, Cunha C, Morrill H, et al, editors. Antimicrobial stewardship: principles & practice. London (United Kingdom): CABI Publishers; 2016. p. 334–41.
61. DiDiodato G, McArthur L, Deyene J, et al. Evaluating the impact of an antimicrobial stewardship program on the length of stay of immune-competent adult patients admitted to a hospital ward with a diagnosis of community-acquired pneumonia: a quasi-experimental study. Am J Infect Control 2016;44:e73–9.
62. Broom J, Broom A, Adams K, et al. What prevents the intravenous to oral antibiotic switch? A qualitative study of hospital doctors accounts of what influences their clinical practice. J Antimicrob Chemother 2016;71(8):2295–9.
63. Schlick W. The problems of treating atypical pneumonia. J Antimicrob Chemother 1993;31:111–20.
64. Trad NA, Baisch A. Management of community-acquired pneumonia in an Australian regional hospital. Aust J Rural Health 2015. [Epub ahead of print].
65. Piso RJ, Arnold C, Bassetti S. Coverage of atypical pathogens for hospitalized patients with community-acquired pneumonia is not guided by clinical parameters. Swiss Med Wkly 2013;143:13870.
66. Dunne WM Jr, Picot N, Van Belkum A. Laboratory tests for legionnaire's disease. Infect Dis Clin North Am 2017;31(1):167–78.
67. Elverdal PL, Jorgensen CS, Krogfelt KA, et al. Two years' performance of an inhouse ELISA for diagnosis of Legionnaire's disease: detection of specific IgM and IgG antibodies against *Legionella pneumophila* serogroup 1, 3, and 6 in human serum. J Microbiol Methods 2013;94:94–7.
68. Mykietiuk A, Carratala J, Fernandez-Sabe N, et al. Clinical outcomes for hospitalized patients with *Legionella* pneumonia in the antigenuria era: the influence of levofloxacin therapy. Clin Infect Dis 2005;40:794–9.
69. Den Boer JW, Yzerman PF. Diagnosis of *Legionella* infection of Legionnaire's disease. Eur J Clin Microbiol Infect Dis 2004;23:871–8.
70. Filice GA, Drekonia DM, Thurn JR, et al. Diagnostic Errors that lead to inappropriate antimicrobial use. Infect Control Hosp Epidemiol 2015;36:949–56.
71. Cunha BA. Characteristic predictors that increase the pretest probability of Legionnaires disease: "Don't order a test just because you can" revisited." South Med J 2015;108:761.
72. Cunha BA. Severe *Legionella* pneumonia: rapid diagnosis with Winthrop-University Hospital's weighted point score system (modified). Heart Lung 2008; 37:312–21.
73. Cunha BA. The diagnostic significance of relative bradycardia in infectious disease. Clin Microbiol Infect 2000;6:633–4.
74. Cunha BA. The clinical diagnosis of Legionnaires disease: the diagnostic value of combining non-specific laboratory tests. J Infect 2008;56:395–7.
75. Cunha BA, Wu G, Raza M. Clinical diagnosis of legionnaire's disease: six characteristic criteria. Am J Med 2015;128:e21–2.
76. Wozniak MA. The clinical efficacy of fluoroquinolone and macrolide combination therapy compared with single-agent therapy against community-acquired pneumonia caused by *Legionella pneumophila*. Br Inf Soc 2009;10:222–4.

77. Cao B, Qu J, Yin Y, et al. Overview of antimicrobial options for *Mycoplasma pneumoniae* pneumonia: focus on macrolide resistance. Clin Respir J 2015. [Epub ahead of print].
78. Jones RN, Sader HS, Fritsche TR. Doxycycline use for community-acquired pneumonia: contemporary in vitro spectrum of activity against *Streptococcus pneumoniae* (1999–2002). Diagn Microbiol Infect Dis 2004;49:147–9.
79. Fogarty C, Goldschmidt R, Bush K. Bacteremic pneumonia due to multi-drug resistant pneumococci in 3 patients treated unsuccessfully with azithromycin and successfully with levofloxacin. Clin Infect Dis 2000;31:613–5.
80. Kelley MA, Weber DJ, Gilligan P, et al. Breakthrough pneumococcal bacteremia in patients being treated with azithromycin and clarithromycin. Clin Infect Dis 2000;31:1008–11.
81. Lonks JR, Garau J, Gomez L, et al. Failure of macrolide antibiotic treatment in patients with bacteremia due to erythromycin resistant *Streptococcus pneumoniae.* Clin Infect Dis 2002;35:556–64.
82. Musher DM, Shortridge VD, Jorgensen JH, et al. Emergence of macrolide resistance during treatment of pneumococcal pneumonia. N Engl J Med 2002;346: 630–1.
83. Hoefken G, Talan D, Larsen LS, et al. Efficacy and safety of sequential moxifloxacin for treatment of community-acquired pneumonia associated with atypical pathogens. Eur J Clin Microbiol Infect Dis 2004;23:772–5.
84. Yu VL, Greenberg RN, Zadeikis N, et al. Levofloxacin efficacy in the treatment of community-acquired legionellosis. Chest 2004;125:2135–9.
85. Pedro-Botet L, Yu VL. *Legionella*: macrolides or quinolones? Clin Microbiol Infect 2006;3:25–30.
86. Sabria M, Pedro-Botet ML, Gomez J, et al. Fluoroquinolones vs macrolides in the treatment of Legionnaires disease. Chest 2005;128:1401–5.
87. Ramirez JA, Cooper AC, Wiemken T, et al. #08 Study Group. Switch therapy in hospitalized patients with community-acquired pneumonia: tigecycline vs. levofloxacin. BMC Infect Dis 2012;12:159.
88. Dunbar LM, Khashab MM, Kahn JB, et al. Efficacy of 750 mg, 5-day levofloxacin in the treatment of community-acquired pneumonia caused by atypical pathogens. Curr Med Res Opin 2004;20:555–63.
89. Burdet C, Lepeule R, Duval X, et al. Quinolones versus macrolides in the treatment of legionellosis: a systematic review and meta-analysis. J Antimicrob Chemother 2014;69:2354–60.
90. Cunha BA. Severe community-acquired pneumonia. J Crit Ilness 1997;12:711–2.
91. Avdic E, Cushinotto LA, Highes AH, et al. Impact of an antimicrobial stewardship intervention on shortening the duration of therapy for community-acquired pneumonia. Clin Infect Dis 2012;54:1581–7.
92. Lattimer GL, Rhodes LV 3rd. Legionnaires disease. Clinical findings and one-year follow-up. JAMA 1978;240:169–71.
93. Woodhead MA, Macfarlane JT. The protean manifestations of Legionnaires disease. J R Coll Physicians Lond 1985;19:224–30.
94. Woodhead MA, Macfarlane JT. Legionnaires disease: a review of 79 community acquired cases in Nottingham. Thorax 1986;41:635–40.
95. Cunha BA, Cunha CB. Legionnaire's disease mimics: a clinical perspective. Infect Dis Clin North Am 2017;31(1):95–109.
96. Cunha CB. Infectious disease differential diagnosis. In: Cunha CB, Cunha BA, editors. Antibiotic essentials. 15th edition. New Delhi (India): Jay Pee Med Pub; 2016. p. 474–506.

97. Cunha BA. Empiric antimicrobial therapy of community-acquired pneumonia: clinical diagnosis versus procalcitonin levels. Scand J Infect Dis 2009;41:782–4.
98. Hasali MA, Ibrahim MI, Sulaiman SA, et al. A clinical and economic study of community-acquired pneumonia between single versus combination therapy. Pharm World Sci 2005;27:249–53.

Index

Note: Page numbers of article titles are in **boldface** type.

Infect Dis Clin N Am 31 (2017) 193–202
http://dx.doi.org/10.1016/S0891-5520(16)30127-1
0891-5520/17

S

T

U

V

W

Moving?

Make sure your subscription moves with you!

To notify us of your new address, find your **Clinics Account Number** (located on your mailing label above your name), and contact customer service at:

Email: journalscustomerservice-usa@elsevier.com

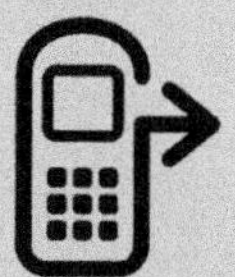

800-654-2452 (subscribers in the U.S. & Canada)
314-447-8871 (subscribers outside of the U.S. & Canada)

Fax number: 314-447-8029

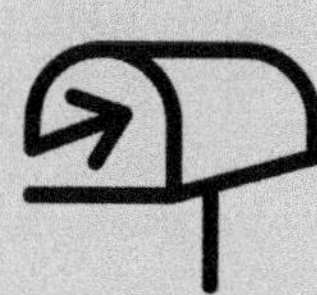

Elsevier Health Sciences Division
Subscription Customer Service
3251 Riverport Lane
Maryland Heights, MO 63043

*To ensure uninterrupted delivery of your subscription, please notify us at least 4 weeks in advance of move.

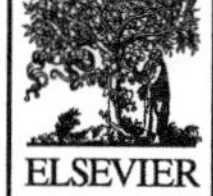

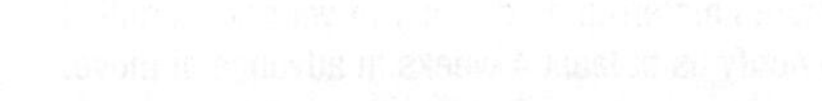

Printed and bound by CPI Group (UK) Ltd, Croydon, CR0 4YY

08/05/2025

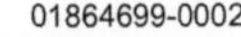

01864699-0002